AF413458

In the
SHADOW
of the NOBEL
PRIZE

In the SHADOW of the NOBEL PRIZE

Gösta Gahrton

Karolinska Institutet, Sweden

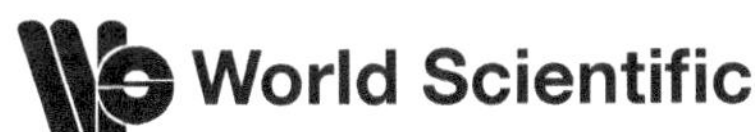

World Scientific

NEW JERSEY · LONDON · SINGAPORE · BEIJING · SHANGHAI · HONG KONG · TAIPEI · CHENNAI · TOKYO

Published by

World Scientific Publishing Co. Pte. Ltd.

5 Toh Tuck Link, Singapore 596224

USA office: 27 Warren Street, Suite 401-402, Hackensack, NJ 07601

UK office: 57 Shelton Street, Covent Garden, London WC2H 9HE

British Library Cataloguing-in-Publication Data
A catalogue record for this book is available from the British Library.

IN THE SHADOW OF THE NOBEL PRIZE

ISBN 978-981-12-9535-5 (hardcover)
ISBN 978-981-12-9536-2 (ebook for institutions)
ISBN 978-981-12-9594-2 (ebook for individuals)

For any available supplementary material, please visit
https://www.worldscientific.com/worldscibooks/10.1142/13905#t=suppl

Contents

Prologue

I was leaning back in my chair and relaxing after a tough day at the Karolinska University Hospital, Huddinge, south of Stockholm City, when my office phone rang. An unstable, apparently confused, voice said: *"I do not feel well"*. I soon realized that it was my previous boss at the Nobel Institute, Torbjörn Caspersson, speaking. He managed to clear his voice a little and we chatted for a short while. Then there was another voice on the phone. It was the carer from the home where Torbjörn, by now an old man, lived. She told me that he had not felt well for a few days, but she did not believe that it was serious. The next day he was dead.

Torbjörn Caspersson was 87 years old when he died and his funeral was attended by a few faithful pupils and previous collaborators. There were no big headings in the newspapers for this giant among professors. Some of his PhD students, including me, wrote a 300-word obituary for the newspapers. His memory will never fade among his contemporaries, but most of the new generation, even at the Karolinska Institutet, have never heard of him.

At his height, this giant of medical research could sometimes be seen in the press and for a short time he was a superstar. In the 1950s, the Swedish weekly journal *SE* featured his picture on its front page, together with three additional persons claimed to be among the 100 most important people for the future of mankind.[1] The other photos were of Dwight D Eisenhower, Albert Einstein and Josef Stalin. But Caspersson's name disappeared from the

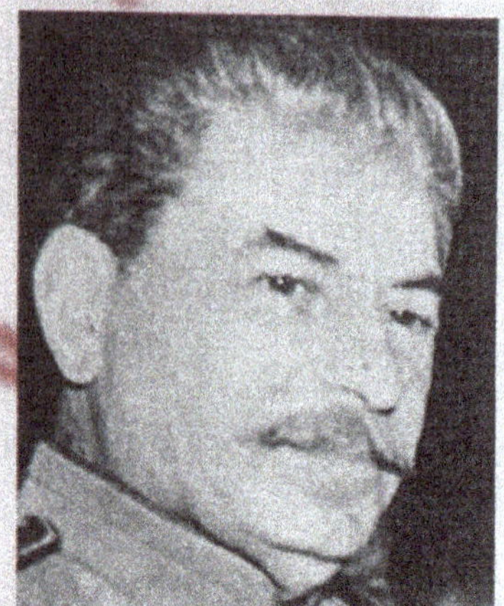

KAN ENDAST DÖDEN HEJDA JOSEF STALIN?

Än har ingen förmått stoppa hans marsch mot världsherra-välde. Tsarernas polis försökte. Trotsky försökte. Röda armén försökte. Hitler försökte. Alla misslyckades. I dag är han 73 år och hans ord lag för 800 miljoner människor.

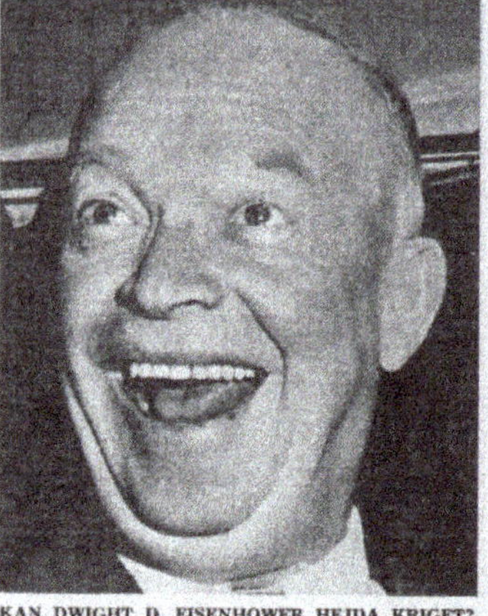

KAN DWIGHT D. EISENHOWER HEJDA KRIGET?

Okänd överstelöjtnant 1939. Exempellös karriär som diplo-matisk soldat. Kallad »vår tids störste strateg» av Sov-jets ÖB i andra världskriget. Satte Atlantpakten i funk-tion. 62 år. Tyngsta ansvaret väntar som USA:s president.

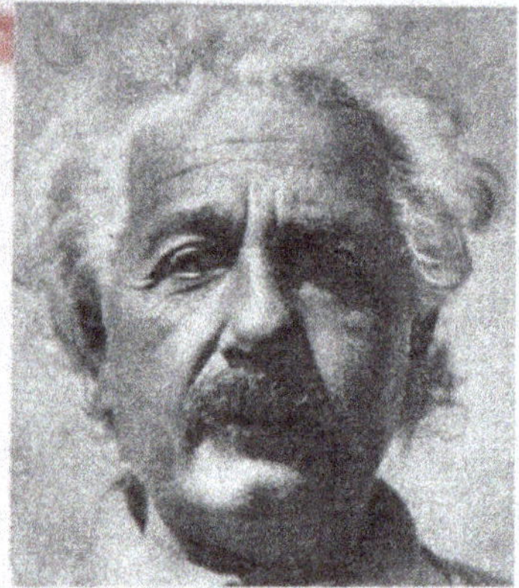

ALBERT EINSTEIN VET MEST OM UNIVERSUM

Hans relativitetsteori ändrade världen och lade grunden till atomåldern på gott och ont. Med penna och papper som enda vapen angriper 73-åringen ännu större problem, vilkas lösning kan sprida ljus över universums djupaste gåtor.

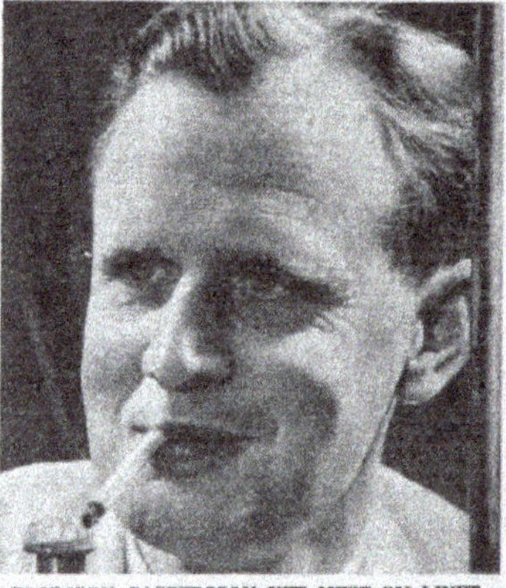

TORBJÖRN CASPERSSON VET MEST OM LIVET

Svensk cellforskare och professor, 42 år. Har fört veten-skapen närmare svaret på frågan: Vad är liv? Utarbetat me-toder för kartläggning av cellernas kemiska substans. Hans rön kanske ger nyckeln till livets och värandets läs.

n är samtidens största, mest
egåvade och heroiska gestalt?
ston Churchill, svarar den ame-
ke författaren Donald Robin-
ilken i en nyutkommen bok
100 Most Important People in
World Today». Pocket Books
fängslande porträtterar 100 nu
le personer som under de se-
15 åren format vår värld och
ikt avgör dess öde ytterligare
framåt.
sta geniet? Einstein. Ädlaste
ilighet? Albert Schweitzer. Mo-

DE 100

SOM FORMAR VÅR VÄRLD

digaste? Taha Hussein, blind eg
ljusspridare. Skarpaste insikt?
rand Russel. Mest inspirerande
niska? Toscanini. Slugaste?
Omänskligaste? Beria, chef för
hemliga polisen. Största bluff?
forskaren Lysenko. Mest tragi
gur? Atomspionen Fuchs.
Urvalet är gjort ur ameri
perspektiv, men greppet är fris
personteckningarna   högintre
SE presenterar dem med ens
i översättning och bearbetni
K. E. Hillgren och Gunnar Isa

In 1952, Torbjörn Caspersson was listed as one of the most important people for the future of mankind, along with Josef Stalin, Dwight D Eisenhower and Albert Einstein, in Donald Robinson's book *The 100 Most Important People in the World Today*.

newspaper headlines. The more that I contemplated the limited publicity that the most important scientists that change the world receive, the more I felt I needed to write this book. Why are soccer players, tennis players, music writers and pop singers more important than scientists? I admit that there are exceptions, for example when the Nobel Prizes are awarded for the most excellent discoveries. Some of them will remain in many people's memories for most of their lives. Who does not know about Albert Einstein or James Watson and Francis Crick? However, most of the great discoveries and their inventors receive limited publicity. At least that is the situation with the so-called Swedish Public Service, which comprises tax-funded, half-monopolized media that dominates all national channels with their own views or those of the Swedish Government. Although media outlets seem to be somewhat different in countries where free media compete with each other, like CNN, CBS and Fox News in the USA, scientists receive limited publicity overall.

The aim of this book is not to tilt against windmills. It is part of my own story and I focus on my encounters with the important medical scientists that I got to know. Some of them became Nobel Laureates and some did not. I want to raise those that I rate highly to the level where I feel they should be, Nobel Laureates or not. I must also admit that I cannot resist mentioning a few that rated themselves higher than I did. This endeavor was relatively easy, because I have a clear memory and an extensive archive of my correspondence, which covers some 40 years. I sent and received approximately 3,000 letters a year and they were numbered chronologically by my outstanding secretary Åsa Johansson, archived in 250 A4 folders and stored on more than 20 meters of shelving. The references listed at the end of the book were put together with the help of the fabulous PubMed database. My wife Astrid helped me to expand on the personal background I have included in this book, thanks to the valuable lessons she had learnt while researching her family background in the Österreichisches Staatsachiv (Austrian Governmental Archive) in Vienna and the City of Amsterdam archives in the Netherlands. Amazingly, I also found important information about my own background by using these sources.

1 Visiting Paris

I woke up on a train sleeper on my way to Paris from Lund in Sweden. The year was 1960. I felt that I had come to a dead end in my research. I was attempting to study the color that neutrophil leukocytes turned, by using a chemical method called the periodic acid-Schiff (PAS) reaction, which turned them various shades of red. The theory was that I could rank the intensity of the stained cells, according to a scoring system, by looking at them under a microscope. This was to form the basis of my doctoral thesis, but it was looking doubtful at that time.

By that stage I had worked as a clinician in the Department of Medicine at the University Hospital in Lund and had only published two scientific articles. One was in the Swedish *Läkartidningen* journal and was about a drug used by obstetricians. The other was about cardiology and was published in the international scientific journal *Acta Medica Scandinavica*. I had long since made up my mind to devote my life to clinical hematology, but now I was stuck with working on the PAS reaction. I had read about Professor Torbjörn Caspersson, who was based at the Karolinska Institutet in Stockholm and had developed a method, called microspectrophotometry, which could measure substances in single cells. I thought it would be useful to try and join his institution for some time. But first I had to study more about histochemistry and cytochemistry, to learn more about the science behind the chemistry of tissue and single cells. I decided that visiting the 1960 International

Histochemistry Congress in Paris would enable me to bring my knowledge up-to-date and discover the frontiers that were being researched in the field. That is how I found myself on a train on my way to Paris.

When I woke up, I looked around in the sleeper. People slept in their clothes, because the sleepers were for both sexes. A young man who was my age had just woken up and we started to chat about where we were going. Yes, he was going to participate in the Histochemistry Congress. Oh, so was I. Where did he work? At the Karolinska Institutet. OK, but in which institution? At the Medical Nobel Institute, Department of Medical Cell Research and Genetics. The head was Professor Torbjörn Caspersson. My sleeper friend was Nils Ringertz, who later succeeded Torbjörn Caspersson. What a coincidence!

2 Alfred Nobel's Will

When Alfred Nobel (1833–1896) died, the prize that was named after him was detailed in his will. *"All of my remaining realizable assets are to be disbursed as follows: the capital, converted to safe securities by my executors, is to constitute a fund, the interest on which is to be distributed annually as prizes to those who, during the preceding year, have conferred the greatest benefit to humankind. The interest is to be divided into five equal parts and distributed as follows: one part to the person who made the most important discovery or invention in the field of physics; one part to the person who made the most important chemical discovery or improvement; one part to the person who made the most important discovery within the domain of physiology or medicine; one part to the person who, in the field of literature, produced the most outstanding work in an idealistic direction, and one part to the person who has done the most or best to advance fellowship among nations, the abolition or reduction of standing armies, and the establishment and promotion of peace congresses. The prizes for physics and chemistry are to be awarded by the Swedish Academy of Sciences; that for physiological or medical achievements by the Karolinska Institute in Stockholm; that for literature by the Swedish Academy in Stockholm; and that for champions of peace by a committee of five persons to be selected by the Norwegian Storting (Parliament). It is my express wish that when awarding the prizes, no consideration be given to nationality, but that the prize be awarded to the worthiest person, whether or not they are Scandinavian."*[2]

This excerpt of Alfred Nobel's will was translated from Swedish to English and can be read on the website www.nobelprize.org. Much of the text on that site was written by Professor Nils Ringertz. After he retired from the Karolinska Institutet he was employed by the Nobel Foundation to build a virtual museum, which was his own idea. In his will, Nobel specified that the remainder of his entire fortune, after specific allowances to relatives and other named beneficiaries, should be used for *"prizes to those who, during the preceding year, have conferred the greatest benefit to humankind."*[2]

Nobel had made an enormous fortune from businesses and inventions. The most important one was dynamite, a mixture of nitroglycerine and diatomite, namely diatomaceous earth or kieselgur, which was patented in 1867. Dynamite is an explosive in which the nitroglycerine is stabilized by the kieselgur. Its uses include mining, construction and demolishing buildings. Nobel's other inventions resulted in 355 patents and, by the time he died, he owned 90 factories in 20 countries.

He was unmarried and had no children. If Nobel had not decided to leave most of his fortune for the Nobel Prize awards, it would have mainly been split between his brothers and their children.

Nobel wrote at least three last will and testaments, all in Swedish, and the excerpt cited above was from his third and final one. The others were destroyed before his death on the 10 November 1896.

Before his death Nobel had made two of his engineers, Ragnar Sohlman (1870–1948) and Rudolf Lilljequist (1855–1930), the executors of his will. Their job was not easy. Most of Nobel's assets were deposited in French Banks and their first task was to remove all the important valuables, including share documents, and transport them to Sweden. There was a danger that they would be embargoed by the French authorities. The two executors loaded the documents onto horse driven carriages and then hurried, armed with guns, to the Gare du Nord railway station in Paris. The numerous valuable packages were then sent to Sweden by train.

Sohlman and Lilljequist eventually managed to overcome the obstacles to realizing Nobel's will. They reached agreements with Alfred's brothers, and the other heirs mentioned in the will, and were finally able to establish the Nobel Foundation, so that Nobel's fortune could be used for the prizes in line with his wishes.

The Nobel Foundation received around 31 million Swedish crowns, which today would be worth about 2,346 million Swedish Krona or about 230 million US dollars. It was an enormous amount of money at that time. The stipulation in Nobel's will, that the money should be placed in safe securities, could have ruined the fortune. However, this request was later ignored by the Foundation and the assets are now mainly in shares on the world market. By 31 December 2022 the market value of the Nobel Foundation was 5,799 million Swedish Krona, which was about 600 million US dollars.

There are five Nobel Prizes, plus a prize that is funded by the Swedish Central Bank (Riksbank) in memory of Alfred Nobel. Each prize has the same value, but this has varied over time. It is based on the value of the assets of the Foundation. It was originally about eight million Swedish Krona, translated from the monetary value on 31 December 2021. Over the years it increased to 10 million and then fell to less than that. Today it is back to 10 million Swedish Krona.

The five Nobel Prize committees work independently of each other. My experience is based on the Nobel Assembly of the Karolinska Institutet, and its working body the Nobel Committee, who award the Nobel Prize in Physiology or Medicine.

3 The Nobel Assembly and the Nobel Committee of the Karolinska Institutet

Each of the five Nobel Prizes, and the Swedish Central Bank prize in memory of Alfred Nobel, are run by separate prize award organizations. The prizes for chemistry, physics and economics are handled by independent committees under the umbrella of the Swedish Academy of Sciences, which decides who will receive them. The prize for literature is awarded by the Swedish Academy and the peace prize is awarded by the Norwegian Parliament.

The prize in physiology or medicine is awarded by the Karolinska Institutet or, more precisely, by the Nobel Assembly at the Karolinska Institutet in Stockholm, Sweden. The members of the Assembly are all full professors at the Karolinska Institutet. Originally, all the Karolinska professors, about 50 in the 1980s, were members, but the increase in the number of academics holding the title professor would have created an Assembly of some 400 members today. This made it necessary to limit the number. In the 1980s, the Assembly took the decision that it should only include 50 members and that is still the number today. New members are elected by the Assembly and need to leave when they retire from the Karolinska Institutet. This means there is a continued renewal of competence. The Assembly is led by a chair and a new one is elected each year.

Although the Nobel Assembly is the decision-making body for the prize, it is not responsible for all the hard work, as the Assembly elects five members from their ranks to form the Nobel

Committee. The five Committee members are elected for a three-year term, with the option of being re-elected for a consecutive three-year period. After a wash out period of one year, they can be re-elected for two more three-year periods, but this is extremely rare. The chair of the Nobel Committee is elected for a three-year term and so is the vice chair. There is no direct line from being vice chair to chair, as each one is independently elected.

The Assembly and the Committee have a joint secretary, who is elected for a six-year period and can apply to be re-elected for one more term. The secretary keeps the threads together and is a full member of both Assembly and Committee. The importance of this role can hardly be overestimated.

The Nobel Committee is the working body for the prize. Every year the Nobel Committee is expanded by the appointment of another 10 adjunct members, so that the nominations for the Prize can be handled efficiently. They are elected after the usual five Committee members have seen the nominations, which should arrive before the end of January the same year. Five Committee members scan some 200 to 400 nominations every year, including some submitted in previous years. They then recommend that the Assembly elect adjuncts, who are experts on the research areas covered by the hot nominees that year. These adjuncts can be found within the Assembly or recruited from outside, but they are usually professors at the Karolinska Institutet. The Assembly almost always elects the adjuncts recommended by the Committee. The identities of these adjuncts are open to anybody, but, amazingly, these details are scarcely used by the media when they try to guess the prize winners before the names of the winners are announced. Looking at the research areas covered by the adjuncts provides hints about the hot nominees.

The interface between the Nobel Committee and the Nobel Assembly is similar to the relationship between a country's elected government and its parliament. The Nobel Committee does all the work and the Assembly takes the decisions based on the Committee's proposals.

The timeline for this Nobel work is as follows. In September of the year before the Nobel Prize winner is announced, the secretary issues invitation for nominations, on behalf of the Assembly. There are eight categories of individuals who can put forward nominations. The most important ones, in my opinion, are the previous Nobel Laureates, as many of them are very active and understand Alfred Nobel's will. Other important individuals are full professors at the numerous medical faculties around the world, who have been selected by the Nobel Assembly, and all the full professors at the faculties of medicine in the Nordic countries. Members of the Nobel Assembly and the Nobel Committee are also invited to put forward nominations, but rarely use this right. This option is mainly used if an individual has been frequently nominated in the past, but has not been nominated in the year when the Committee would like to propose him or her for the prize. The Assembly has the right to invite any scientist that it considers appropriate, in addition to the eight specified categories.

The real work of the Nobel Committee starts in early spring, when the adjuncts are in place. Each nomination is considered and allocated to one of four categories. The first option is to do nothing, because the nominee has previously been proposed and reviewed and was not considered a top candidate. The second option is a protocol note, which means that this is the first time the candidate has been nominated and the proposal does not seem right for the particular year, but may be reviewed further in another year. The third option is a first short preliminary investigation of the candidate by an expert, to see if a further, deeper investigation should be carried out. The fourth option usually applies to candidates who have been nominated in previous years and are now considered to be possible top candidates. One or more experts in the field then write a special investigation report on the research area and of the contribution that the candidate or candidates have made to the field. What did the candidate discover and how did it relate to discoveries by others in the same field? How important was the discovery and was this field a priority? Several fields may be investigated in the same year and several important candidates from each of them may be considered.

The Committee has a continuous dialog with the Assembly at joint meetings. The Committee informs the Assembly about the special investigations and proposes the top candidate or candidates for the Nobel Prize at the penultimate joint meeting. If there is no opposition or counter proposals from the Assembly, the Committee assumes that the Assembly will support their proposal at the last joint meeting in October. This is followed by a press conference at the Karolinska Institute, when the winner or winners and the media hear who has won the Nobel Prize.

The strength of the selection process lies in the procedure. The Nobel Committee proposes the winner or winners to the Nobel Assembly and does not make the decision themselves. This forces the Committee to carry out a very extensive investigation of the proposed candidate or candidates. The arguments must be crystal clear. All the voting is closed and secret, which means there is little risk for inappropriate influencing. This does not prevent members from openly taking a stand and sharing their views. Having an open discussion is very important for the chairman of the Committee, who eventually has to put forward the final proposal to the Assembly, so that an anonymous decision can be made about who should be awarded the Nobel Prize.

My 10-year journey through the Committee and Assembly started in early 1988, when I was asked to join the Committee as an adjunct and was then formally elected to the Assembly in the next year. In the early days of the Assembly I would have qualified for automatic membership when I was appointed a full professor of medicine of the Karolinska Institute in 1985, but by then the number of members was limited to 50. After I started working for the Committee, I was elected to the Assembly, based on my assumed competence in the field, which was at the top of the list at that time. I am not revealing any secrets, as my expertise was clearly reflected by the 1988 winners. Two of the three prize winners were Gertrude Elion and George Hitchings who had discovered, among other drugs, 6-mercaptopurine, which was important in the treatment of acute leukemia.

Following my election to the Assembly, I was again elected to the Nobel Committee. I served for some years as an adjunct and for five years as a full member. I was then elected vice chair and finally became the chair.

When I first entered the Committee, the Chairman was the Nobel Laureate Professor Bengt Samuelsson. He was also the President/Rector of the Karolinska Institutet. His successor in both positions was Hans Wigzell, a well-known immunologist and co-discoverer of the natural killer cell. He was succeeded by the Professor of Medicine Göran Holm, who held the equivalent post to me at the Karolinska University Hospital at Solna. At the time I was at the Karolinska University Hospital at Huddinge, then known as the Huddinge Hospital. When I started, the Secretary of the Committee was Jan Lindsten, Professor in Medical Genetics, but he had to step down after serving both the Committee and

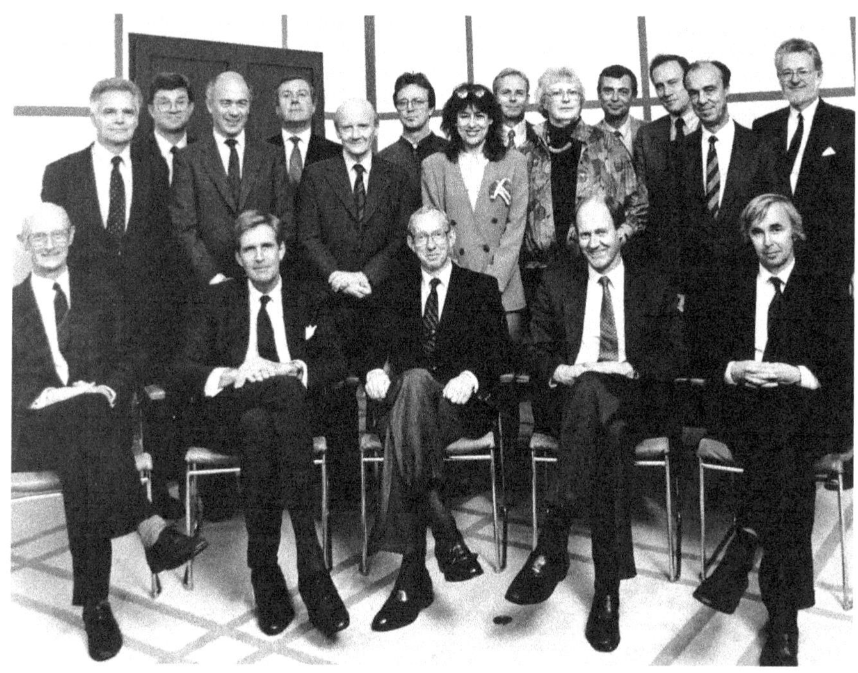

The Nobel Committee in 1988.

The ordinary members (sitting) are left to right: Jan Wersäll, Sten Orrenius, Bengt Samuelsson (Chairman of the Committee and Nobel Laureate), Thomas Hökfelt, Hans Wigzell.

The adjuncts (standing) are left to right: Gösta Gahrton (the author of this book), Sten Grillner, Alf Lindberg (later Secretary of the Nobel Committee), Folke Sjöqvist, Viktor Mutt, Göran Akusjärvi, Anita Aperia, Göran Holm, Kerstin Hall, Bertil Fredholm, Nils Ringertz (later Secretary of the Nobel Committee), Erling Norrby (later Secretary of the Swedish Academy of Sciences), Jan Lindsten (Secretary of the Nobel Committee).

Assembly for 12 years, as the new rule meant he had served the maximum number of years in the position. His successor for only two years was Alf Lindberg, who was succeeded in 1992 by the friend I had met on the sleeper train to Paris, Nils Ringertz (Chapter 1). His service has probably never been surpassed. When he died at 69 years of age in 2002, his successor Hans Jörnvall claimed that Ringertz had participated in the selection of close to one-third of the Nobel Prize winners in Physiology or Medicine. Ringertz received an obituary in the *New York Times*.

4 My Background on My Father's Side

My grandfather was a farmer. He owned a small farm of 75 acres in southern Sweden, with the best soil, according to my father. His father and grandfather were also farmers. The earliest known ancestor on my father's side was Trued Troppman, who was apparently a soldier. It was a much-needed profession in the 18th century during the wars against Denmark and Russia. I met my grandfather shortly before he died. I was four years old and he was 89. I met my grandmother about twice a year until she died at the age of 95, when I was 15 years old. She lived about 60 miles south of our home, but close to my grandparents on my mother's side, who we visited frequently. My paternal grandma was cared for by her daughter, my father's sister Hilma, until she died. Hilma was a laboratory assistant at the Department of Physiology at the University of Lund when she was younger. According to my father, she performed all the Nobel Prize worthy experiments, planned by her boss, Professor Torsten Thunberg, for 25 years. However, Thunberg was never awarded the prize, despite being nominated 15 times (Chapter 35). Hilma died at the age of 104.

5 My Father

My father was a physician who specialized in internal medicine. When he was 14 he told my grandfather that he would never take over the farm, as he wanted to pursue an academic career. My grandfather sold the farm and spent his money on my father, who studied medicine at the University of Lund. Halfway through his studies, he was allowed to take a break and he used his father's money to visit the USA and widen his views. He managed to get a job at a laboratory in New York and was offered both a job and the chance to continue his studies. However, he later told me that he returned to Sweden after eight months to take care of his mother. He graduated as an MD from the University of Lund and was offered a position at the Department of Surgery by the legendary Professor Gustaf Petrén. He turned the offer down, to the great astonishment of the professor. My father had decided to specialize in internal medicine. It did not take long before he received a second offer, this time from an even better-known professor, Gustaf's brother Karl Petrén. He was not just Professor of Internal Medicine and Head of the Department of Medicine, but also the Head of the entire University Hospital of Lund. My father had to work hard day and night and lived at the hospital. After a few years he became a specialist in internal medicine. Only three physicians at the department were specialists, including my later boss Haqvin Malmros. Many years later Malmros followed Sven Ingvar, Karl Petrén's successor, to become Head of the Department of

Medicine. In my father's time, the specialists and residents were required to get involved in research projects and produce theses on them. Karl Petrén initiated the projects and was the formal tutor for all of them. My father started a project about the nature and treatment of multiple sclerosis, but got tired of it after a couple of years. One reason might have been that he had met my mother and wanted to marry her. It was impossible to feed a family on the lousy salary he got for his job at Lund. Another reason, which he frequently explained to me, was that Karl Petrén was a poor tutor. Whatever the true story, he went to Karl Petrén and told him that he wanted to resign from the department and give up his academic plans. He wanted a position at a hospital where he could use his competence and receive a salary that could feed a family. Petrén was a powerful man and it was said that he decided who should fill all the positions in internal medicine in southern Sweden. *"Well"* Petrén said *"you may want to get the position as head of the new hospital for epidemic disorders in Kristianstad?"* The new position was 80 kilometers north of Lund. My father, who was well trained in the field, thought about the consequences of moving from the city where he was educated for a while and then accepted. He married my mother, Asta de Sharengrad (Chapter 7), who was now a physiotherapist and gymnastics director after studying at the South Swedish Institute for Gymnastics in Lund. They moved to Kristianstad and my father became the Head of Epidemisjukhuset, the hospital for epidemic disorders. He was the only physician and was assisted by several nurses and secretaries. Patient histories were dictated to an assistant nurse, who took notes at the bedside. When he needed to, he could refer patients to the adjacent hospital, which provided most of the other specialties, such as internal medicine, surgery, ear disorders and eye disorders. Epidemic disorders, like polio and scarlet fever, were supposed to be admitted to special hospitals, due to risk of infection. So-called epidemic hospitals were erected in close vicinity, but not in the same buildings, as departments for other diseases.

My father was a hard worker. His job at the hospital took about one to two hours a day between 9am and 10/11am. Before 9am he performed his role as a military doctor and after 10/11am to 12 noon he was a doctor for workers employed by the railway authorities in the city. In the afternoon he worked in his private practice. This was in the building where we lived, but in a separate apartment. He regularly visited patient's homes and helped to provide emergency services in the city at night.

Remarkably, my father did not seem to be exhausted by his demanding job schedule. On the contrary, he seemed to love it. He did not have to think about running our household, as that was my mother's job. She was assisted by a cook and there was a nanny to take care of us children. My father came home at 10am or 11am for a break and was served a boiled egg, tea and toast. At 12 noon he had lunch with the family and then joined us for dinner at 5.30pm. This meant that, despite his hard work, we saw him at least twice a day. During the weekends we would frequently hurry out to the countryside, where my father hunted and the rest of us picked mushrooms, depending on the time of year. His influence on us children was probably greater than we would admit. He disliked politicians in general, but particularly the socialists. He was skeptical about the press, but in general liberal. He loved America. The country where he had spent eight months of his life undoubtedly had a profound influence on his view of the world.

Although he was a physician, my father admired engineers, particularly those who developed the mines in northern Sweden.

These mining engineers enjoyed high prestige and he thought that the future was in their hands. He advised me to try and get into the prestigious Kungliga Tekniska Högskolan (the Royal Technical High School) in Stockholm and study engineering. I was amazed that he did not advise me to enter the medical school at the university. I knew that he loved his work, but sometimes I felt that he did not think that I was tough enough for medicine. And then there was his failure to finish his thesis, although he tended to blame Karl Petrén for that, saying that he was not the tutor he should have been. Whatever the reason, engineering was the top profession for me as far as he was concerned. My final school grades needed to be as high for both professions and he advised me to work hard.

6 My Background on My Mother's Side

My mother was a Swedish citizen, but she had an unusual background. Her father, Wilhelm de Sharengrad, was the son of a Croatian immigrant called Karl, later known as Carlos. Karl was an adventurer, who ended up working as a photographer in Malmö, Sweden. He was from a Croatian military family in the Austrian Empire. Croatia was part of Austria at that time. Although Karl's father was a low-ranking officer, who defended the borders to Serbia, Karl and his brother were admitted to the best school for Austrian officer education, which was located in Olmütz, Czechoslovakia, which was also part of Great Austria. However, Karl was a young revolutionary, who believed that Croatia and Serbia should be amalgamated to create a Great Serbia. After he reached the rank of a cadet, he was accused of treason and sentenced to death. He managed to escape and joined the freedom fighter Giuseppe Garibaldi in Italy, where he joined his famous red shirts, who united Italy and fought the Austrians. However, Garibaldi's army was dispersed after the peace treaty in Aspromonte in northern Italy. Karl was now known as Carlos and was using the new last name of de Sharengrad, copied from the castle ruin Sharengrad, located close to his hometown of Ilok in Croatia, and lost his military role. Garibaldi helped him find another military job in London, where the British Government was planning to help the Poles in their rebellion against the Russians in Poland. However, before the warship he was on had reached the Polish coast, the rebellion was over and the ship ended up in Malmö, Sweden. It was taken into custody by the Swedes and the officers on the ship were treated as guests by Swedish families. Carlos was now 28 years old and tired of life in the military. He fell in love with a German teacher working in Sweden, eventually married her in 1863 and settled down in Malmö. He taught himself photography, which was new at that time, and managed to capture a photo of the Swedish King Karl XV being carried on a bier after his sudden death in Malmö on 18 September 1872. He became famous for his photographic skills, and was named "Hovfotograf", photographer to the King. However, he died suddenly from a stroke in 1877, when he was only 43 years old and my grandfather Wilhelm was only seven years of age. His mother Cathinka died when my grandfather was only 15 years old, leaving him without parents at this young age. However, when his mother knew that she was dying she instructed him on how to handle the situation after her death. He was taken care of by a famous industrial man in Malmö, Rolf Fredrik Berg, whose nickname was the King of Limhamn, who planned his education as an engineer in Germany. My grandfather was apparently a bright person and Berg noticed this and helped him throughout his life. Wilhelm returned to Sweden, where he became the chief executive officer of a brick factory outside Malmö. He held the same position in a marketing organization, Cementa. He was also chairman of the employer's organization in Malmö and finally he built up the Scandinavian Eternit factory. Eternit is a fiber cement that contains asbestos. Wilhelm died in 1955, happily unaware of the hazardous effects that the asbestos dust spread by this material had on human health.

Although my maternal grandfather was born in Sweden, he was not a real Swede. Both his parents were born abroad. This applied even more to my grandmother. She was a German, born in

Strasbourg, which at that time was a German city. Her grandmother was originally a Jew, born into a business family in Amsterdam, the Netherlands. She met a German lawyer, converted to his Protestant religion and settled down in Mainz, Germany. They had four children, including my great grandmother Rosette Hernsheim. She married a journalist called Friedrich Thiel, who was the son of a German lawyer and a cousin of a well-known German politician and government member in Prussia, Hugo Thiel, who gave his name to Thiel's Park and Thiel's Platz in Berlin. Thiel planned and built the Dahlem suburb, which was the home of culture and education and included the Free University of Berlin.

Friedrich was journalist during the 1870–1871 French–German war. He was captured by the French six weeks before the war ended and then he was released.

Rosette's brother Edward Hernsheim was a master mariner and entrepreneur who helped to colonize the islands in what is now western Papua Guinea, New Britain and New Ireland, around the Bismarck Archipelago. He and his brother Franz built a company on the small island of Matupi, close to Rabaul, that exported copra to Hong Kong, Sydney and Singapore.

During one of his early voyages to China, in the Robertson sailing boat, he and his team got caught up in a typhoon. One man died and the boat was shipwrecked on the coral reefs outside the Miyako-jima island. The rest of the crew, 12 seamen and himself, were saved the next day when the local islands sent canoes to their rescue. After some months on the island, he managed to borrow a new ship to take him first to Formosa, now Taiwan, and then back to his trading post at Matupi.

The story was later reported by a Japanese journalist, as an example of philanthropy, and resulted in a book that was used in Japanese schools. A monument was later erected on the shore of the island where he was shipwrecked. It was delivered by a German warship in 1876, by order of the Emperor, Wilhelm I. The story about the shipwreck and the rescue operation by the islanders is recorded on the monument in both German and Chinese, as the island was not under Japanese rule at that time. Later, the event was recorded in a museum on the island, housed in a copy of the Marksburg Castle in Germany. A full-sized statue of Edward was erected at the entrance to the museum and, to this day, a wall is covered with pictures describing the event. A model of the Robertson ship is displayed in a showcase.

In 2007, my wife Astrid and I visited the island and were met by the fifth-generation natives, who knew all about the story and how their ancestors had rescued the German crew. A village had been built around the recreated castle and called Ueno, or German village, and a Japanese–German Society had been created to remember the philanthropic event. The Society hosted a dinner in our honor, as we were the relatives of the famous Eduard Hernsheim. A 20-minute movie about the event, with professional actors, was shown at the dinner. It described the whole story, the shipwreck, the rescue and how the islanders helped the German crew. As guests of honor, we were interviewed by Japanese Television and we saw the program the next day at a restaurant on Okinawa on our way back to Tokyo (Chapter 50).

Eduard's copra trading went very well after that and he brought back ethnographic items to museums in Europe, particularly to Mainz, the city where he was born, and to Hamburg, where he had lived. He became well known in the scientific community. In 1882, when he was visiting his home country after 11 years abroad, he was invited to meetings with famous scientists. They included Rudolph Virchow, who was one of the most important pathologists ever, and who had discovered new diseases, such as acute leukemia. A dinner with 12 scientists was held after one of these meetings and there was a debate about a scientific work that had recently been published by Virchow about the reason for the bush-shaped hair growth on natives from Papua New Guinea. Virchow had claimed that it was inherited, while Eduard argued that it was due to the external use of calcium carbonate, based on information he had got from a scientist and friend in Hong Kong. Eduard did not know the people around him and argued heavily with the man sitting next to him. *"You just believe it because Virchow has claimed it"* he said. The man sitting on the other side kicked his foot under the table and whispered *"You are talking to Virchow"*. After the dinner, Virchow came up to him and presented himself in a friendly way, saying *"Fine, now we know each other"*. Virchow was later nominated for the Nobel Prize in Physiology or Medicine three times, twice for the first ever prize in 1901 and once in 1902. However, he died on 5 September 1901, a month before the Nobel Assembly at the Karolinska Institutet made their decision. In 1901 the prize went to Emil von Behring for his work on serum therapy and in 1902 it went to Ronald Ross for his work on malaria.

Eduard's trading post on Matupi was later taken over by my mother's uncle Max Thiel. Together, Eduard and Max supported German museums, particularly in Hamburg, Stuttgart and Berlin, by donating numerous ethnological items, including masks, spears and shields. However, many of these objects from the Bismarck Archipelago ended up in my mother's parental home in Lomma, outside Malmö, Sweden. The walls in their grand veranda room were covered with ethnographic objects from New Britain and other islands around the Bismarck Archipelago. Part of the collection eventually ended up in my home. However, our walls were not protected when our children and their friends were innocently playing or having parties. Spears were thrown into the garden and one valuable boomerang did not return as it should have done. Beautiful clothes were eaten by insects. Our ignorance of the value of these objects came to an end when my cousin sold a small statue of a witch doctor for more than 100,000 US dollars.

7 My Mother

My mother was relatively ignorant of her marvelous family history. Her father Wilhelm eventually became a wealthy man. As the chief executive officer of Cementa, he had a 20-room house with a large garden and servants, including a housekeeper, gardener, chauffeur, cook and nanny. This was my mother's childhood home. She was born in 1903, went to a school for girls in Malmö and, after she completed her exams at 17 years of age, she spent one year in a private French-speaking school for girls in Saltsjöbaden, outside Stockholm. She was already bilingual, as she spoke German as well as Swedish. Now she spoke French well, but not fluently. Her interest in gymnastics brought her back to Lund, close to her parental home, where she spent three years at the private Sydsvenska Gymnatik Institutet (South Swedish Institute for Gymnastics). This provided her with the skills she needed to be both a physiotherapist and gymnastics teacher. She longed to work abroad and speak French and she found a job at a military hospital in Antwerp, Belgium, where she spent one year. In the fall of 1924, she returned to Lund after she received an offer from the head of the school where she completed her gymnastics education. Josef Gottfrid Thulin asked her to work as his assistant in the Institute, which he had founded with his wife Emy. Thulin was very dominating, but respected, and was never called by his first name. He was referred to as Major Thulin or just Majoren, which was the rank he had risen to in the military. My mother only spent a year at the Institute, but during that time she organized an international camp in Ljungbyhed, in southern Sweden, where her students took part in great gymnastics shows that were established by Crown Prince Gustav Adolf.

She then met my father, fell in love, married him and followed him to Kristianstad and was called Doktorinnan, the wife of the doctor. Her professional career ended, as my father did not think that she should work professionally. He felt her role was to help him to establish their new home and be head of the household. She accepted and raised four children in a liberal atmosphere and employed servants, as her mother had done in her childhood. My mother engaged in the city's cultural life and became chair of the local Alliance Française. During World War II she became a volunteer car driver for the Bilkåren military organization. All she needed was her driver's license. She was a loving, and loved, mother, who wrote a book with photographs about each of her children. She developed breast cancer in 1943, when she was 40 years of age and had just given birth to my youngest sibling. Surgery was the only treatment at that time. She had her breast and local lymph nodes removed and, after five years of good health, she was considered cured. However, four years later an X-ray showed that she had lung metastasis. She died after several months of terrible suffering.

8 My Childhood

I was born on 20 December 1932. My parents had lived in Kristianstad for four years and I was their second child. My sister Anita was born on 9 June 1930 and was more than two years older than me.

Kristianstad was a small city of about 40,000 inhabitants and was called Little Paris because the center was surrounded by four boulevards. Our first home was a rented apartment in the Östra Boulevarden (eastern boulevard). We later moved to the Västra Boulevarden (west boulevard), with a railway in front of our home and a popular park and the Helge River behind it.

I started elementary school at six years of age in the fall of 1939. I liked school from the beginning. I was already getting very good grades in my first class, I loved my teachers and I made very good friends among my classmates. I was one of the shortest pupils in my class, but also the youngest, since I was born at the end of the year. I learned to cope with this, because I was popular, not the least with the girls, even though I was often shorter than them.

In 1934, when I was two years of age, my parents bought a nice summerhouse 17 kilometers outside Kristianstad. From then on we spent the summer holidays, which were more than two months long, there. Although the house was relatively big, with four bedrooms and a large, combined drawing and dining room, it was only half furnished. This meant that furniture, and even a piano, was transported back and forth from Kristianstad every year, first on a horse and carriage and later on a truck. The house was nicely located on the top of a hill, with a splendid view over the Baltic Sea.

On 1 September 1939, my mother was very unhappy. She was standing at the top of the stairs leading down to the beach and she told me that war had broken out in Germany. I was only six years of age and I did not fully understand what it meant, but I felt that something terrible had happened because mother was so upset. I still remember exactly how she stood at the top of the stairs and what she said. *"War has broken out in Germany"*. She did not say that the Germans had invaded Poland. In retrospect, this is very easy to understand. My mother's sister Karin had married a German officer employed by Wehrmacht, the German army, many years earlier (Chapter 6). The family, including my three cousins, lived in Lindau at Lake Bodensee in southern Germany. My maternal grandmother, who I already loved and had visited numerous times in Lomma, outside Malmö, was born a German. Her family had numerous relatives all around Germany. Although my mother's great grandmother had converted to Protestantism after she married a Protestant lawyer, she was born into a Jewish family. It is not difficult to understand my mother's concern about the future. To make things even more complicated, her brother was married to an English lady from Brighton and her father was a consul to Italy, with a German mother and a father who was Austrian-Croatian and thought to be Serbian at that time (Chapter 6). My father was an admirer of the USA and in fact had some distant relatives there.

I understood why my mother was unhappy. I do not think that she thought about the consequences for our family in Kristianstad, after all Germany was on the other side of the sea, but she was afraid about what would happen to her sister and her family in

Germany. Her father, my grandfather Willy, had other concerns. He did not want political issues to split his larger family in Sweden. He decided that talking politics should be banned, or at least avoided, at the frequent family reunions at his home in Lomma.

My mother's German-style upbringing had made her love the German culture, including the music and literature. Her sister had ended up in Germany because she attended a bookbinding school and had met her destiny there, a German officer. This did not diminish my mother's affection for her older sister and thus for Germany. During the first year of the war my evening prayer included *"Good Lord please make the Germans win the war"* because of my aunt Karin and my cousins. However, as increasing information emerged about what was happening during the war I changed this plea to *"Good Lord please make no one win the war"*. During the latter part of the war, I abstained from prayers and from any kind of stand on the issue.

9 My Youth

I spent four years in elementary school. This was during the breaking point between the old and the modern way of living. At least in a small community like ours. There was a horse market outside our apartment and the horse sellers ran back and forth with the horses to show that they were fit. They exposed their teeth to show that they were healthy. The horses were used by the farmers for hard work and even to transport our goods, for example taking our furniture to our summer house (Chapter 8).

The war was raging outside our country, but was always close. When Denmark and Norway were invaded by the Germans, we were alerted that the Hanö Bay, where our summer house was located, was the ideal part of the coastline if Hitler wanted to invade Sweden. Our defense was not as strong as our Prime Minister, Per Albin Hansson, claimed that it was. On the radio, he said that the military had to work hard to cover our beaches with barbed wire to prevent the Germans from invading us. However, the wire was not strong enough to stop me and my eight-year-old best friend Lennart Pettersson from crawling through it to reach the water for a swim.

Although the war never reached us, it was always present. Convoys of merchant ships followed the coast, just within neutral Swedish territory, in an attempt to avoid enemy torpedoes. They were always escorted and protected by destroyers. We were able to follow it all with our binoculars from our excellent position on the house on the hill. Fortifications with coastal artillery were built all along the coast and there are remains on the sand dunes outside our house. However, we did not refrain from staying in Åhus every year during the two summer months, despite our location being the optimal beach for an invader, and despite frequently hosting relatives dressed in military outfits and with military equipment. We were confident that we would not get involved, although my father spent time in unknown places as a military physician. Our Prime Minister delivered reassuring messages on the radio, and we tended to believe him, not knowing that he was compromising on many controversial issues with the Germans.

Then the war came closer. One day a damaged German submarine entered Åhus Harbor. My father bought a large pair of binoculars from the captain, as he did not need them anymore. We treasured them for the rest of the war and used them to follow what happened on the sea outside our summer house.

Kristianstad was not the center of the world, but it was my center during the school years. After four years at elementary school, there was an entrance exam for the school for higher education (Högre Allmänna Läroverket). After another five years there was an exam called realexamen. Then students had the chance to continue in the gymnasium (upper secondary school) at the same school, ending with matriculation, which was the entrance ticket to a university or comparable schools for subjects such as engineering.

I liked to go to school, most of the time, as I got good grades. I got special rewards every year, as I was one of the top pupils in the class. The reward was usually a book, but could be money, such as 50 crowns, which was about 10 US dollars at that time.

I loved my teacher in the lower elementary school and I liked many of those I had later. We received grades in every subject from the first school year, when I was seven years of age, to the last one, when I was 18. I liked the grades. You knew if you had done well or if you had to work harder to obtain grades to continue the path to matriculation.

The discipline at school was sometimes tough, but in general not difficult to follow. Most teachers showed authority and were respected. However, one day in the third year at elementary school I became very disappointed with one of my best teachers. I was 10 years of age. On the beach at Åhus there were certain stony spots where you could find amber, which were small, yellowish shiny stones. I had become good at finding them. Sometimes they were bigger than a pea or a bean. I wanted to show one of them, a big one, to my teacher and my class. So I brought one of them to school and asked my teacher if I could show him and the class my amber. He looked at it and said to me, and to the whole class, *"but this is just a piece of glass"*. The authority had spoken. But I knew that it was amber. I knew more than my teacher.

I passed the four years in elementary school without problems. There was an entrance exam giving access to Läroverket, and the first part, which was called Realskolan (high school). It was relatively difficult for a 10-year-old youngster and it was also psychologically demanding. Only about half of the pupils in elementary school would be able to progress to higher education after passing year four. The rest had to continue for another two, or even five, years, depending on whether they managed to enter "Läroverket" at their second attempt after year six in elementary school.

I completed the exam without any great problems and started at the new school in the fall of 1943, when I was 10 years old. There were two groups during those first years. The one that lasted five years was for those of us who had entered after four years in elementary school, the one that lasted four years was for those who had entered after six years in elementary school. The idea was that those who had entered after six years would have the chance to catch up and only lose one year until they entered the gymnasium that started after the end of high school.

I had a particular interest in chemistry, but was also interested in important training subjects like gymnastics and music. I managed well and got awards every year, including a special award in gymnastics and music. It turned out that I was the best male gymnast and my only competition was a girl who later participated in the Olympic Games. I was very interested in classical music and received an award for playing the piano. I don't think I was worthy of an award and probably got it because I took private piano lessons from our music teacher.

As in elementary school, I liked most of my teachers in the new Realskolan. However, there were some exceptions. An artwork teacher called Ludde struggled to handle the class and we often threw rags and water cups at each other and sometimes at him. Ludde sometimes reported the incidents to the class teacher, who stopped us. One Monday morning, in front of the whole class, the class teacher asked me with a harsh voice what I had done yesterday. I was in the first class in the new school and I was 11 years old. I was totally unprepared and surprised. I stuttered something like "*I picked mushrooms with my parents in the woods*". The class teacher called me a liar in front of the whole class. He said that I had followed Ludde from a distance on a street and had shouted swear words at him. I was angry and firmly denied it, but he did not believe me. Then something happened that I will never forget. One classmate, Kaj Holmberg, raised his hand and admitted that it was him. There was immediate silence in the class. The class teacher had obviously got confused and fell silent for half a minute. Then he just continued teaching without any further comments. I did not respect this teacher, but I admired Kaj's courage. I thanked him afterwards, but I do not think that he realized that I would remember him throughout my life, although I have lost contact with him since then. Fortunately, I got a new class teacher the next year.

I have a daughter who is a high school teacher and I generally admire teachers. They have one of the most important jobs and that is to make educated citizens out of children and youngsters.

After five years in high school I entered the gymnasium. There were two main groups, for natural science and humanistic studies. Of course, I took natural science, as this was the only one that could lead to university courses in natural science, medicine and engineering.

We had to work much harder from the first day, which I had not fully understood. I started out taking it relatively easy and my results started to decline, particularly in mathematics. My mathematics teacher was a man called Brunnström, but known as Brunte by the pupils, which was the name of a horse, due to his incompetence in mathematics. He quickly spotted my laziness, but knew that I had done well in high school. After I scored poor results in a mathematics test he said in front of all classmates *"Gahrton should not believe that he can live on his antecedents"*. I had to ask my mother what antecedents meant, but I still understood that I had to do better at school.

Eventually everything got better. I took private lessons in special mathematics from Borg, who was the best mathematics and physics teacher at the school. He was my class teacher for physics and I admired him. There was a rumor that he had to help Brunte with his mathematics classes. Borg was able to explain the most difficult mathematical problems. I had to do better in special mathematics to get enough high grades to enter the KTH

(Royal Institute of Technology) in Stockholm, which provided the most highly rated education in engineering in Sweden. Therefore I took a private lesson from Borg just before one of the last and most important tests in special mathematics. We usually had to solve eight mathematical problems over four hours on the day of the test. Borg showed me eight mathematical problems and explained them to me and I understood them all thanks to him. A few days later we had our official class test in special mathematics. To my amazement, I recognized the principal issues in each mathematical question. They were not the same as the ones that Borg had explained to me, but they were similar. Right or wrong, I scored 90% and my final matriculation grade was good enough for me to enter the chemistry class at KTH. I never told anybody about Borg's help, until now, but my conscience was not totally clear.

There were a few student associations at the school. There was an Association for Natural Sciences and I was its Chairman for a couple of years. There was also a very active association for humanities called Atheneum. I was a member, but not a very active one. My sister Anita was the Secretary for some time.

I met a clever and very spiritual boy called Nils Åslund at the Association for Natural Science, He was one year older than me and was not a classmate. He often sat at the back of the meeting room and his natural humor made us laugh. Having passed matriculation, he entered KTH and developed the confocal microscope, which made it possible to view fluorescence marked cells in three dimensions. It was an outstanding achievement. Eventually, he became a member of both the Swedish Royal Academy of Sciences and the Academy of Engineering Sciences. Our paths crossed again many years later, when he was collaborating with the Karolinska Institutet, where he eventually became an honorary doctor.

One of my mother's concerns about me was that I was careless. I was often late for my first school lessons and I tended to forget my schoolbooks and meeting times. One year I missed morning prayers before ordinary lessons three times and risked losing the normal final A grade of the year for the Order subject. We had morning prayers in a great hall at 8am every other day, as it could only accommodate half of the classes. The prayers lasted for 15 minutes before the ordinary lesson. The big entrance doors to the school closed at exactly 8am and did not open until the first lesson had started, which meant that you could not be on time if you missed prayers. Late arrivals received special remarks in the teacher's class book and three remarks triggered a warning message about the reduced Order grade. Your parents were alerted about this a month before the end of the school year. The warning needed to be signed by one of your parents and returned to the class teacher. My mother decided that my father should sign it and he did so angrily. I understood how serious it was and managed to be on time for the rest of the school term.

During the last year in the Realskolan, the teacher providing lessons in Christianity ran an extra course, outside the school curriculum, called confirmation. At about 15 years of age all Swedes were supposed to learn more about their Lutheran religion and this ended with an exam and communion. An important part of this was to know, read and believe the creed. I did not like it and felt that I was a non-believer. I particularly disliked the claim that there was only *"one holy general church"*. Why should I believe that there could not be other churches than ours? Despite that, I took the course, passed the exam and took the communion.

I was probably affected by my mother, who skipped the Christmas morning communion in the church in Lomma. For her, Christmas was more an important tradition than a religious holiday. She advised us that we should not hesitate to take communion, although she did not feel that she wanted to do it herself. My father usually managed to avoid Christmas morning at church. He believed in nature, not in a particular God.

After I had taken my confirmation, and ended school, it was summer. The two and a half or three summer months were very important for all Swedes, after several dark and cold months. That is why I had forgotten that I had accepted an almost compulsory invitation by the confirmation teacher to a dinner for all those who had taken their confirmation. This was held in his home at the beginning of the summer and I just failed to appear. My mother was angry and made me write a nice letter to the teacher apologizing for my poor behavior, which of course I did. My religious story deteriorated after that. We got a new teacher, but it did not help. I could not resist arguing when he claimed that when we eventually got married, it was God who had selected our wives. My final grade in Christianity was the worst one of all. Remarkably, it counted as much as history or English language for entering University or KTH.

The last year at school was very tough. We had to get good enough grades to enter higher education at KTH or University. A couple of months before matriculation, I understood that my final grades would be good enough to enter the chemistry course at KTH. However, I had started to rethink my future. I did not want to be a chemistry or mining engineer, which were the professions that my father liked so much. I wanted to study medicine. He did not protest. In fact, I soon realized that he liked it.

After matriculation, every male in Sweden had to do military service before entering KTH or other professional schools. I had already been assigned to the engineering troops after having declared my intention to study engineering. Military service lasted for many months, or even more than a year, but there was a special schedule for those who entered medical school, so that it did not infringe on how long their studies took. This was considered reasonable, because it took longer to study for a medical degree than other degrees. Therefore, you had to spend your summer holidays in the military over a period of years. I served for a total of 450 days. I had to write a formal letter to Your Majesty the King to change my military service from the engineering troops to the marines for medical students. The first three years were educational ones, but as soon as I had finished my courses in internal medicine and surgery at the university I was given a temporary license to serve as a doctor in the military. In the 1950s Sweden was strengthening its defenses and new destroyers were being built. My most enjoyable assignment was when I was a temporary physician in chief on a new destroyer, Halland, during its initial gyro probes. This ended with a lobster dinner at the most fashionable restaurant in Gothenburg. The job was easy, because everybody on the ship was in good health.

The time I spent at the Läroverket school was, in addition to my schoolwork, a time of fellowship and love affairs. I was part of an unofficial group of boys and girls that socialized a lot and had parties at our homes at the weekends. The composition of the group varied, but some core youngsters were the same and I was one of them. I have since wondered about the feelings of those who never belonged to our group. My own opinion was that I treated all human beings in a similar way without any kind of discrimination. However, I later understood, when our class gathered for reunions, that some classmates that did not belong to our selective group may have felt otherwise.

10 Summer Work and Holidays in England

After a couple of years in high school my father decided that I could not spend the whole summer holidays just having fun. It was reasonable that I worked and made some money for part of the summer. When I was 13 years old, I got my first paid job, helping a gardener at a market garden between Kristianstad and Åhus. The work was mainly to remove weeds around the flowers. The pay was five cents an hour. The more experienced gardeners earned five times as much, namely 25 cents an hour, and I and a couple of my classmates who worked there considered that this was unfair. In July, we thought that we had the right to steal some strawberries from a lot that was not far from where we worked. There was a hedge close to the strawberries where we could hide. When the coast was clear, we rushed out into the strawberry lot and picked as many berries as we could in a few minutes, before rushing back to our hiding spot. Then, one day when I was removing weeds, the 80-year-old mother of the owner visited the strawberry lot, picked a small basket of strawberries and approached me where I was working. She said *"Please take this basket with the strawberries, you are working very well and hard"*. I felt very ashamed, but of course I took the basket and thanked her. Those are events that you remember.

My father had a weird idea about what I should do one of the following summers. He thought that it was important to learn about car mechanics. He had to use charcoal-driven cars during the war and felt hampered because he did not have the knowledge he needed to fix frequent minor mechanical problems with his cars. He had to rely on a car mechanic who had a garage in Åhus. He arranged for me to work with the mechanic for three weeks and I was paid 25 Swedish crowns, which was about five US dollars, a week. At that time, I was still planning to work as an engineer and I could have used what I had learnt during those educational three weeks. However, it turned out that my employer, Tage, was one of the worst alcoholics in Åhus. He did not teach me anything. Instead, he used me to repaint an old truck and a fence around his garage, which he was forced to do by the village authorities. Åhus was going to celebrate its 800 year history in 1949 and the village needed to look nice and clean. After the three-week period I knew about as much as my father about car mechanics and it has stayed that way throughout my life.

A couple of years after the end of World War Two, schools were able to arrange exchange trips with pupils from some foreign countries. In 1949 it was possible to go by ship to Great Britain. I and one of my classmates went to England on the ship Suezia to visit two different families for three weeks. Then a youngster from those families came to Sweden for a three-week stay. We were very disappointed when we first arrived in a small town called Ashington in Northumberland, which was surrounded by pit heaps. Everything was gray and dust covered the houses. Furthermore, the British boys were only 13 and 14 years of age, while we were 16 and 17. However, we soon changed our opinion, due to the kindness and great hospitality shown by our host families. We learned to master the English language relatively well, which was the main objective of the exchange, and one day we were taken to the coast, which was only a short bus drive away, and had wonderful beaches. With the exception of an earlier short visit to Copenhagen, this was my first visit abroad and I liked it a lot. We became very good friends with our younger exchange companions and enjoyed their return trip to Sweden. Although we spent a lot of time talking about sea mines that had not yet been recovered, we were able to reassure our friends that the captain of the ship they travelled on was in control. We had travelled on the same ship when we visited them. The boys were very excited about coming to Sweden as it was also their first trip abroad. They seemed to appreciate Sweden during the three weeks they spent with us and returned home happy, as far as we could tell.

11 My French Period

My mother was the Chairperson of the French-inspired society Alliance Française in Kristianstad. She spoke French well, as she had attended a French-speaking girls' school in Saltsjöbaden (Chapter 7) and worked in Antwerp. At this time, any upper class, well-educated lady in Sweden was expected to be able to speak French. This was an old, but slowly disappearing, tradition in Sweden, which may have remained from the time of Gustav III, a French inspired Swedish king in the 18th century. My older sister Anita was good at speaking both German and French and she got an au pair job in France after she matriculated in 1949. Although it was quite clear to me that English was the most important language for whatever I was going to do, I started to see French as an interesting option. I had only studied French for two years at school and realized that my knowledge of the language was very poor. I could understand text relatively well, but could hardly speak or understand the language when people spoke to me. I decided it would be fun to learn French, and the family my sister was working for offered me the chance to work on a farm owned by a friend of theirs for two months in the summer of 1950. The farm was located in Touvaux, Boigneville, 80 kilometers south of Paris and was owned by Count d'Abovilles. I was not offered a salary, but I received free accommodation and meals and the opportunity to speak French with the family members. However, I was expected to work all day, as I arrived in July when the harvesting had just started.

My parents planned to take a car trip to Germany and France to pick up my sister, who had spent half a year in the French village of Chevigny, and drop me at the farm for my two-month stay. When we arrived at the agreed meeting point, a person who we believed to be an employee arrived in a Cinq Chevaux Citroen that looked ready for the scrap yard to pick me up. It turned out to be the Count. I said goodbye to my parents, transferred my small luggage to the Cinq Chevaux and we drove away. The Count was talking eagerly, probably about what I was going to do, but I understood absolutely nothing.

It turned out that the farm that the Count owned had been part of his father's large property holdings. His parents' home, which I later visited, looked like a castle, while my host lived in a smaller house with his young wife, two children and a stagiaire, Michel Degroote, a trainee who like me was employed, and treated as a family member. Michel became my friend for life. He knew a lot about farming and was practicing his skills while he waited to take over a farm in Normandy that he had inherited from his father. It was being restored after suffering severe damage during the war by the invading allied forces.

I started to work the next day. *"Rammaser des bottes!"* was my job for two months and this involved picking up the wheat-sheaves produced by a self-binder that was drawn by two horses. I picked the sheaves and placed them against each other to build small cottage-like heaps for drying. The field was eventually filled with the small drying heaps that later provided grain for meals.

I worked with a Polish guy in the field, which did not help my French, but during the two-hour lunches and dinners both the Countess and Michel were extremely helpful and patient in their attempts to teach me French. My language skills improved rapidly. Two or three glasses of wine with every meal helped a lot. Now and then Michel and I slipped away in the evening to a bar and had a glass of Pernod, which improved my French even more.

After the two months in Touvaux, Michel offered me the chance to spend some time in an apartment that his family owned in Paris. He thought that I should do some sightseeing in the capital before leaving France. He was unable to keep me company, as he had to work, but his family had employed an old maid to take care of the apartment and she looked after the household while I was staying there. I spent five days looking around in Paris, lived a life of luxury, went to Grand Opéra and was taken care of by the family's faithful old servant. And I spoke French.

Michel told me before I left that he was going to take over the farm in Normandy as soon as it was restored and then he would invite me to visit him. Michel was the youngest child in a wealthy family and he had, together with his 10 sisters and brothers, inherited their deceased father's fortune. His father had been a successful brewer, who had built up his fortune between the two world wars. He had expected new wars between the old enemies of Germany and France in the late 1930s, but thought that there were less likely to be battles in Normandy. That is why he bought farms in Normandy that could be taken over by his sons. Michel had inherited a mid-sized farm, one-eleventh of his father's fortune and a castle-like building. The predicted location of the future battle fields could not have been more wrong. During the allied invasion in World War Two, the farmhouses in Normandy were heavily damaged or destroyed. The big mansion house that Michel had inherited had been used as a store house by the military and was heavily damaged by artillery fire. The restoration took many years. In the meantime, Michel was working as a stagiaire at different farms. At the start of 1953 he was working in a large, modern farm, close to the one that he had inherited, and living in a small house with his wife Annicke. I think that when he invited me to work with him, he thought that he would have taken over his own farm by then, but for some reason that had not happened. I stayed with him and Annicke and worked at the same place that he did on the same conditions as a few years earlier in Touvaux. The only difference was that my host family was the Degroote family. Michel and Annicke did not think that I should work too much and that I should have time to study French. Thus, Annicke became my unofficial teacher, while Michel was working, and I only spent about half my time in the fields.

That was a wonderful summer. I was trained to write and speak French when I was not working in the fields and Annicke corrected my writing. The field work was totally different and heavier than in Touvaux. We still took care of the harvest, but with a modern combined harvester. My job was to load a cart with the heavy pressed straw rest from the harvester. However, I did not suffer as I only spent half my time doing that. Sometimes in the evenings we drove to the casino in Deauville and lost some money. And my French improved.

12 My Early Medical Studies with Nobel Prize-Worthy Teachers

Carl Herman Hjortsjö was Professor of Anatomy at the University of Lund. He occupied himself with bones and eventually became famous for his anthropological investigations of the Catholic Saint Birgitta from Sweden, as well as the Swedish King Eric XIV and Queen Kristina from the 16th and 17th centuries, respectively. When I started my studies in medicine at his institution, he was also the main teacher for the 30 young students. Each of us were given a box containing human bones and we were required to learn their Latin names, as well as each little structure, groove or elevation. There were regular intermittent examinations and most of these were conducted by ambitious older students who had been employed as an amanuensis, which was a part-time position. After about a month we were split into groups of four and each group received half a dead human to dissect. We were expected to identify each little nerve or vessel. We worked on this in parallel with our lectures for about six months and the course ended with a final examination in anatomy. The next course was histology, which involved carrying out microscopic investigations of all the structures in the body. As with our anatomy classes, there was only one Professor of Histology. Gösta Glimstedt[3] was not the brightest professor during my time as a student, but he was a meticulous man and researcher. However, he was widely surpassed in science by his closest subordinate, Nils Åke Hillarp, who was a prosector, which meant he was second in line and responsible for preparing dissections for demonstrations. Hillarp was an eccentric and unconventional person who would examine his students wearing a swimsuit and sun hat, if the weather permitted. Together with his closest collaborator and doctoral student, Bengt Falck, Hillarp developed a technique using fluorescence to visualize some of the most important substances in the human nervous system under the microscope, namely noradrenaline, dopamine, adrenaline and serotonin[4]. Some of his other doctoral students became famous and the most successful one was Arvid Carlsson, who received the Nobel Prize in Physiology or Medicine in 2000 (Chapter 35). Hillarp became world famous much earlier and was recruited to the Chair in Histology at the Karolinska Institutet in 1962. Sadly, his time in Stockholm was short. He died from a malignant melanoma in 1965 when he was only 49 years old, before the knowledge that too much sunshine was an important risk factor had emerged. Hillarp never received the Nobel Prize, but his research was immensely important for later scientists who did. In 1970, Ulf von Euler, a Professor in Physiology at the Karolinska Institutet, received the Nobel Prize with Bernard Katz and Julius Axelrod *"for their discoveries concerning the humoral transmitters in the nerve terminals and the mechanism for their storage, release and inactivation"*. von Euler repeatedly mentioned Hillarp's groundbreaking work in his Nobel lecture and said it has inspired some of the work he had done himself. Hillarp could have been a candidate for the Nobel Prize with Ulf von Euler in 1961–1965, but the latter was the secretary of the Nobel Committee at the time, which made it impossible for the Committee to propose them. So even though Hillarp was worthy of the prize, he did not survive long enough to receive it (Chapter 35).

I received a very good grade for my medical chemistry course and these followed the good grades in anatomy and histology. I appreciated my teachers, but they were not exceptionally good. The rumor was that many were excellent researchers and were apparently more interested in their own science than in teaching. However, never in my wildest fantasies did I think that two of them would be Nobel Laureates and that one teacher, who was two years younger than me, and entered the institution as I left, would join them. Sune Bergström had the chair in medical chemistry and was the department head. He has signed my examination in this subject *"with praise approved"*. Sune was a boring teacher, but his subordinate Arvid Carlson was somewhat more inspiring. Bengt Samuelsson entered the institution after I had left and then he joined Bergström in his research. The later destinies of these exceptional scientists are worthy of some comments at this point. They will also feature in later chapters, due to my collaboration with them many years later, not in science, but on other issues.

Bergström discovered the prostaglandines[5,6] and Carlson discovered the dopamines[7]. Samuelsson discovered prostaglandins with Bergström[6] and also discovered the leukotrienes[8]. All these substances were eventually used to develop therapeutics for various diseases. Both Bergström and Samuelsson later became the President/Rector of the Karolinska Institutet. Carlson moved to a chair in pharmacology at the University of Gothenburg. In 1982, Bergström and Samuelsson received the Nobel Prize together with John R Vane, and in 2000 Carlson received it together with Paul Greengard and Eric Kandel.

Bergström was probably the most unique of the three. My later boss, Gunnar Birke, Professor of Medicine at the Karolinska Institutet (Chapter 27), was the Head of the Huddinge Hospital, now the Karolinska University Hospital, Huddinge, south of Stockholm when Bergström was President of Karolinska Institutet. It meant that they worked closely together. Gunnar used to say that Bergström had his office in his head. It was very practical, because he didn't need to be bothered by too much paperwork. This was before the computer era.

After Bergström's death, it emerged that he had secretly been supporting a son that he had with Karin Pääbo, an Estonian chemist who had worked with him for some time. None of his friends or social circle appeared to know about it. It seemed somewhat strange, but Bergström did not talk about himself much. Whatever the reason, his son, Svante Pääbo, became a world-famous scientist like his father. In 1984 he managed to isolate DNA from a 2,400-year-old Egyptian mummy[9]. He also collected DNA from extinct animals, like a 200,000-year-old mammoth. In 1997, he managed to sequence mitochondrial DNA from a Neanderthal, which led to the conclusion that there was some interbreeding between Neanderthals and the ancestors of present-day Eurasian humans. Amazingly, a small number of genes from the Neanderthals appeared to be important for sensitivity to virus disorders i.e., COVID-19 infection. Eventually, he discovered a third human-like race, the Denisovans, that also seemed to have migrated north from Africa at a different time tens of thousands of years ago.

In 1997, Svante Pääbo became the Head of the newly established Department of Genetics at the Max Planck Institute for Evolutionary Anthropology in Leipzig, Germany. He became an internationally leading researcher in the field and is known as a founder of paleogenetics. He has received numerous internationally important awards. In my first (nonpublished) edition of this book, I wrote *"but he has not received the Nobel Prize yet. I would not be surprised if he eventually receives the award, like his father, because he is a worthy candidate"*. He got it in 2022 and I had the privilege to listen to his fascinating Nobel lecture. This was after the death of his father, who would then hopefully have been proud of his denied son.

My course in medical chemistry was followed by courses in general and special pathology. For the first time, we were confronted with patients who had died from their diseases during the last 24 hours. The Head of the Department of Pathology at the University Hospital in Lund was Carl Gustav Ahlström or CG as we called him. He was an excellent teacher and managed to provide demonstrations of the causes of death in the finest detail. For example, if a patient died from cardiac infarction, CG showed us the very spot where the coronary artery stenosis has occurred. It was fascinating, but of course it was also frightening. Just a few millimeters had closed and stopped the blood that should have provided the heart muscles with oxygen and the patient had died.

A few years later, when I had passed my examination in pathology with an excellent grade, CG offered me a position as an amanuensis, or part-time assistant, initially for three months. I became rather skilled in performing autopsies and finding the cause of death, but I soon realized that I was more interested in working with living patients than dead ones. After the three months had passed, I left CG and pathology, but we remained friends.

My real clinical education started at the Department of Lung Disorders. It was a small department that was headed by Eric von Rosen, who was just a docent in lung disorders, which was less than a full professor. He was a vain man of the old school, who knew all the special sounds you could hear when a stethoscope was attached to the back or chest. For example, there were numerous different sounds for the special stages of tuberculosis. In the short time we spent with him, he did not manage to teach us more than a fraction of them. The advancement of X-ray diagnostics made a lot of these sounds irrelevant. Of course, it was important to recognize the typical sounds of pneumonia, but all the ones that were considered typical of the stages of tuberculosis were, in my opinion, obsolete.

von Rosen was not highly rated by us students. He was very proud of being of noble heritage. However, when my friend Erik Leijonhufvud, who belonged to an old Swedish noble family, was called Baron Leijonhufvud, while we were called candidate, followed by our surname, even Erik thought that was ridiculous.

In 1954, after nearly three years of studies, we started working close to the patients. The course in internal medicine was very practical. Every student was assigned to an in-patient ward and there were usually two students on the same ward. It was the students' responsibility to take and record the patients' disease history and suggest the diagnostic and therapeutic plan for them. This was checked and corrected by the responsible physician. The head of the course and the whole Department of Medicine was the Professor of Medicine at the University of Lund, Haqvin Malmros. He was well known internationally for his research in diabetes and the important role that it played in coronary heart disease. He was a good friend of my father since they had worked together under Karl Petrén in the 1920s (Chapter 5). When my father moved to Kristianstad, Malmros remained in Lund and passed his thesis in 1928, one year after the death of Petrén. In 1935 Malmros was appointed Head of the Department of Medicine in Örebro in central Sweden. He continued his research and in 1950 he returned to

Lund as Professor of Medicine after a tough competition. Malmros was a modest person, who was not very inspiring as a teacher, but I felt he was a hardworking scientist and clinician and underestimated as a researcher. He saw the connection between saturated fat in food, high cholesterol in the blood and coronary heart disease at an early stage. He performed large clinical trials to prove the case, which is hardly debated today. However, many other scientists worked in parallel with him in this field and Malmros was never a Nobel Prize candidate.

Malmros brought a controversial physician with him from Örebro as his closest subordinate. Docent Åke Nordén was in charge of patients with hematologic disorders and he later became both my tutor and, remarkably, he was later the opponent when I defended my thesis (Chapter 19).

The most internationally well-known of my teachers was a Professor of Renal Disorders called Nils Alwall. He competed with Willem Kolff to be called the father of hemofiltration and was responsible for the first workable artificial kidney. He had his own department and worked independently of Malmros, but participated in teaching renal disorders. It is no secret that both Alwall and Kolff were repeatedly nominated for the Nobel Prize (Chapter 48).

13 Mountain Climbing

By 1954, I had caught the mountain climbing bug. My first climb was not planned. It happened when I teamed up with three school friends for a trip around Europe, after I had managed to convince my father to let us borrow his car, a well-used Vauxhall. After many adventures we ended up at Franz Josef Höhe in Austria, at the foot of the highest mountain in the country. Grossglockner was 3,798 meters high. As we sat in the hotel restaurant eating breakfast we looked up to the mountain and discussed how difficult it would be to reach the top. I was bold and youthful and claimed that it would probably not be extremely difficult. After some polarizing discussions, we agreed that Sture Svantesson and I would try to climb to the top, while our companions Lennart Pettersson and Christer Håkanson took a trip to Italy and picked us up at the hotel after a couple of days, when we had hopefully returned alive. We rushed to a store to rent crampons, namely climbing irons, and ice axes, despite the fact that we had no idea how to use the equipment. We were asked whether we wanted to rent a rope, but as we did not know how to use it, we just said that we did not need it. We passed a glacier on ski boots, without using the crampons, and amazingly managed to reach a manned cottage at a height of 3,000 meters, where we got food and stayed overnight. We were informed that two professional mountain climbers were offering tourists the chance to climb with them to the top early in the morning, with three tourists on each of the two ropes for security. We learned the essential skills of attaching the crampons and handling the ice axe and reached the top in heavy fog early in the morning, after a couple of hours' climbing. Having passed narrow passages, and seen the frightening abysses on both sides of our path, we were happy when we were back alive and in the cottage. We were warned about overhangs and glacier cracks going down from the cottage to the hotel without security ropes. However, we wanted to hurry down to meet our friends and that is what we did. After only one overnight stay on the mountain, we were back. This was the start of the mountaineering bug, which was to last many years.

I got the chance to combine my interest in mountain climbing with speaking French the next summer, which was 1955. In addition to previous courses in pathology, medical students were required to spend two additional months at a pathology institution and were encouraged to do it abroad. We had to arrange it ourselves, but it had to be approved by the Chair in Pathology at our university, which in my case was CG Ahlström. I had heard that the French-speaking University Hospital in Lausanne, Switzerland, had an excellent Department of Pathology and allowed students at my level to participate in the activities at no cost. I wrote to the chair and, with support from CG, I was admitted for two summer months.

Of course, I did not tell them that the possibility to reach the highest mountains in the Swiss and French Alps from Lausanne was a great incentive. I loaded my travel equipment onto a second-hand Vespa motorbike and started my trip south in the early summer. It took three days to reach Lausanne from Lund. I slept in haystacks and in the forest under the Vespa cover that I had brought with me. Nobody disturbed me. I had arranged to rent a room in a property owned by a nice old lady close to the hospital.

I soon found friends who were interested in mountain climbing and joined a course a few hours away that arranged climbing in the Swiss mountains. I set off on my Vespa and we climbed every weekend during the two months I spent at the Institution of Pathology. It was like a drug. We constantly had to climb and reach new peaks, which we did. A girl on the course told me that her father had been an enthusiastic climber but fell from a cliff. He survived, but sustained brain damage, and hemiplegia prevented him from climbing again. But she still climbed. Our base was usually at a village called Martigny, which provided access to many climbing areas. We climbed Les Diablerets, les Ecandies and many more mountains. I learned all that I should have done before my friend and I had tackled Grossglockner, such as rock climbing, glacier climbing, how you secure your friend on your rope and how you can descend rapidly on the snow without the high risk of ending up in glacier cracks.

After the course I wanted to do more difficult climbing. The course leader had an assistant who was an excellent rock climber. He had not yet climbed the highest mountains in Switzerland and I convinced him that we should climb the Jungfrau, a 4,158 meter mountain that was not too difficult to climb. There was also a railway station at 3,454 meters, which we could reach by a mountain train and a hotel at Jungfraujoch, from which we could start our climb. We stayed overnight in the hotel and planned to reach the peak early the next morning. We started out in fair weather, but when we were approaching the peak, the weather deteriorated and there was a terrible thunderstorm. Lightning struck all around us, electricity sparkled in the crampons and in the ice axes and it started snowing. We tried to find cover behind a rock but were only half successful. The peak was only a couple of hundred meters in front of us, but my friend decided that we had to return. Amazingly enough I was not afraid, but I was disappointed that we had to return without reaching our goal. However, my experienced friend knew better. This was life threatening. With sparkling crampons and ice axes we climbed down as quickly as we could. The weather got worse, but we managed to reach the hotel without coming to any harm. We took the mountain train back to civilization the next day.

However, I had not given up on my ambition to reach the highest peaks in Europe. I tried to convince my friend that we should climb Mont Blanc, which at 4,810 meters, was the highest mountain in Europe at that time. Now it is supposed to be Elbrus in the Caucasus. He accepted with some hesitation. To reach the peak of Mont Blanc we mainly had to climb and walk on glaciers, but he was a typical rock climber. However, he was obviously as keen as I was to reach the highest peak in Europe. We started in Chamonix in France and planned to stay overnight in an old cottage, Les Grand Mulets, at 3,051 meters. It was built in 1896, was in poor condition and unmanned. We reached it by traversing a somewhat difficult glacier, Les Bosson. We arrived without problems in the evening to find the cottage occupied by a group of alpine hunters, who had started to cut wood from the run-down cottage to make a fire. Les Grand Mulets has now been rebuilt several times, and since 2006 it has provided an excellent, modern overnight facility that is perfect for starting the last climb to the top of Mont Blanc. We made friends with them, and they let us use their fire to do some cooking and eat a poor meal. Eventually, we found some space to sleep in our sleeping bags until very early in the morning, when we started our attempt to reach the top. However, after some hours, when we had reached about 4,300 meters above sea level, my friend started to have difficulty breathing. He had got mountain sickness, which is fairly common if you have not spent enough time adapting to the high altitude before attempting to reach the highest peaks. Luckily enough there was, and still is, a large 35 square-meter aluminum house called Refuge Vallot with four beds at 4,350 meters. It is used as a meteorological observation station and a rescue station for alpine climbers in trouble. We had to stay overnight until my friend had recovered enough to descend to Chamonix the next morning. Thus, we had failed in another attempt to reach one of the 4,000 meters plus peaks in the Alps.

We reached Chamonix without problems, and we had dinner at the lodge with a Catholic church party that were going to climb to the top the next day. They planned to do exactly what we had intended to do the day before, go to Les Grand Mulets, spend the night there and then climb to the top early the next morning. We told them about our failed attempt and the conditions at Les Grand Mulets. They sensed that I was very disappointed and probably strong enough to reach the peak and perhaps they thought that I could be of some value in directing them to Les Grand Mulets. Anyway, they offered me the chance to be the number four in one of their three ropes. My friend encouraged me to join them. He preferred to stay and have fun in Chamonix for the two days that I was supposed to be away. I packed for another climb and was happy. The next day I was on track again, this time with a religious group. To my amazement, an enormous avalanche had blocked the track we had taken the day before on our descent. I was happy that we had passed it before it had happened. We reached Les Grand Mulets as planned, slept a few hours, and then started our climb at 2am with headlamps. Early morning was the safest time if we wanted to avoid avalanches. We proceeded slowly over the steep glacier slopes, looking down into deep valleys. Every step above 4,200 meters was like lifting a stone, even though I was very well trained. We reached the top well before noon after some nine hours' climbing. The clouds obstructed the view completely. My friends arranged a table out of pins and a cloth and held a Catholic Mass. We did not stay for long and started our descent to reach the valley before the afternoon when the avalanches usually raged. We took another track down and had just passed below the famous peak, Aiguille du Midi, when our leader shouted, *"heads down against the mountain"*. His warning had come just in time, as enormous rocks came bumping down the steep mountain wall above our bodies. Fortunately, none of us were hurt, and we reached our base after a few hours. My friend was already there and the next day we went back on our motorbikes to Lausanne.

My climbing eventually stopped, and my last climb was after a hematology congress in Vienna in 1961. I took a train to Hoher Dachstein in Austria, hired an experienced mountain guide and reached the narrow peak after steep rock climbing. Looking around, and down into the valley a couple of thousand meters below, I got that strange feeling of wanting to fly off the peak a little bit, just like the Dohle, a black bird we frequently saw in the mountains. By then I had a wife and children. It was time to stop climbing.

14 Exchange Student in Zürich with Guido Fanconi, Manfred Bleuler and Sven Moeschlin

My tennis partner in Lund had academic degrees in the German language. He told me that there was an exchange program between Sweden and the University of Zürich, whereby you could apply for a one-year stay and your free choice of studies at any faculty. Normally, students had to pay significant fees for each course, but there was no limit to the number of free courses that exchange students could attend. The Faculty of Medicine had some of the best teachers in Europe and you got a grant to cover your food and housing. I was tempted to apply, despite only having about a year and four courses until my final examination. I spoke to three professors in Lund and one in Stockholm about what they would require if I had passed the courses in Zürich. The Lund professors were Erik Essen-Möller in psychiatry[10], Torsten Krakau in ophthalmology[11] and Hjalmar Koch in otorhinolaryngology[12]. They each required one months' service in their departments and then an examination. The rumor was that the Head of Pediatrics in Lund, Sture Siwe, did not like the star in pediatrics in Zürich, Guido Fanconi. It was possible that this was because Fanconi had written one of the best textbooks worldwide in pediatrics, together with Siwe's better-known competitor, the pediatrician, Professor Arvid Wall-gren, who retired from the Karolinska Institutet in Stockholm in 1956. As far as we knew, the professor in Stockholm in 1958, Professor Curt Gyllensvärd at the Crown Princess Lovisa's Hospital for Children, was on good terms with Fanconi. I approached him and he enthusiastically approved my plan and promised me that I only had to spend one month in his departments when I returned and then he would examine me himself.

I applied and got the grant. I joined all the necessary courses, and a few unnecessary ones that I found interesting and that were led by important teachers.

I arrived in Zürich well in time for the start of the courses. I had some friends who were engineering students at the important Eidgenössische Technische Hochschule and they had promised that I could spend some days in their rooms until I found a place to stay. This was easy in Zürich. I rented a room from a very nice old lady, who frequently invited me to have lunch with her.

Medical education in Zürich was very different from Sweden. Most of it took place in the lecture hall and you were not assigned a specific department where you were responsible for writing patient histories or examining patients. The lecture halls looked like amphitheaters and you had an excellent view down to the teacher, and, most important, to the patient that the teacher used for the lecture. The lack of ward work was very much compensated for by the excellent lectures and demonstrations in the lecture hall. The teacher was usually the professor who headed the specific department. I must admit that some of my teachers in Zürich were not surpassed in excellence by any of those I had at Lund or after that point. The most brilliant was no doubt Fanconi in pediatrics, closely followed by Manfred Bleuler in psychiatry.

Fanconi[13] was Professor of Pediatrics and Head of the Children's Hospital at the University of Zürich. He was born in 1892 in a small village called Poschiavo in the Canton of Grisons. In 1920 he was admitted to the hospital as a young doctor after his medical education, mainly in Lausanne. He stayed at the Children's Hospital throughout his medical career. In 1929 he succeeded his mentor Professor Emil Feer as Professor of Pediatrics and head of the hospital.

Fanconi has been called the father of modern pediatrics. He described several diseases and the most well known is an inherited blood disorder, named after him, called Fanconi anemia[14]. It is a homozygous disorder, meaning that each parent has one abnormal gene, without having the disease, and the affected child has the misfortune of inheriting an abnormal gene from each parent. The disease is characterized by bone marrow failure, resulting in thrombocytopenia, anemia and leukopenia. This means that the most important blood cells, which are responsible for preventing bleeding, providing oxygen support to the body and preventing infections, are not produced in enough numbers. The children suffer from bleeding, infections, fatigue and powerlessness. In addition, they have malformations, particularly in the radius in the forearm. There is an increased risk of developing leukemia and myelodysplastic syndrome, a leukemia-like disease. Fanconi anemia is extremely rare, as the prevalence is about one in 1–3 million. Modern molecular techniques have shown that the disorder involves mutations in several genes named after Fanconi, including *FANCA* and *FANCB*. The only treatment is a hematopoietic stem cell transplantation, and this is not without its risks (Chapter 29).

Fanconi described several other disorders, particularly renal ones, but it is difficult to determine what part he played, because other scientists also described these. The Swedish pediatrician Rolf Zetterström reviewed Fanconi's life and scientific contributions and asked Guido's son Andreas Fanconi, later Professor of Pediatrics in Zürich, how he rated his father's scientific contributions. This is how Zetterström cites Andreas[15]: *"Fanconi anemia is a rare but very interesting disease, which has found new interest in the last years because of the chromosome breakages. This term is firmly established in paediatric haematology. I would not consider the Fanconi–Lignac syndrome, an eponym no more used. However, Fanconi–Debré–de Toni syndrome or 'Fanconi syndrome' as used in the English language would be worthwhile considering, as this denomination is currently used for the global insufficiency of the proximal renal tubule. It is interesting to see that amongst his discoveries, these rare diseases or syndromes have kept his name, whereas the much more frequent and important disease, cystic fibrosis, also first described by Guido Fanconi 1936, is no more associated with his name."*

During his 40 years as Head of the Children's Hospital, Fanconi made it world famous and comparable to university hospitals like the Children's Hospital in Boston, USA. In addition to his outstanding contribution to medical research, as administrative head of the hospital and an active and excellent physician who saw patients most days of the week, he managed to write a textbook with Arvid Wallgren and be an excellent teacher. Without doubt, he was the best teacher in clinical medicine that I ever had. His demonstrations with patients were outstanding. He kept his audience engaged with a marvelous combination of to-the-point conversations with patients, X-ray findings, microscopic bone marrow patterns shown on a screen and summarizing his diagnosis and suggestions for treatment.

Fanconi retired in 1962, only three years after I left Zürich. Many of his students and collaborators became outstanding pediatricians. One of them became his successor and that was Andrea Prader, endocrinologist and co-discoverer of Prader–Willi syndrome, another genetic disorder due to aberrant genes on chromosome 15. Prader gave a few lectures during my time in Zürich, as a private docent, but these were far less inspiring than those by Fanconi.

With all his discoveries, you would assume that Fanconi was an excellent candidate for the Nobel Prize. However, as seen in Chapters 2 and 3, discovering a new disease is not enough to win this award. Even discovering many diseases is not enough. Discoveries only qualify if they change the principle or view of how people see diseases. The term paradigm-shifting is frequently used. Still, until 1972 Fanconi was nominated once in 1967 i.e., many years after his main scientific discoveries and as long as you are allowed to reveal nominations. He died in 1979.

Manfred Bleuler, Professor of Psychiatry, was another famous teacher, who gave brilliant lectures. He was the son of an even more famous father, Eugene Bleuler, who had been Professor of Psychiatry in Zürich before Manfred. He created the word schizophrenia and believed the cause was a primary brain dysfunction due to an inherited disposition. However, he also pointed out that biographical and environmental factors could play a role in the etiology. His most important original work was probably describing schizophrenia symptoms and defining them as one disease[16]. It appears that his work is still of value and relevant for present schizophrenia research[17]. Eugene Bleuler was nominated for the Nobel Prize in 1930, but never received it.

Manfred did not intend to follow in his father's footsteps, as he wanted to specialize in surgery. However, after a serious accident he decided to specialize in psychiatry and eventually, in 1942, he became professor at the same university his father had worked at. He continued his father's research on schizophrenia and made a number of important contributions, in particular about defining the difference between acute and chronic schizophrenia and how to treat the disease. Manfred is still best known for his teaching capabilities and for continuing writing new editions of the textbook in psychiatry that was first published by his father. When he died in 1994, at the age of 91, there had been 15 editions. My edition was number nine, which was the version available in 1958.

Manfred Bleuler liked to create drama during his lectures. I still remember how a woman entered the amphitheater on a rolling bed and Bleuler deliberately provoked a seizure. Four students were asked to rush to her bedside to try make her pupils contract using a flashlight. They were told that if they did not contract it indicated an epileptic seizure. However, the lucky students were able to inform their peers in the auditorium that her pupils had contracted normally, and this meant it was probably a hysterical seizure and not epilepsy. I wonder what an ethical review board would have thought about the drama today, although it was without risk.

Manfred Bleuler received some awards for his scientific and teaching contributions in psychiatry, including the Stanley R Dean Award. Unlike his father, he was never a candidate for the Nobel Prize.

I had agreed with the Swedish professors that I would pass a number of courses in Zürich. I also signed up for an additional course in bone marrow examination and my teacher was the world-famous hematologist Sven Moeschlin[18]. The rumor was that he had lost the competition to become the chair in medicine at the University of Zürich to a nephrologist called Jean Rossier and that their relationship was not very good. Moeschlin, therefore, moved to a head position in medicine at the hospital in Solothurn, a medium-sized historical city about 94 kilometers west of Zürich. The hospital served the whole canton of Solothurn, with some 80,000 inhabitants. However, he was still allowed to lead the course in bone marrow examination in Zürich.

Sven Moeschlin was born in 1910, the son of the famous Swiss author and journalist Felix Moeschlin and his wife, the Swedish artist Elsa Sophia Hammar. Felix lived and worked in Sweden as a journalist from 1909–1914 and Sven was born there. The family then moved to Felix's home country of Switzerland. Sven had learnt Swedish during his childhood and spoke it throughout his life, although following the death of his mother he had no opportunities to speak it at home. Sven had noticed that I was from Sweden, and it was obvious that he was very happy to speak Swedish with me. We became very good friends and I returned to Switzerland many years later for a two-month stay in Solothurn, where I looked through the microscope at his exclusive collection of spleen smears, to learn how to use the cytological picture for diagnostical purposes.

However, this turned out to be much less important than what I learned during his course in bone marrow examination, which is the most important diagnostic tool for discovering all sorts of hematologic disorders, including leukemia and aplastic anemia.

In 1958 Sven Moeschlin was one of the leading hematologists in the world after his discoveries of the cause of drug-related agranulocytosis a few years earlier. He could show that some drugs induced antibodies against the patient's own white blood cells, namely leukoagglutinines[19]. Agranulocytosis is a life-threatening disorder. The granulocytes, or neutrophil leukocytes, disappear from the blood and the patient, who now has no defense against bacterial infections, develops a high fever and other severe symptoms of infection. Sven showed that the cause was not a primary deficiency of the bone marrow to produce the granulocytes. It was drug-induced damage to those cells that made the immune system see them as foreign. Antibodies were developed against them and destroyed them. I viewed this fundamentally important discovery, which was made in 1952, as a forerunner to the later discoveries of the H2 complex by George Snell and the HLA (human leukocyte antigen) system by Jean Dausset, who were awarded the Nobel Prize in 1980 (Chapter 42). Sven was never a candidate.

After he left Zürich to go to Solothurn, Sven devoted himself to the clinic and to writing textbooks. I later stayed with him in Solothurn. In addition to my studies on spleen smears, I followed him on his rounds, when he carried out individual investigations and decided on the treatment of all of the visited patients. This took the whole morning and after lunch he went to his private outpatient clinic. He was a knowledgeable and excellent clinician. Sven Moeschlin retired from the hospital in 1976, but continued writing educational other books for many years. He died in 2005 when he was 95 years old. Unfortunately, I had lost contact with him many years before that.

After an eventful and, from an educational point of view, most rewarding year at the University of Zürich I returned to Sweden. I finalized the courses and services I had agreed to in Lund and Stockholm, i.e., ophthalmology, otorhinolaryngology, pediatrics and psychiatry. I passed the examinations in all of them. Six months after my return I also passed the examination in internal medicine, which was the most extensive subject during all of my studies.

15 My Time as a Physician in Lund

I passed the examination in internal medicine with the second highest grade that you could get. The highest one was only used in exceptional circumstances, for example if you had previously started scientific work within the department. The examiner was the Head of the Department of Medicine, Professor Haqvin Malmros. The examination took all day. I was assigned a patient with breathing difficulties. I took the patient history and carried out a physical examination, just using my stethoscope and a percussion hammer. After that, I had to suggest diagnoses, further investigations and alternatives for treatment. I had a couple of hours to work and talk with the patient, who was fully informed that this was an academic examination. I wrote the patient history, noted the physical findings and suggested my diagnosis, which was heart failure. Then I discussed the possible treatment alternatives. The examination consisted of two parts. One was the examination and the discussion about the patient and the other was an oral examination that could include anything related to internal medicine. I decided to be particularly prepared in diabetes and heart disorders for the second part of the examination, because I knew that Malmros was particularly interested in those diseases. However, my intuition was totally wrong. After answering questions about the patient to his satisfaction, he asked about the treatment of leukemia. This was the favorite subject of his associate professor,

Åke Nordén, and my own main interest at the time. I think I knew more about it than my examiner.

After the examination, Malmros asked if I would consider work in his department. If so, I would be responsible for the propedeutic medicine course, under the Head of Cardiology, who was Inge Edler. This was exactly what I wanted.

I started to work as a qualified physician in the Department of Medicine in September 1959. In later years I tried to persuade myself that the offer from Malmros was due to my excellent examination, but I still had a faint suspicion that my father's old friendship with him, when they worked in the same department under Karl Petrén in the 1920s, may have played a role. However, my life went in the right direction.

The propedeutic course was very much focused on physical diagnostics. Edler and his collaborators were excellent teachers. My job was to administrate the course. In addition, I was a resident in Malmros' private ward and participated in the emergency service at night.

I told Edler from the beginning that I did not intend to be a cardiologist. I had already decided to devote myself to hematology. However, as I was going to spend at least a year in the cardiology department, he suggested that I should devote myself to a small cardiology project that could be finished in about six months. He suggested that I should try to clarify the reason for electrocardiographic (ECG) abnormalities seen in patients with pectus excavatum, also known as funnel chest. This is a congenital disorder in which the chest bones form an inward groove that does not usually cause symptoms. It was unclear why there were ECG changes in these patients, although they generally did not show cardiac symptoms. I was eventually able to show that the

ECG changes were due to the rotation of the heart, because of the deformities of the chest, but that they did not indicate damage to the heart. My results were published in the international journal *Acta Medica Scandinavica*, which is now the *Journal of Internal Medicine* (Chapter 38). This was my entry into the international scientific world[20]. However, it was far from the revolutionary work that Edler had started with his well-established clinical scientific group.

16 Inge Edler and Echocardiography

Inge Edler was born in 1911. He started his career in cardiology in Malmö but moved to Lund after a few years. There were unconfirmed rumors that this was due to some difficulties with his much more famous head, Jan Waldenström (Chapter 18). Edler became Head of the section of Cardiology at the Department of Medicine under Professor Haqvin Malmros. By the start of the 1950s, Inge had decided to develop non-invasive methods, such as radar, to diagnose valve disorders of the heart. He thought that it could be possible to visualize abnormalities in the movements of the heart valves, which would be very important, because such abnormalities were life threatening and could be corrected by heart surgery.

Edler made contact with the physicist Hellmuth Hertz. He was interested in the possibility of using ultrasound for practical purposes and suggested to Edler that they should work together to try to develop an ultrasound device that could be adapted to heart investigations. Hertz belonged to a well-known family of physicists. His father, Gustav Ludwig Hertz was a Nobel Prize winner in physics in 1925 with James Franck *"for their discovery of the laws governing the impact of an electron upon an atom"*. It is interesting to note that he was nominated by Albert Einstein, who had been awarded the prize in 1921. Gustav's uncle, Heinrich Hertz, would probably have been an equally worthy candidate for a Nobel Prize if he had not died in 1894, before the prize was established.

He had proved the existence of electromagnetic waves and given the name hertz to the frequency of these waves.

Hellmuth Hertz now constructed a device that could take pictures from inside the heart, just by attaching it to the front wall of the chest. He and Edler tested the apparatus for the first time in 1953 on a patient with heart valve failure[21]. The investigation was completely safe because the ultrasound device was just pressed against the chest while Edler held it. However, it produced poor quality pictures, and it was impossible to identify the valves or the other structures in the heart. Edler was disappointed, but he did not give up. Hertz tried to improve the ultrasound device and Edler was thinking about how to create an experimental model that could follow the ultrasound through the heart and then prove its anatomical path.

When I arrived at Edler's department in the fall of 1959, he, and his closest collaborators Arne Gustafsson, Tord Karlefors and Birger Christensson, had decided to experiment on a heart harvested from a calf. They attached it to a water pipe system so that they could open and close the valves of the heart by opening and closing the water flow. The aim was to recreate what happened in a living animal. The movements of the valves were registered on an electrical printer and so were the echoes obtained by the ultrasound device.

One day in the autumn of 1959, when everything was set up in the rinsing room, Edler asked me to come and participate in the first experiment. They needed an assistant. How was I to know that I was going to be involved in a crucial and historical event in the development of ultrasound? This was to become the most important method for diagnosing abnormalities of the heart, including heart valve abnormalities, such as mitral stenosis, that could be surgically corrected. I was given a 20cm long steel pin and told to direct it exactly against the ultrasound device adapted to the heart by Edler. Forcing the pin through the heart from the opposite side showed the anatomical path of the ultrasound. The ultrasound pictures could then be analyzed. The pin was forced through the mitral valve and Edler was able to show that the ultrasound pictures visualized the movements of the valves. The findings were published by Edler and his group in 1961[22]. Further work identified many valve abnormalities and other heart failures. Today, ultrasound is probably the most important method for diagnosing and following up heart diseases.

Edler and Hertz never received a Nobel Prize, but they were awarded the next most important prize in medicine, the Lasker Prize. History will tell why. To my great joy, Edler was in the audience when I had the honor of being invited to give a lecture at the Department of Medicine in Lund in the late 1990s. This time the

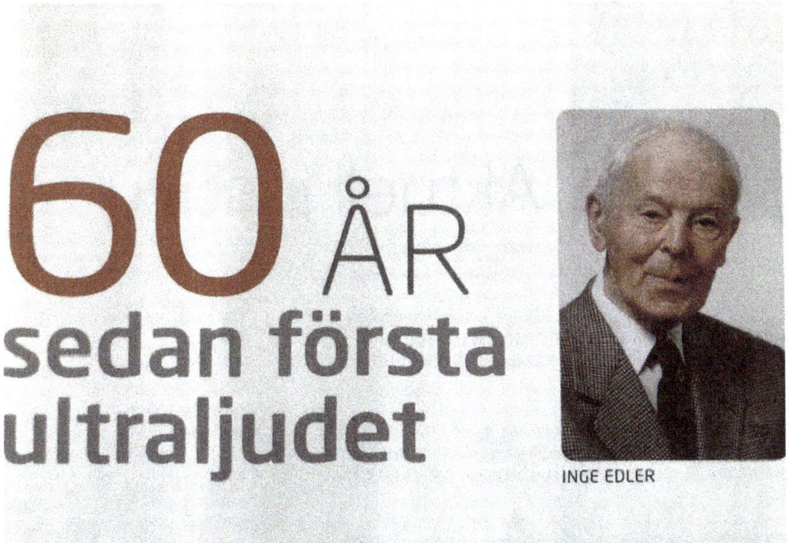

Inge Edler (pictured) and Hellmuth Hertz were the fathers of echocardiography. The 60-year anniversary of the first echo was celebrated in Lund, Sweden, with a lecture by Professor Joseph Kisslo of Duke University, USA.

focus was on my own research in gene transfer and hematopoietic stem cell transplants for multiple myeloma, which was very different from echocardiography. But Edler was there and that was a great honor. He passed away in 2001, only a few days before his 90th birthday.

17 Stig Radner and Heart Catheterization

"Gösta, this is not a heart infarction, it is a perforated gastric ulcer". I did not feel responsible for the wrong diagnosis. The patient had arrived from the emergency department to the private ward where I had just started my service as a young and inexperienced doctor. A patient who had arrived at the emergency department had been given a preliminary diagnosis and was then transferred, as soon as possible, to the ward that handled that disorder, so that they could receive immediate care. The patient had just arrived, and I had not even had time to carry out an investigation when Stig Radner arrived at the ward and made the comment. The wrong diagnosis had been made on the emergency ward. When Radner happened to pass the ward, the patient was still in the corridor, and I was just going to start my investigation. I told Radner that I had received a patient from the emergency department, who was experiencing great chest pain and the preliminary diagnosis has been heart infarction. I intended to give him morphine. Radner looked at the patient, put his hand on the upper part of his stomach and showed me that it was as hard as a board. Hence his comment. I confirmed the finding. I knew that it was a perforated gastric ulcer and that transfer to the surgical department was imminent.

Radner was a brilliant clinician. When you were on call you always felt safe when Radner was backing you up as the responsible senior doctor, which he seemed to be seven days a week. You could always call him for advice.

Radner was born in 1913. He studied medicine in Lund and qualified as a doctor in 1941. He passed his thesis in 1951, which was the same year that I started my medical education. Radner was an innovator and showed early interest in improving all kinds of diagnostic approaches that could be carried out using catheterization and needle punctures of organs, particularly in combination with X-rays. By 1945, he had already managed to visualize the coronary arteries, by introducing a catheter through the groin into the venous system and up to the heart. He then injected dense X-ray contrast into the vessels before taking X-ray pictures. The discovery was first published in *Acta Medica Radiologica*[23] and later commented on in the *American Journal of Medicine*, which was also known as the green journal. When Radner showed the pictures to his boss, he said that they were very nice, but then asked what they should be used for. I thought about this comment and Radner's discovery 58 years earlier, when I was lying on an operating table viewing my own coronary arteries. One was occluded but was opened through a catheter and cured by a stent.

Radner continued his work on catheterization in the 1940s and this led to the discovery of new brain areas. Once the catheter slipped into a new vessel that had never been visualized before, namely the vertebral artery, the X-ray pictures discovered new vessel trees in the brain[24]. This discovery later became important for brain surgery.

In 1951, Radner went to USA for further education in heart catheterization. He was based in the laboratory run by André Cournand, who would go on to win the Nobel Prize in 1956 with Werner Forssmann and Dickinson W Richards *"for their discoveries concerning heart catheterization and pathological changes in the circulatory system"*. Forssmann had courageously inserted a catheter into his own veins in 1929, but it took some years before Cournand started a program of diagnostic catheterization in humans at Bellevue Hospital in New York in 1941. When Radner joined Cournand, he had already gained important experience in heart catheterization. Catheterization was invented when Radner made his own important discoveries in the 1940s, but I think that his contribution to science has been underestimated. Nobody in the field really knows about him outside Lund, not even in other parts of Sweden. Should he have been a Nobel Prize candidate? No, that would be an exaggeration. However, his discoveries have proven to be immensely important.

Radner continued his research in Lund after his stay at the Bellevue Hospital. He usually started out in the Department of Pathology and worked on deceased patients. He inserted needles through the large vessels around the heart and into the chambers of the heart. When he was certain of the anatomy, he did the same for diagnostic purposes on patients and could measure, with just one puncture, the pressure in the aorta, the artery to the lung and the left atrium of the heart. This provided important information on how the heart surgeons approached the patient during their operation. He called the method *suprasternal puncture*[25]. He was often called Stickan, because his first name, Stig, was similar to the Swedish word sticka, which means to insert a needle.

Radner was one of the most original people I have ever met. He was an excellent artist and created wonderful paintings and posters for the student musicals, theaters and performances. One of the posters adorns my study at work. I acquired it much later, when I gave a lecture at the Department of Medicine in Lund.

I have been told that the Professor of Medicine in Uppsala, Erik Ask-Upmark (Chapter 50), tried to persuade Radner to become a Professor in Neurology or Diagnostic Radiology in Uppsala. These two posts seemed rather different at first glance. Radner was considered competent for both posts, but he declined them. He eventually received the title of professor at Lund, which was exactly what he wanted, but without any administrative responsibilities. Administration was not his favorite activity. Radner died at 96 years of age.

18 Jan Waldenström and the Discovery of Macroglobulinemia

Jan Waldenström is probably, from a global perspective, the most well-known hematologist and internist in Sweden. He discovered at least three diseases and one of them was named after him: Waldenström's macroglobulinemia[26].

These patients bleed from their nose and mouth, have enlarged lymph glands and sometimes anemia, an enlarged spleen and liver and various neurological symptoms. Laboratory investigations show high erythrocyte sedimentation rates, abnormal lymphocytes and high viscosity in the blood. These symptoms could be explained by the presence of a protein in the blood, which Waldenström called macroglobulin due to its high molecular weight. It causes high viscosity and is produced by the abnormal lymphocytes. The disease is a chronic hematologic malignancy and eventually kills the patients. However, with optimal treatment, most of them can live for a very long time and have a good quality of life.

Waldenström encountered two patients with these symptoms in 1942. He lived close to Arne Tiselius, the 1948 Nobel Prize Laureate in chemistry, who had developed ultracentrifugation and discovered immunoglobulins. He took patients' blood to the Department of Physical Chemistry at Tiselius Laboratory in Uppsala, where Kai Pedersen, one of his gifted collaborators, performed the ultracentrifugation and identified the macroglobulin that is now called IgM. Waldenström became world famous after he described the first two patients with this previously unknown disease in 1944[26].

However, Waldenström's interest in immunoglobulins also led him to another discovery. He saw that the sharp band in the electrophoresis found in patients with multiple myeloma could also be found in normal individuals. He called the band monoclonal and the condition benign monoclonal gammopathy[27]. Most of these individuals never developed any disease. This sharp band in the electrophoresis contrasted with the broad band found in rheumatoid arthritis and autoimmune disorders that he called polyclonal.

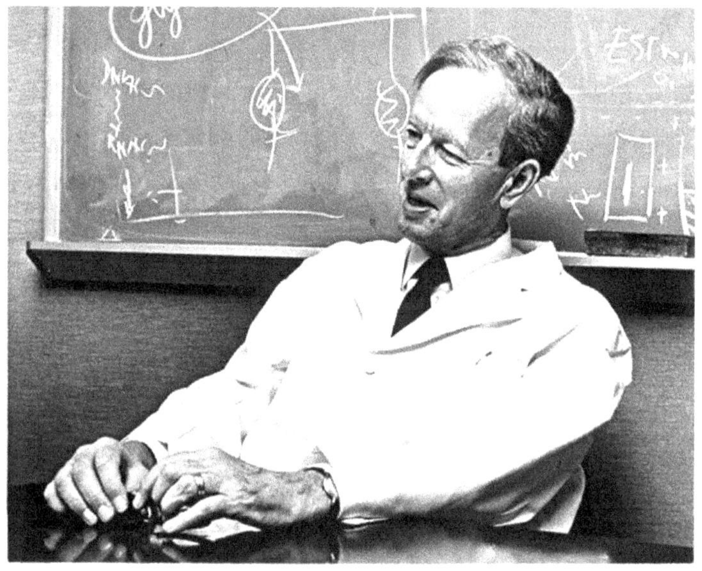

Professor Jan Waldenström discovered the disease Waldenström macroglobulinemia.

Today, benign monoclonal gammopathy is called monoclonal gammopathy of undetermined significance and every year about 1% of individuals with this abnormality will develop a malignancy, which is usually multiple myeloma. Waldenström's discovery was the start of the process to sort out the differences between monoclonal and polyclonal abnormalities and research their importance.

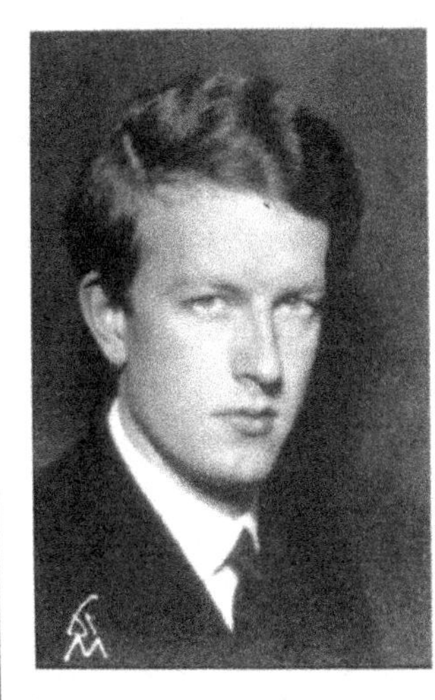

The young Jan Waldenström discovered what he called benign monoclonal gammopathy in contrast to polyclonal hyperglobulinemia seen in nonmalignant disease.

Waldenström had already described an unusual disorder in his thesis and that was acute intermittent porphyria, which was characterized by bouts of acute abdominal pain and excreting red urine. It was known to exist in families in northern Sweden and was called Arjeplog disease. By investigating a number of these Swedish families, he was able to show that it was an autosomal dominant inherited disorder. He also clarified the pathogenesis and biochemistry of the disease and defined certain proteins of importance, including porphobilinogen, which was previously unknown.

Waldenström was born in 1906 and became Professor of Theoretical Medicine at the University of Uppsala in 1947. When his antagonist, Erik Ask-Upmark, was appointed Professor of Medicine and Chair of the Department of Medicine in 1949, Waldenström moved to Malmö General Hospital in southern Sweden, where he was Head of Medicine and Professor of Medicine at the University of Lund.

The University of Lund had two Professors of Medicine who were heads of the clinical departments in Lund and Malmö, respectively. The two cities are only about 20 kilometers apart. Waldenström's counterpart in Lund, Haqvin Malmros (Chapter 15) was a relatively shy person, who liked to keep out of the spotlight, unlike his more famous colleague in Malmö. In contrast, Waldenström was a globetrotter and highly visible at international congresses. Maybe the differences in their personalities were why they seemed to get along very well with each other, unlike the situation that Waldenström had experienced in Uppsala. Both were excellent clinicians, with great knowledge in medicine, with Waldenström focusing on hematology and Malmros on diabetes and cardiovascular diseases.

My first contact with Waldenström was by letter. In 1960 I had started to work with Åke Nordén (Chapter 19) in the hematology section. My early research on the periodic acid-Schiff (PAS) reaction in neutrophil leukocytes had stalled. I had read that Ludwig Heilmeyer, the famous hematology chief in Freiburg, Germany, had an associate called Hermann Merker who was involved in cytochemistry research, by studying the PAS reaction. I wanted to visit him as I hoped that this would help me to solve some of my problems. I asked Malmros for a one-week leave of absence so that I could go to Freiburg. *"You need a letter of recommendation"* he said *"I do not know Heilmeyer, but I will ask Jan Waldenström if he can help you. I am sure he knows Heilmeyer"*. After a few days I got a letter from Waldenström to Heilmeyer that was written in German. He said: *"I know that Gösta Gahrton is a very talented physician, who is particularly interested in hematology. Thus, it is obvious that he wants to study at your department. Yours affectionate Jan"*.

The letter revealed a good relationship between Heilmeyer and Waldenström, as well as Waldenström's generosity in supporting a young researcher that he only knew because his counterpart in Lund had recommended him. I am thankful to both Waldenström and Malmros. The doors in Freiburg were wide open when I arrived. I spoke to Heilmeyer and planned my visit together with his associate Hermann Merker. It became clear to me that I needed to leave Lund and move north if I wanted to continue with my PAS project (Chapter 19).

My path crossed with Waldenström's on many occasions. He called me after I had completed my five theoretical years at the Nobel Institute at the Karolinska Institutet, gained my thesis with the highest grade and spent six clinical years at the Department of Medicine at the Karolinska Hospital. By that time, I was a specialist in internal medicine and hematology and a docent, also known as an assistant professor. Waldenström asked if I would consider being the faculty opponent to a thesis written by one of his pupils, Jörgen Malmquist. I was honored to be asked by the most influential Professor in Medicine in Sweden. I accepted without knowing exactly what the thesis was about, but I remembered his letter of recommendation in 1960 and he was someone I trusted. However, Waldenström had one more question. After the 1968 student rebellions, the Government had revised the instructions for dissertations and opponents. Grading a thesis was not allowed. You were no longer allowed to write down your opinion about the quality of the thesis or the defense. The only option was to approve the thesis or reject it, which was something that practically never occurred. Before the Government changes there had been five grades upwards from approved. That elitist approach was now viewed as outdated. Waldenström asked his question with caution.

Would I consider writing down what I thought about the thesis, for his eyes only? He would hide my evaluation in his pocket, and it would never be official. I was flattered that he valued what I thought about his student's work. Wonderful. I understood that we had the same type of thoughts. I put a lot of effort into my evaluation of the thesis, and I graded it as I had done when I had undertaken a number of opponent assignments before 1968.

I met Waldenström before the dissertation and he asked me if I had written down my evaluation. I took two pages out of my pocket, and he let them slip down into his own. My grading was that it was a very good, but not excellent, thesis. *"Thank you"* he said, *"it will never be official. I will read it later"*. Waldenström never revealed to me what he thought of my evaluation. Perhaps he just wanted some guidance to confirm his total appreciation of his student.

Throughout my career I felt that Waldenström practically always supported me. In 1969, when I returned from a year of researching in USA, I wanted to start some prospective randomized studies, which had never been performed with cancer patients in Sweden. This had been happening in USA for many years and the pharmaceutical industry knew that, in most cases, a new drug would only be approved by the Food and Drug Administration (FDA) and reach the market if randomized studies had been carried out. A new drug had to be tested on animals, then for toxicity in Phase I patient studies, then smaller Phase II patient studies and finally in a comparative, randomized Phase III trial. During the last stage, patients were randomized to receive the new drug and their outcomes were compared with another group that had received the best treatment to date without the new drug. This had to happen before they were approved by the FDA in the

USA. The same process applies today to the FDA and European Medicines Agency. However, Waldenström was old fashioned. He always claimed that studies on drug effects should be based on observations in single patients. At first, Peter Reizenstein, who was my boss at that time, did not want me to present the project. He thought that Waldenström would turn it down and that would have been the end of it. However, he eventually agreed. In 1970 I attended a national congress in Gothenburg and presented a proposal for a randomized study on acute myeloblastic leukemia. The aim of the study was to test the efficacy of adding l-asparaginase to current treatment[28]. Waldenström was in the audience. After I finished my presentation, I waited anxiously for him to comment. After a while he raised his hand and gave me his support. *"The time has come for new approaches to investigate the efficacy and toxicity of drugs in patients"* he said, *"Randomized studies are here to stay"*. This meant that the study could start, and it would be the first one of its kind in Sweden (Chapter 25). Waldenström showed that he was broad-minded and could change his views when he was presented with good arguments. The findings of the study were published in the American scientific journal *Cancer* in 1974[29].

My friend Sixten Franzén, the father of fine needle aspiration cytology, gathered 12 of Waldenström's friends in Stockholm to a dinner to celebrate his 80th birthday. It was held at the famous Opera Cellar restaurant, and he asked each of us to tell a short story about our relationship with Waldenström. Mine was obviously the introduction letter he wrote to Heilmeyer on my behalf.

There were many stories about Waldenström and some of most common ones were risky. One person asked *"Who takes care of your department during your frequent travels abroad?"* Waldenström's answer was *"the same people as when I am at home"*.

This attitude made Malmö General Hospital one of the leading university hospitals in Europe.

Waldenström was active to his last day. In the 1970s and 1980s, long after his retirement, he was asked by Professor Jerzy Einhorn from the Department of Oncology at the Karolinska Hospital in Stockholm to give lectures for doctors and students. He was a brilliant teacher. However, Waldenström was an anti-bureaucrat and he only accepted if he was not offered a fee, as he didn't want any problems with the tax authorities.

As late as in the 1990s, I meet him at congresses or conferences about multiple myeloma, which was a common interest of ours. He delivered inspiring historical lectures about Waldenström's macroglobulinemia or benign monoclonal gammopathy.

Waldenström's interests were not limited to medicine. He was a skilled and enthusiastic botanist. In The Swedish Society of Hematology's 50-year Jubilee book, Ingemar Turesson, his friend and former student, described how he drove Waldenström to a parking lot close to the bridge joining Sweden and Denmark, when he was old and no longer able to walk or drive. Suddenly, Waldenström asked him to stop because he saw an unusual orchid. It filled him with joy[30]. Waldenström passed away in 1996 when he was 90 years old.

Waldenström received many honors and prizes, but he never received the Nobel Prize. However, until 1972 he was nominated five times, according to the available records, for his outstanding discoveries. They could, in my opinion, best be compared to those of Guido Fanconi (Chapter 14). Both physicians were brilliant clinicians and teachers. They initially made their discoveries at the bedside and then developed them to reveal, characterize and define diseases, which was a prerequisite for later treatment approaches.

Both had diseases named after them: Fanconi's anemia and Waldenström's macroglobulinemia. However, describing a new disease did not merit a Nobel Prize *per se*. To be worthy of an award, a discovery needed to point to a new view on diseases or how to treat them. Maybe both Waldenström and Fanconi were close to doing that. But convincing the Nobel Committee is not easy.

19

Torbjörn Caspersson and Chromosome Banding

After I had spent about one year with Inge Edler at the Department of Medicine in Lund in 1959–1960, I asked to switch to hematology, under Associate Professor Åke Nordén. He was also in charge of patients with diabetes, which was a strange combination. However, perhaps this was the reason that he had started a program on cytochemistry, which involved studying single cells under the microscope after having induced an interpretable chemical reaction. He was working on the periodic acid-Schiff (PAS) reaction, which under certain conditions could indicate the amount of glycogen in leukocytes. He had the idea that it could be possible to demonstrate increased amounts of glycogen in the neutrophil leukocytes in patients with diabetes. This would indicate that these cells were involved in the pathogenesis of this disease. My own interest came from the discoveries by Frank Hayhoe at Cambridge, which suggested that the pattern of the reaction in single cells could differentiate acute myeloblastic and acute lymphoblastic leukemia. I was interested in using it in diagnostic and pathogenetic studies of other hematologic disorders, like chronic myelocytic leukemia (CML). For unknown reasons, cytochemical methods had shown that the neutrophils in CML were low in alkaline phosphatases, in contrast to the high levels in polycythemia vera. Maybe the PAS reaction could be the next step in clarifying what happened in the cells and perhaps shed some light on the pathogenesis of the disease. This was long before the discovery of specific chromosomal aberrations.

Nordén had a technician called Ingrid Gärtner, who looked at the neutrophils under the microscope and tried to grade the intensity of the beautiful red staining in each of them. She used three grades: +, ++ and +++, where +++ indicated the highest intensity[31]. The neutrophils with the highest grade were supposed to have the largest amount of glycogen. I immediately realized that this was a most uncertain interpretation, because the cells flattened more when the blood or bone marrow were smeared on glass, and they looked larger at the tail end of the smear. Consequently, they displayed a less intensive stain than those in the middle, without necessarily having less substance. I came to the conclusion that estimating the amount of a substance in single cells could only be performed accurately by using an instrument for single cell light absorption measurements. Such instrumentation was only available in Sweden at the Karolinska Institutet in Torbjörn Caspersson's laboratory.

When I returned home from the histochemistry and cytochemistry congress in Paris (Chapter 1), I decided to leave Lund for some time. Nils Ringertz had assured me that there were good opportunities for me to start a research project using Caspersson's microspectrophotometers, particularly if I arrived with my own research grants in place. My feeling was that Nordén would support my education and use of the technique for a PAS project.

Everything went fine. I successfully applied for a four-year PhD stipend from the University of Lund. After some preparatory work by Nils Ringertz, I and Nordén met Caspersson at the Nobel Institute at the Karolinska Institutet in Stockholm. After a short discussion about the project, we agreed that I should start work in Stockholm in September 1961. All the necessary equipment for the project was provided by Caspersson. I would not receive a salary from him and would need to live on the Lund stipend. I had to do all practical work myself, but I would get support and advice from his engineers on the methodology.

After much help from my new friend Ringertz, I moved my family to a four-room apartment in Hägernäs, a suburb about 15 kilometers north of central Stockholm. I started my work as planned and a very knowledgeable and friendly Polish engineer called Jan Kudynowski trained me to perform measurements using one of the microspectrophotometers.

The short name for Caspersson's place was the Cell Research Institute, and it was based in half of a three-story house on the Karolinska Institutet campus. Its full name was the Institute for Medical Cell Research and Genetics, Medical Nobel Institute, Karolinska Institutet.

The Nobel Foundation had established the Nobel Institutes that would help the process of selecting Nobel Prize winners and the Karolinska Institutet got one of them. These Institutes were allowed to carry out research activities that were partly supported by the Nobel Foundation. The Nobel Institute at the Karolinska Institutet was split into three institutes. Caspersson was the Head of Cell Research, the 1955 Nobel Laureate Hugo Theorell was the Head of Biochemistry and Ragnar Granit, who became a Nobel Laureate in 1967, was the Head of Neurophysiology. The joint venture with the Karolinska Institutet was why Caspersson's department had such a long name.

Caspersson and Theorell shared the same three-story house with their teams and many felt that an iron curtain existed between the two halves. It was only partly true since there was some collaboration between Ringertz and researchers in the other institution. Caspersson and Theorell may not have been the best of friends during the most active parts of their lives, but Theorell was an honored guest when Caspersson celebrated his 70th birthday in 1980, after receiving the prestigious Balzan prize.

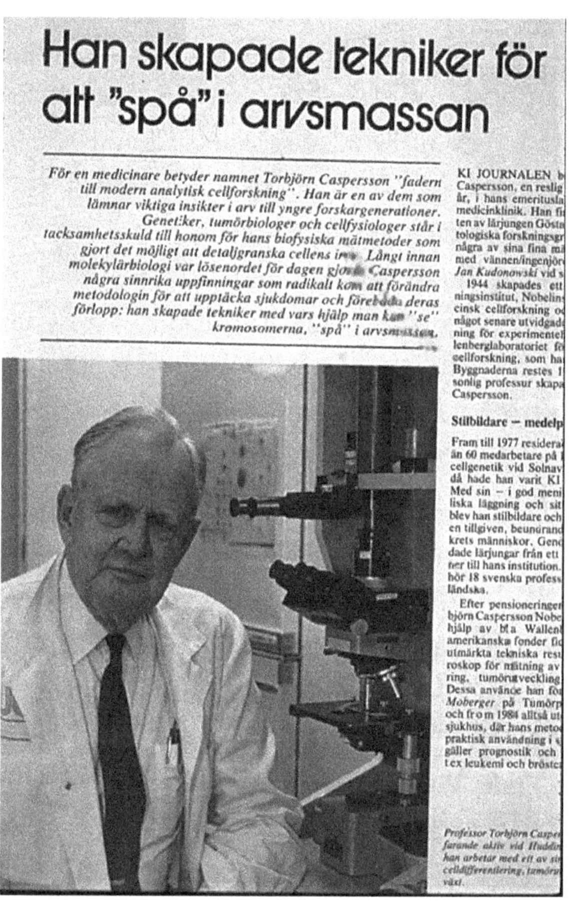

Han skapade tekniker för att "spå" i arvsmassan

För en medicinare betyder namnet Torbjörn Caspersson "fadern till modern analytisk cellforskning". Han är en av dem som lämnar viktiga insikter i arv till yngre forskargenerationer. Genetiker, tumörbiologer och cellfysiologer står i tacksamhetsskuld till honom för hans biofysiska mätmetoder som gjort det möjligt att detaljgranska cellens inre. Långt innan molekylärbiologi var lösenordet för dagen gjorde Caspersson några sinnrika uppfinningar som radikalt kom att förändra metodologin för att upptäcka sjukdomar och förebåda deras förlopp: han skapade tekniker med vars hjälp man kan "se" kromosomerna, "spå" i arvsmassan.

KI JOURNALEN b
Caspersson, en reslig
år, i hans emeritusla
medicinklinik. Han fi
ten av lärjungen Gösta
tologiska forskningsgr
några av sina fina mä
med vännen/ingenjör
Jan Kudonowski vid s
1944 skapades ett
ningsinstitut, Nobelins
cinsk cellforskning oc
något senare utvidgad
ning för experimentel
lenberglaboratoriet fö
cellforskning, som ha
Byggnaderna restes 1
sonlig professur skapa
Caspersson.

Stilbildare — medelp

Fram till 1977 residera
än 60 medarbetare på
cellgenetik vid Solnav
då hade han varit KI
Med sin — i god meni
liska läggning och sit
blev han stilbildare och
en tillgiven, beundranc
krets människor. Genc
dade lärjungar från ett
ner till hans institution.
hör 18 svenska profess
ländska.
Efter pensioneringer
björn Caspersson Nobe
hjälp av bl a Wallen
amerikanska fonder fic
utmärkta tekniska res
roskop för mätning av
ring, tumörutveckling
Dessa använde han för
Moberger på Tumörp
och fr o m 1984 alltså ut
sjukhus, där hans meto
praktisk användning i s
gäller prognostik och
t ex leukemi och bröste

*Professor Torbjörn Caspe
farande aktiv vid Huddin
han arbetar med ett av si
celldifferentiering, tumöru
växt.*

The headline states that Professor Torbjörn Caspersson "created the technique to tell the future by analyzing the genome".

By the 1930s, Caspersson had predicted, and showed, that nucleic acids were keys for protein synthesis. In the late 1960s, he invented the chromosome banding technique, used to order all chromosomes and identify chromosomal aberrations.

Torbjörn Caspersson was born 1910 in Motala, a small town 240 kilometers south-west of Stockholm. He studied medicine at the Karolinska Institutet and, during his studies, he worked as an amanuensis, at the Department of Medical Chemistry, an unpaid or low-paid position for students who wanted to do research. The Head of the Department was Einar Hammarsten (1889–1968), who was an internationally well-known professor and a member of both the Royal Akademie of Sciences and the Nobel Committee at the Karolinska Institutet. He had studied microanalysis of organic substances at a laboratory in Graz, Austria, run by Fritz Pregl, who won the 1923 Nobel Prize for chemistry. Hammarsten applied this technique to his study of nucleic acids in tissues.

Encouraged by Hammarsten, Caspersson made his first internationally recognized discoveries about the structure of nucleic acids in the 1930s, by showing that the molecules were much larger than previously thought. They were called polymers[32]. He continued his research by developing microspectrophotometry, which made it possible to measure substances in single cells. This showed that the nucleus, and particularly the nucleolus, contained large amounts of ribonucleic acid. Caspersson claimed that ribonucleic acid determined the synthesis of proteins and cell growth, which was a revolutionary discovery that the established scientific community found difficult to accept[33]. Earlier researchers thought that proteins were the key substances for cell growth, not nucleic acids. These discoveries were made long before the 1962 Nobel Prize winners James Watson and Francis Crick made their fundamental discoveries concerning the molecular structure of deoxyribonucleic acid (DNA)[34], and also considerably predated the discoveries that DNA provides the genetic material and ribonucleic acid (RNA) copies the codes for the production of specific proteins.

The Cell Research Institute, led by Caspersson, became the world leader in nucleic acid research in the 1930s and 1940s. The machines he used to carry out single cell measurements of nucleic acids were unique. The possibility of determining other substances in single cells was in the pipeline at this stage. Caspersson summarized his pioneering discoveries in 1950 in the book *Cell Growth and Cell Function*[35].

When Watson and Crick published their discovery about the structure of DNA in 1953[34], and its importance as genetic material, it eclipsed Caspersson's work. Although he had understood that nucleic acids were key to protein structures and synthesis, he did not seem to understand, or show, that DNA was the key factor and RNA was just an intermediate.

When I arrived to work with Caspersson in 1961 he had partly changed the direction of his research. He wanted to apply the microspectrophotometric method to diagnostic approaches. His hypothesis was that the interindividual variability in the cellular amounts of nucleic acids, proteins and other substances was larger in cancer cell populations than in normal cell populations. This variability could be of diagnostic importance. Most pathologists and cytologists were not impressed, as they argued that it was possible to see these variations just by looking under a microscope.

I was happy that my project was different. Although my plan was to measure the amount of substance that single cells contained for diagnostic purposes, I also wanted to find the metabolic differences between specific cells, namely the neutrophil leukocytes from leukemia patients and healthy individuals. This in turn could perhaps provide clues about the treatment of hematologic malignancies, which at this time was still almost rudimentary.

Torbjörn, as we were all allowed to call him, seemed relatively uninterested in my project. His focus was still on nucleic acids. Sometimes he asked if I was still occupied with my small *"red balls"*, which is what he called my PAS-stained neutrophil leukocytes. Perhaps he wanted me to become one of the many collaborators that worked with him on his nucleic acid research. At the same time, he was keen to ensure that I got all the help and advice I needed from his skillful engineers, Leon Carlson, Gösta Lomakka and Jan Kudynowski. After some time, I realized that, despite his seeming lack of interest in my research, he recognized that it could expand the use of his sophisticated machinery to other areas. Caspersson was a machine freak and knew all the technical details at least as well as his engineers. I was the only qualified Swedish doctor, except for him, among the students, technicians, engineers and others at his institution. I enjoyed good collaboration with the physicians at the Karolinska Hospital on the other side of Solna Street, that divided the Karolinska Institutet from the Karolinska Hospital. I got all the clinical material I needed from the hospital. This meant I was part of his plan to expand his methods to the Karolinska clinics. Sometimes I felt prioritized.

While Caspersson could be very demanding with his closer collaborators, I was not approached by him very often in the beginning. However, when I began to show results, after about a year, he became more interested in my work. I could show nice absorption curves from PAS-stained single cells, and I had developed a model system that could measure the weight and the glycogen content in single neutrophil leukocytes. Once day he asked if I would allow him to use my slides, showing absorption curves and other results of my measurements of the neutrophils, for a presentation at an international conference. It made me happy.

This was the proof I needed that he appreciated the work I had done. He never asked to be a co-author on my work. I knew that he always claimed that authors on joint publication should be presented in alphabetic order, meaning that he was almost always the first author. He never was, and never claimed to be, a co-author on my PAS publications.

Caspersson had started a collaboration with one of the leading figures in cancer research in the USA, Professor Sidney Farber. He was Professor in Pathology at Harvard Medical School and Head of Pathology at Children's Hospital in Boston, Massachusetts (Chapter 21). The collaboration enabled Caspersson to receive funding from the USA for his research. It also meant he could send his associates to Boston to work at the Children's Cancer Research Foundation (CCRF), a research establishment that Farber had built next to the Children's Hospital. Caspersson was also supposed to spend a couple of weeks every year at the CCRF to initiate collaboration projects with researchers there.

Caspersson was still enjoying his fame in the 1940s and 1950s, when the Boston collaboration started, but I felt that his fame had diminished during my first stay at the CCRF in 1963–1964 (Chapter 20). However, it was still a great advantage to be Caspersson's *"boy"* when I approached people for contacts. Doors opened and I always felt welcomed. The best time was when Caspersson came for his yearly two-week visit to the CCRF. He was then invited to give lectures at other institutions or to attend parties held in his honor. I was always at his side, and I felt that I was accompanying a King. People invited both of us. Torbjörn Caspersson had arrived!

During my second visit to the CCRF in 1968–1969, Caspersson presented his second breakthrough, the banding technique, during a lecture at CCRF. As far as I know, this was the first time he revealed this discovery.

I am convinced that Caspersson understood that his attempts to use his machinery for diagnostic purposes, by studying the inter-cellular variability of weight and nucleic acids, was a dead end. Few people believed that this approach would result in important diagnostic tools. Now Caspersson had the idea that he could use the machines to determine the way cytotoxic drugs bind to chromosomes. He had managed to build machines that could measure fluorescence in single cells, and he thought that he could adapt them to single chromosomes. He argued that if he could find a fluorescent substance that could be bound to a cytotoxic drug, maybe he could identify the binding locus on the chromosomes. He had a skillful cytogeneticist working with him at the Cell Research Institute that he wanted to work on the project. Lore Zech was an immigrant from Germany, and she mainly worked with plant chromosomes, but now on Caspersson's request had to switch to work with human chromosomes. The two key issues for the project were to select the most suitable cytotoxic drug and to find a fluorescent substance by which the drug could be labeled.

Caspersson discussed the idea with the chemist at the CCRF, Ed Modest, who suggested that he used the cytotoxic drug nitrogen mustard, which had proved effective treating Hodgkin's disease, a cancer of the lymph glands. Caspersson asked how nitrogen mustard could be made fluorescent so that it could be measured in the microfluorimeter? Ed pointed up to his shelf and said that he had quinacrine, which could easily bind to nitrogen mustard. Ed synthesized quinacrine mustard (QM) and Caspersson's most brilliant technician, Evy Simonsson, developed a staining method that could identify QM on chromosomes prepared by Zech and his technicians. His engineers worked on the development of the machinery for measuring the fluorescence elicited by the chromosomes. They started by analyzing large chromosomes from plants.

To their astonishment they did not find specific spots on the chromosomes that indicated QM binding. Instead, they found numerous fluorescent transverse bands on them. When I spoke to members of Caspersson's team at a much later date no one knew for sure who first saw the pattern. They said it was so easy to see. Maybe it was Zech who first identified the bands and saw that the chromosomes could be paired by looking at their appearance, fluorescent intensity, and thereby put a number on the chromosomes. Two chromosomes always had identical banding patterns, and these were different for all the pairs. It was obvious to Caspersson that this was a breakthrough that could lead to the differentiation of all chromosomes. However, he was not satisfied to just look at the chromosomes. He used a microfluorimeter to measure the fluorescence over the length of the chromosome and create a reproducible picture of the banding pattern.

Eventually Caspersson, Zech and his team identified the specific patterns on all the 46 human chromosomes, which differentiated them from each other, and gave them numbers from 1 to 22 plus X and Y[36]. The old groups, such as A, B and C, were gone forever. The starting point for identifying aberrations in diseases had been reached. The race for defining association with genetic disorders, cancer and other diseases was suddenly ongoing.

When I visited CCRF for the second time in 1968–1969, Caspersson arrived for his two-week visit. He was asked to give a lecture at one of the weekly conferences. The first bands on plant chromosomes had just been identified in Stockholm. No one in Boston knew about the progress of the project. Caspersson started by talking about the use of his machines for diagnostic purposes and he showed a number of pictures showing the intercellular variability in weight and nucleic acids and discussed the possibility of using the results for diagnostic purpose. The audience seemed less than interested and some seemed to fall asleep. Everybody seemed to wake up when one of the last slides showed a banded chromosome and Caspersson explained the potential. A lively discussion started and Caspersson was once again a star.

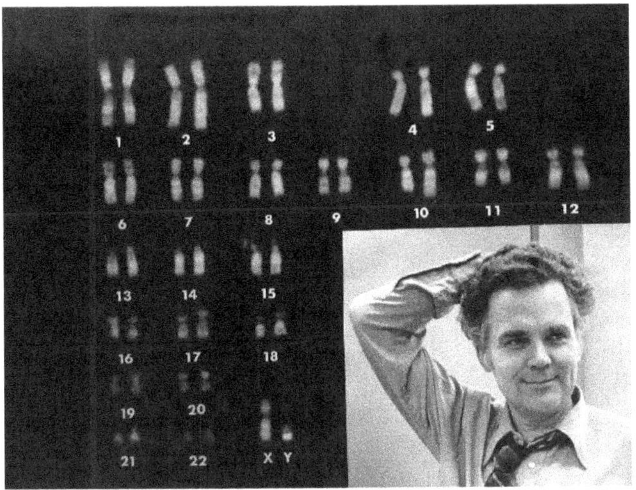

The author and his chromosomes ordered from 1–22, X, Y with the help of Caspersson's banding technique.

Many researchers have wondered about who first identified the bands on the chromosomes. It is quite possible that it was Zech. At least that is what she claimed. However, she was not involved in the first part of the project, and she was only engaged by Caspersson to do part of the work, namely preparing the chromosomes involved in the analysis. Any cytogeneticist could have done that, even a technician. She did not even know how the staining procedure was applied when I asked her. That was planned by Caspersson and developed by his head technician, Simonsson, and possibly some of his other technicians. Zech was an important person in the project, but it was Caspersson's vision, persistence in developing the ideas for practical projects and engaging the right people for each part of it that made it successful. Caspersson's group made many new discoveries related to disease before this novel banding method became part of every cytogeneticist's tools. The first important discovery was related to two disorders, chronic myelocytic leukemia (CML) and Down's syndrome. Down's syndrome is an inherited disease with an extra number 21, small trisomic chromosome, and this had been seen before the banding technique. Down's was associated with a higher incidence of acute leukemia. Since the Philadelphia (Ph) chromosome in CML was defined as a deleted chromosome 21, the speculation was that there was an association between CML and leukemia development in Down's. However, banding made it clear that the trisomic chromosome in Down's syndrome was different from the one that was partly deleted in CML which was subsequently redefined as number 22[37]. This ruled out a connection between the two disorders and provided one example of the clarity that banding could provide.

Later, other staining methods were developed that could also show similar bands e.g., the Giemsa method. Measurement in the microspectrofluorometer was soon shown not to be required for the discovery of new chromosomal aberrations. Observations in the microscope were sufficient.

Caspersson's discovery made me change the direction of my research and I collaborated with Zech to use the banding technique to define chromosomal aberrations in hematologic malignancies. We predicted that the deletion in CML may have been a translocation instead. However, Zech thought that the deleted part of the chromosome, which we had defined as number 22, or the Ph chromosome, and not number 21 as previously thought, was too small to be identified on an unknown receiver chromosome. I foolishly agreed and decided instead to investigate inherited fluorescent satellites on the chromosomes to show that the Ph chromosome positive cells developed from a single cell, so-called clonal development. In each patient these cells are always derived from a chromosome that was inherited from either the mother or the father. There was never a mixture of cells from both parents[38]. Although we published this discovery in the prestigious scientific journal *Blood*, it never became a big hit[39]. We had failed to identify the translocation between chromosome 22, the Ph chromosome and chromosome 9. That discovery was made two years later by Janet Rowley, who went on to become the world star in cytogenetics. I can only blame myself for this. My technicians claimed afterwards that if I had asked them to look for the deleted piece of number 22, they would have seen it easily.

We took some revenge in the 1980s, by identifying the first chromosomal aberration in chronic lymphocytic leukemia (CLL). This had been difficult up to that point, because it had not been possible to induce mitotic figures in CLL cells, which was a prerequisite for chromosome analysis at that time. I collaborated with Karl-Henrik Robert on this project. He was one of the most brilliant doctors and clinical researchers in my department and he developed the method to induce growth and division of the cells. We could, for the first time, show that chromosomal aberrations were present in CLL and appeared to have prognostic importance. Trisomy for chromosome 12 was present in about 30% of the patients and we also identified aberrations on chromosome 14, as well as on some other chromosomes[40,41]. Patients with these aberrations tended to have worse prognoses than those with a normal karyotype. This was just the beginning of identifying specific chromosomal aberrations in CLL and seeking a prognostic impact. The research field later exploded.

After a few years, Caspersson's band-producing QM method, and similar ones that did not use his machines, became the standard procedures in cytogenetics. However, after a while some researchers seemed to forget who had made the original discovery, even when they delivered historical lectures at international congresses.

In 2011 I visited the Congress of the American Society of Hematology in the USA. Rowley was due to give one of the prestigious lectures, which was about the history of discoveries in CML. The disease had gone from a 100% death rate to being completely eradicated in most patients, due to the molecular discoveries that had been made possible by the banding technique. Rowley had studied the banding technique in Zech's laboratory in Stockholm but preferred the Giemsa variant to using fluorescence. She described the progress that had been made since 1960, when Nowell and Hungerford discovered the minute chromosome, known as number 21 or the Philadelphia chromosome. Rowley continued her presentation with her own discovery of the translocation. She did not mention Caspersson and Zech and said nothing about the banding method or our original studies that defined the position of the chromosome as number 22 and the clonal development of the Ph positive cells. I was very disappointed, because I had met her several times and had appreciated her outstanding skills as a cytogeneticist. After some hesitation, I could not resist commenting on her presentation in front of the 3,000 people in the audience. I thanked her for her brilliant lecture and congratulated her on her important discoveries and said I felt that those who had made her discoveries possible would wish to send their greetings to her. Torbjörn Caspersson, who had died, and Zech who was still alive. Some people came up to me after the lecture and complemented me on my comment. After all, without Caspersson's banding method, she would not have made her most important discovery of the translocation of t(9;22)(q34;q11), as it is now called. On the way home I wrote a letter to the journal *Cancer Genetics*, which was published under the headline *Historical note on the discovery of the Philadelphia chromosome*[42].

In 1979, Caspersson had received the prestigious Balzan prize, mainly because of his work on chromosomal banding. He received many other prizes but was never awarded a Nobel Prize. Due to the 50-year secrecy rule for Nobel Committee members, it is not yet possible to describe the later discussions about a Nobel Prize for Caspersson. However, until 1972 he was nominated seventeen times for the prize in physiology or medicine and once for the one in chemistry. He was nominated for the prize in physiology or medicine as early as 1945, for his discoveries about nucleic acids as initiators of cellular protein synthesis. This was before the discovery of banding. You can hardly imagine how many times he was nominated after 1972. By coincidence, I found that my host in Freiburg in the early 1960s, Professor Ludwig Heilmeyer, was one of the nominators in 1953.

So why didn't Caspersson ever receive the Nobel Prize, having already been considered worthy of the prize for his discoveries of nucleic acids as initiators of protein synthesis? Without revealing any secrets, it is obvious that the discovery of the banding on chromosomes was well worth a Nobel Prize.

The reason why he wasn't awarded a Nobel Prize for his early discoveries was no doubt because by the time he had reached the top of the priority list in 1953, Watson and Crick had described the structure of the DNA molecule and showed that DNA was genetic material. Caspersson's discoveries became obsolete. By the time Crick, Watson and Wilkins won the Nobel Prize in 1962 *"for their discoveries concerning the molecular structure of nucleic acids and its significance for information transfer in living material"* Caspersson's contribution had been forgotten.

I cannot discuss why Caspersson did not receive a Nobel Prize for his banding method, as I served on the Nobel Committee for 10 years as both its vice chairman and chairman. That would violate the secrecy rules for members of the Committee. When I joined the Committee in 1988, nearly 20 years had passed since Caspersson's original discovery. Although I recognized that the banding method started the use of molecular methods in chromosome studies, an analysis of the list of Nobel Laureates from 1988 clearly shows that other important fields were a priority. Caspersson retired in 1977 and was slowly forgotten, not just by the international community, but by those in the Karolinska Institutet.

Like many other professors at the Karolinska Institutet, Caspersson wanted to continue his research after he retired at 65 years of age. There was an old rule that full professors had the right to have space and a telephone at the Karolinska Institutet to continue their research without a salary, if they could raise their own research money. Unfortunately, Caspersson and his successor, my friend Ringertz, immediately became enemies. Caspersson knew before his retirement that he had to move from his existing workplace. He found space with one of his old students Anders Zetterberg, who was now Professor in Pathology at the Karolinska Institutet. The Institution of Pathology was located only a few hundred meters away on the other side of Solna Street in the grounds of the Karolinska Hospital. Zetterberg and Caspersson arranged to transfer of all his machines to his new workplace before he lost the power to do that. Ringertz had always been critical of his boss and had not used Caspersson's machines. Despite that, he got angry and accused Caspersson of stealing the equipment from his Institute, despite the fact that the transfer was made within the Karolinska Institute. This was a tragic end to a period that had been far more successful than what came after.

At the beginning of the 1980s, Caspersson moved to Rönninge, a suburb south of Stockholm, which was 30 kilometers from the Karolinska Hospital but only 10 kilometers from the Huddinge Hospital. He asked me if I thought that he could secure some space for a couple of his machines and work at the Huddinge Hospital. I was still not head of the department, but I asked my boss Professor Gunnar Birke (Chapter 27) if Caspersson could work there. Birke knew Caspersson from the days when he was famous and from his joint working within the faculty and he responded positively and arranged two rooms for Caspersson to work in. For a few years Caspersson collaborated with the gastroenterologists and wrote a couple of papers, but he did not achieve any breakthroughs during this time.

I invited Caspersson to have dinner at my home in 1985, after I was appointed Professor of Medicine at the Karolinska Institutet and Head of the Department of Medicine at the Huddinge Hospital. He told me that I was the 13th of his docents to become a full professor. This was at a time when there was tough competition for each chair. The Karolinska Institutet had just over 60 chairs, but there were only two in medicine. Caspersson was rightly proud of his success in educating scientists to head positions in both theoretical and clinical medical disciplines.

Caspersson ended his research career in 1992, when he was 82 years of age. He decided to use his time to take care of his wife

Siv, who had been slowly deteriorating from Alzheimer's disease. During our telephone conversation in December 1997, which I describe in the Prologue, I understood that he was seriously ill, but the carer who helped him to contact me did not think it was serious. She had seen him deteriorate in the same way before. There were no newspaper headlines following his death the next day. Caspersson left us at 87 years of age without having been awarded the Nobel Prize.

20 United States of America

The collaboration between Caspersson and Sidney Farber led to an offer for me to spend about one year at the CCRF. The plan was that I would work in the cell biology laboratory headed by Dr George Foley, Farber's closest associate at the CCRF, and my formal position would be Research Associate in the Department of Pathology at Harvard Medical School. The plan was supported by Dr Robert McCarthy, who wanted to build up a microspectro-photometric unit at the CCRF. He had spent one year in Stockholm and had been educated by Caspersson's engineers. It means that I would be able to continue my work on a thesis on the use of microspectrophotometry for diagnostic purposes, particularly studies on the periodic acid-Schiff (PAS) reaction. This was an excellent opportunity to collect clinical material from patients with CML, polycythemia vera (PV) and other disorders of interest from the hospitals that were collaborating with CCRF. I would also be allowed to establish collaborations if I felt that they could promote my research.

I was happy about the offer and accepted with great pleasure. I was offered a much better salary in Boston than the stipend that I received in Stockholm. In the fall of 1963, I went with my family, wife and two children, two-year-old Måns and five-month-old Charlotte (Lotta) to the USA. We had rented a two-room apartment for two weeks at a small pension in Cambridge, close to

Harvard University. It was arranged by my friend, docent Einar Perman, who was a guest researcher at Boston City Hospital. The idea was that during these two weeks I would find a house to rent in Arlington, which was a suburb where other Swedes had lived and thrived. The supply of rented houses was excellent and after about a week I found a nice house. I bought an old Chevrolet for a few hundred dollars, and we were all set.

I soon realized that the work was not what I expected. A microspectrophotometer could not be properly built or correctly used without knowledgeable engineers. McCarthy had not managed to build the equipment and I was not the one to do it. Fortunately, I had continued to employ my skillful technician, Eva Östling, in Stockholm. She was an expert in using both the microspectrophotometer and the microinterferometer. Thus, I concentrated on getting the clinical material and preparing it for measurements. Then I sent the preparations to Eva for measurements.

I managed to collect a large amount of material from patients with three different diseases, CML, PV and paroxysmal nocturnal hemoglobinuria (PNH). I also wanted to see if any abnormal amounts of glycogen in the neutrophil leukocytes would normalize after treatment. An enzyme, alkaline phosphatase, had previously been shown to occur in low amounts in neutrophils in CML, but in high amounts in PV. This was despite the fact that, at that time, these two diseases were supposed to belong to the same type of disorders, the myeloproliferative diseases. PNH was an unusual disease that had low amounts of alkaline phosphatase in neutrophils, and I wanted to see if glycogen also occurred in low amounts. If any differences could be documented, that could lead to the design of further studies on the metabolism in the cells in these disorders. Perhaps such knowledge could then be used to design drugs.

It must be remembered that the treatment of these disorders was extremely poor at this time. All patients with CML died, whatever treatment they received. Usually, the cytotoxic agent busulfan was used and resulted in a median survival of about three years, with occasional long-term survivors of 10–15 years. PV was less severe, but a significant number of patients developed acute leukemia, with short survival. PNH was also a deadly disorder and sometimes turned into leukemia.

Harvard Medical School and CCRF were surrounded by some of the most important hospitals in the world: the Peter Bent Brigham Hospital, the Children's Hospital and the Beth Israel Hospital. This was the place for a young physician who wanted to extend his knowledge of medicine and collect clinical research material. The patients' clinical records were generally excellent and there were high-quality correlations between research results and common clinical parameters. I went on rounds with Professor Frank Gardner at Peter Bent Brigham, who was always questioned by his young resident David Nathan. Many years later, Nathan went on to become the head of CCRF, which by then had changed its name to the Dana-Farber Cancer Institute. The Hospital also provided me with blood and bone marrow for my research.

Boston had many other hospitals of the highest quality, and they were often linked to one or more universities. I belonged to Harvard Medical School, due to its affiliation with the CCRF and Boston Children's Hospital. It had units at many other hospitals, for example the Boston City Hospital through the Thorndyke laboratories, and the Massachusetts General Hospital. Boston had many other hospitals that were affiliated with other universities, including the New England Medical Center, which was associated with the Tufts Medical School. It was world famous for its hematology department, which was led by William Dameshek, who was one of the global leaders of this specialty.

21 Sidney Farber and the First Treatment for Acute Leukemia

When I arrived at the CCRF in August 1963 I was whole-heartedly welcomed by Sidney Farber. I worked in the laboratories run by Dr George Foley, who was a cell biologist and the head administrator under Farber and 100% loyal to his boss. I was allowed to do practically anything that was possible in his laboratory and was supported by one of Foley's technicians. I was welcome to participate in the weekly clinical conferences led by Farber, and I could follow the clinical activities with the agreement of the respective clinicians working in the outpatients' clinics. The clinical departments were happy to support me by providing bone marrow and blood for my research. The doors were wide open because I was Torbjörn Caspersson's *"boy"*. The fact that I was a qualified physician in Sweden was a strength. I got all the offers from Farber, who sat behind his enormous desk in a big room on the top floor of the CCRF building. He radiated authority and spoke slowly in a low voice. Then he asked a few questions about me and my family and the audience was over after about 15 minutes.

Sidney Farber was born in 1903 into a Jewish family in Buffalo, New York[43]. After he completed his academic examinations at the University of Buffalo, he started his medical studies at the University of Heidelberg in Germany. After a year, he returned to USA and continued his studies in medicine at Harvard Medical School in Boston, where he passed his MD examination. He specialized in pathology at the Peter Bent Brigham Hospital and was then employed as a pathologist at the Children's Hospital. In 1948, he was appointed Professor of Pathology at Harvard Medical School and Head of the Pathology Unit at the Children's Hospital.

Farber paid great interest to the biology of cancer cells from an early stage. He had the idea that since these cells needed the vitamin folic acid to grow, a folic acid antagonist would lead to the death of the cancer cells. He established collaborations with the Lederle pharmaceutical company and their chemist Dr Yellapragada Subbarow. He had been working on folic acid antagonists for some time and he managed to produce several variants. The most potent one was 4-aminopteroyl-glutamic acid, also named aminopterin.

Farber received permission to use this drug to treat children with acute leukemia. During the first study it was given as an intramuscular injection to 16 children with the disease. Ten of the children responded with normalization of their high white blood cell counts and their immature abnormal leukemic cells disappeared from their blood and diminished in their bone marrow. The children appeared to be clinically normal or better physically. Farber called the improvement a remission. In 1948, he published the results, together with his clinical collaborator LK Diamond, in the *New England Journal of Medicine*[44]. It provoked an intense debate and some researchers believed that cancer could be eradicated, although Farber had been careful to tell them that the leukemia had returned in all the patients after weeks or months.

Farber became world famous. As a strong and skilled administrator, organizer, and opinion leader he used the results to engage with numerous organizations and raise money for cancer research. One of his leukemia patients appeared on a radio channel using the name *"Jimmy"*, which after a while gave rise to the Jimmy Fund.

In 1947, he persuaded the Variety Club of the Boston Red Socks baseball team to support the Jimmy Fund. The club was very successful in raising money and the Jimmy Fund became the largest financing body for the CCRF building where I worked. In fact, the building was often known as the Jimmy Fund. When I visited the clinic in 1963, it was only for children, but Farber continued his building activity. By the time he died in 1973, he had built and inaugurated the Sidney Farber Cancer Center, for children and adult outpatients and inpatients. After his death, others continued to expand the Center, according to his wishes. The support of the Charles A Dana Foundation led to it being renamed the Dana-Farber Cancer Institute.

Farber was a master in engaging with important people, including politicians, to further cancer research. I have been told that he talked directly with President Eisenhower and managed to convince him that the National Cancer Institute needed substantially more money for clinical cancer research, as well as independence from the National Institute of Health.

Farber lobbied intensively to increase the budget for the National Cancer Institute, with Mary Lasker (1900–1994) and her husband Albert Lasker (1880–1952), who had created the Lasker Foundation and the prestigious Lasker Prize[45]. During their most active lobbying period, from 1957–1967, the National Cancer Institute increased its budget for cancer research from 48 to 176 million US dollars, which was an enormous sum of money at that time.

Many thought that Sidney Farber was worthy of receiving a Nobel Prize and he was nominated five times until early 1973, just before his death. In the special investigation performed by the Nobel Committee member Rolf Zetterström in 1971 he

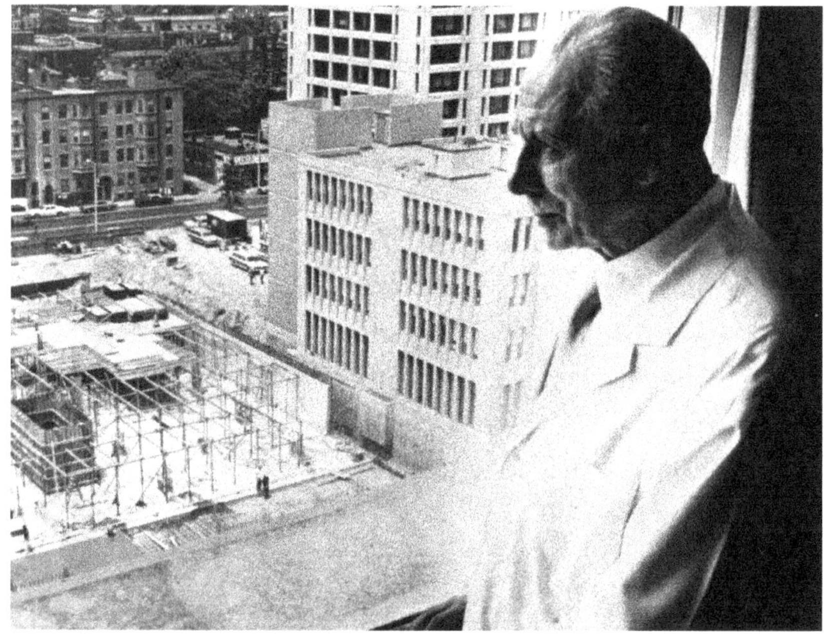

Sidney Farber achieved temporary remission for the first patient with acute lympho-blastic leukemia using the drug, aminopterin. This picture shows him looking out of the window of the Children's Cancer Research Foundation (CCRF) building at the construction of the Sidney Farber Cancer Center, which later became the Dana-Farber Cancer Institute.

was found worthy of the prize, but competition with other candidates in other areas was tough. In 1971 the Nobel Prize was awarded to Earl W Sutherland, Jr. *"for his discoveries concerning the mechanisms of the action of hormones"*, and 1972 it went to Gerald M Edelman and Rodney R Porter *"for their discoveries concerning the chemical structure of antibodies"*, and the next year Farber passed away. Although he was the first to treat patients with an anticancer drug that was effective, at least in short term, it lasted until 1988, when the Nobel Prize was eventually given to Gertrude Elion and George Hitchings for discovering cancer drugs (Chapter 36). However, even without the Nobel Prize, Farber's legacy will always be associated with the first treatment of children with acute lymphoblastic leukemia with an anticancer drug. He created the word remission, which is still used to define grades of response. Cures came later and today we use other drugs and combinations of drugs. Aminopterin, or rather its derivative methotrexate, is still in use. It was used at the CCRF long after other drugs had been shown to be more effective. These days it is mainly used in other disorders, or in association with allogeneic transplants. However, Farber's intuition and driving force to find and use the first remission-inducing anticancer drug was the start of the fabulous developments in cancer treatment that have taken place ever since.

22 William Dameshek and Robert Schwartz

William Dameshek (1900–1969) was born in Voronezh in southwest Russia, at a time when Jewish families like his were being persecuted and even killed. His family emigrated to the USA in 1903 and settled down in Medford, Massachusetts. Dameshek studied medicine at Harvard Medical School and graduated in 1923. He completed his internship at Boston City Hospital and became interested in hematology when he attended a course in laboratory medicine at Tufts Medical School. He got a position as a hematologist at Beth Israel Hospital, but after 10 years he moved to the New England Medical Center, where he established the Blood Research Laboratory. He soon became Head of Medicine at the New England Medical Center and Professor of Medicine at Tufts Medical School.

I called Dameshek some months after my arrival at CCRF and asked him if he would allow me to visit him and his famous department. I had heard from Farber's closest collaborators at the CCRF that Dameshek was not a friend of Farber, so I stressed my Swedish background and my collaboration with Torbjörn Caspersson, who Dameshek knew well. I also said that I had been working at the CCRF for some time as a visitor.

Some years earlier, Dameshek had founded the concept of *"myeloproliferative syndrome"*, which incorporated many malignant hematologic disorders. I had some difficulties buying into the concept, because two of the priority diseases that I studied, CML and PV, were included and I thought that they were very different. The glycogen content in the progeny of the premalignant or malignant immature cells in the bone marrow, the neutrophil leukocytes, had a high glycogen content in PV and was very low in CML, according to my microspectrophotometric measurements. Similarly, the enzyme alkaline phosphatase had been found to be high in PV and low in CML.

Dameshek was a well-known and extremely skillful clinician and he saw patients from all over the world. He was still engaged in important scientific activity and a number of the students in his department went on to become well-known hematologists. In addition to this, he had started *Blood*, the most famous hematology scientific journal, in 1946 and was its Editor-in-Chief. It was an enormously powerful position. Getting a paper published in *Blood* was much more important for a hematologist than being published in any other scientific journal in the field.

My phone call to Dameshek resulted in an invitation to visit him. When I told him about my research on two of the disorders included in his new concept of the myeloproliferative syndrome, he asked if I could give a lecture about my research to his group. Microspectrophotometry was new to him, particularly as a diagnostic tool. I was, of course, proud to receive his invitation and had no intention of trying to crush his concept. However, I was prepared for a tough discussion.

Dameshek was a very informal person. After my lecture, there was a lively discussion among his group of about 25 physicians. One of the people who I particularly remember attending my lecture was Robert Schwartz (1928–2017). He was an immunologist who solved the problem of organ transplants being rejected, by introducing the concept of immunosuppression. Four years before I arrived in Boston, he had written a paper with Dameshek, who was his mentor and collaborator, that stated that using 6-mercaptopurine, and later its derivative azathioprine, could prevent rejection. This was acknowledged by the 1988 Nobel Prize winner Gertrude Elion, who discovered the 6-mercaptopurine with George Hitchings. In her Nobel Prize lecture, Elion stated that *"in 1958 a new horizon appeared"* when Robert Schwartz, who was working with Dameshek in Boston, investigated the effect of 6-mercaptopurine on the immune response. Schwartz was also acknowledged in 1990 by the Nobel Prize Laureate Joseph Murray, who carried out the first successful renal transplant. He stated in his Nobel Prize lecture that: *"the real breakthrough came with the introduction of immunosuppressive drugs by Schwartz and Dameshek in 1959"*[46].

Schwartz received his MD degree from New York University in 1954 and in 1957 he joined Dameshek at Tufts. When I first met him in 1963, he had been a professor at Tufts Medical School since 1961. He was later appointed Head of the Division of Hematology and stayed until 1994. He then became Deputy Editor-in-Chief for the most famous clinical journal, the *New England Journal of Medicine*. He then approached me, more than 40 years after we had first met, and he asked me to write a review of a book about immunology and transplantation for the journal. I did so with great pleasure and ensured that he was correctly cited and appreciated in the book.

Dameshek and his group did not seem to consider my presentation in 1963 as an attack on the concept of myeloproliferative syndrome. Dameshek's students, interns, residents and the others who attended my lecture had no fear of challenging his views, as he seemed to enjoy any attack on himself. This was in very sharp contrast to what I had experienced at the weekly clinical conferences around Farber's oval table (Chapter 21).

Five years later, Dameshek obviously remembered my visit, and the lecture that I delivered in his department, when he was asked by the American President, Lyndon B Johnson, to recommend peaceful activities that could take place in Richland, Washington, where the atomic bomb was born. Dameshek invited me to a symposium about myeloproliferative syndrome, which was still considered a valid concept. I had passed my thesis at the Karolinska Institutet two years earlier and had substantial results that indicated great differences between the two disorders within his concept[47]. The glycogen content in neutrophil leukocytes was high in PV and low in CML[48], but demonstrated similar intercellular variations. I was able to show that the values in CML normalized after effective treatment with busulfan treatment[49]. Dameshek chaired my session. He initiated a lively discussion, just like the one at Tufts in 1963. His ideas about myeloproliferative syndrome prevailed and he stated that there could be variations within it. I once again concluded that Dameshek and Farber, two giants in hematology and oncology were very different personalities.

Dameshek and Schwartz both received many important prizes, but neither of them were nominated for the Nobel Prize before 1972. The discovery of immunosuppression could well have been deemed worthy of a prize, due to the importance for transplantation. However, their work was obviously not prioritized after the 1988 Nobel Prize was awarded to Hitchings and Elion and the 1990 prize was awarded to Joseph Murray and Donnall Thomas.

23 William (Bill) Curry Moloney and Emil (Tom) Frei III

My friend Einar Perman was spending one year at the Thorndike Memorial Laboratory at Boston City Hospital during part of my time at the CCRF. I got to know two hematologists who became my friends through him. Boston City Hospital was associated with three different medical schools: Harvard, Tufts and Boston University. When I arrived in Boston in 1963 William (Bill) Moloney (1907–1995)[50] was Head of Hematology at Tufts Medical School and Louis Sullivan from Thorndyke Laboratories was at Boston University (Chapter 24).

I first encountered Moloney in 1963 and he had already been the Chief Hematologist at the Tufts hematology unit for many years. He was a highly recognized clinician and became famous after he served as the Head of the Hematology Division of the Atomic Bomb Casualty Commission in 1952. This organization had investigated the hematological effects that the atomic bombs that had dropped over Hiroshima and Nagasaki during World War Two had on the Japanese survivors. He was able to clearly document an increased incidence of leukemia among survivors who had received high doses of irradiation. There were concerns about the increase in CML. Moloney was an all-round hematologist and up to that point he had been mainly interested in anemia and other benign hematology disorders, but after his experience in Japan his interest in leukemia grew. He was in demand because he had become one of the most skilled hematologists and was able to diagnose leukemia just by looking at the bone marrow and blood cytology under the microscope. He established close collaborations with the scientists and clinicians at the Thorndyke Memorial Laboratories, including William Castle, who had been working with the 1934 Nobel Prize winners, George Richards Minot and William Parry Murphy. They had received the prize, with George Hoyt Whipple, *"for their discoveries concerning liver therapy in cases of anemia"*.

Castle's main interest was not leukemia and he needed Moloney's expert knowledge to diagnose the many different types that existed. This was important, because new drugs had been developed after Farber first achieved remission with aminopterin in patients with acute lymphoblastic leukemia (ALL), and it was important to choose the right drugs or drug combinations for each specific type of leukemia.

My contact with Perman led to me being invited to give a lecture about my microspectrophotometric investigations of leukemic cells for him and his hematology group on the afternoon of Friday 22 November 1963. I was driving my old Chevrolet down Memorial Drive on the Cambridge side of Charles River at about 12.30pm, listening to the radio. Suddenly, there was a break in the music program and a journalist dramatically reported that there had been a shot fired at President Kennedy in Dallas, Texas. He believed that the President had been hit. I didn't think it was real at first. However, after a short while the journalist returned to the program and said that it was serious. He provided regular updates. About 20 minutes before I had arrived at Boston City Hospital, he claimed that the President had been shot in the head and transported to a hospital and was unlikely to survive. When I arrived at my destination, the news had already reached people at the hospital that the President was dead. I found the Tuft Hematology unit and the lecture room. I met Moloney for the first time and he said that the President was dead. I expressed my condolences and suggested that my lecture should be postponed. Moloney hesitated, but then said that I should give the lecture, as life had to go on. I started my lecture by extending my condolences to my American colleagues. It was my attempt, as a foreigner, to show that I participated in their loss. Then I gave my lecture. The atmosphere was heavy, but my lecture was still well received.

After this meeting Moloney and I became very good friends. When we chatted after the lecture, it turned out that we both were tennis fans. He invited me to play doubles with two of his friends. It turned out that we were evenly matched on the tennis court, and I became a frequent partner and member of his team. It was a good way to get to know each other.

In the mid-1960s, Moloney was recruited by George Thorn[51], then Hersey Professor of Medicine at Harvard Medical School and Chairman of Medicine at the Peter Bent Brigham Hospital. His role was to build a strong hematology unit at this hospital. Moloney stayed on as Chief of Hematology until 1976 and eventually became a full Professor of Medicine at Harvard Medical School. Peter Bent Brigham was close to the CCRF and soon Sidney Farber engaged Moloney's services at the CCRF.

When I returned to the CCRF in 1972 for a two-week follow-up on the clinical records of patients that I had studied, I once again took part in a clinical conference around the oval table in Farber's office. To my great astonishment, Moloney was one of the participants. It was a great reunion and he had important views on one of the patients we were discussing. However, he could not hide that he felt very uncomfortable with Farber's formal style, which I had experienced many years earlier. Moloney and Farber were as different as personalities as Farber and Dameshek. The collaboration between Moloney and Farber was short lived. Farber died in March 1973 and Moloney survived him by 26 years, even though he was only four years younger than him.

Moloney experienced a new period of success building the hematology department at Peter Bent Brigham. After stepping down as the chief, he continued to work and collaborated with the new leaders at the CCRF and Dana-Farber Cancer Center.

In 1972, Emil (Tom) Frei III (1924–2013) was recruited by Farber as the Physician in Chief, when Farber was still the Head of CCRF. Frei received his MD in 1948 after studying medicine at Yale University. In 1953, after his internship and serving in the Navy during the Korean war, he became a resident at Washington University in St Louis, Missouri. It was there that he met Dr C Gordon Zubrod, who introduced him to medical research. When Zubrod got a position at the National Cancer Institute in 1955, he took Frei with him. Frei now decided to focus on hematologic malignancies. In 1958, he had published a paper showing that combining 6-mercaptopurine and aminopterin improved the survival rates for acute leukemia, compared to treatment with just one drug[52]. In 1966, he teamed up with Vincent DeVita and showed that combination chemotherapy was more effective than single drug treatment for Hodgkin's disease[53]. They eventually showed dramatic results with the cytotoxic drug combination of mechlorethamine (Mustargen) hydrochloride, vincristine (Oncovin) sulfate, procarbazine hydrochloride and prednisone, called MOPP for short[54].

Frei then developed a combination chemotherapy for acute leukemia called COAP, which comprised cyclophosphamide, vincristine, cytarabine hydrochloride and prednisone[55]. The results were excellent. This was the start of combination chemotherapy for numerous hematologic and other cancers.

In 1965, Frei moved to the MD Anderson Cancer Center in Houston, Texas, as the Director of Clinical Research and Chairman of Experimental Therapeutics. His friend and collaborator Emil Freireich joined him and their fruitful collaboration on combination chemotherapy in leukemia continued.

This was Frei's background when he arrived at the CCRF in 1972 and I visited my old workplace. It was a privilege to talk with him about his visions for the CCRF and leukemia treatment. Although I knew about his achievements and had already started a clinical project on acute myelocytic leukemia in Stockholm, it was very valuable to hear the views of this giant in clinical leukemia research on the future for leukemia patients.

After Farber's death in 1973, Frei became Head of the CCRF and Professor of Medicine at Harvard Medical School. He remained in his CCRF position until 1980, when there were some complaints about his administration. He stepped down as Head of the CCRF, but continued as Physician in Chief under the immunologist and Nobel Prize winner Baruj Benacerraf (1920–2011). Benacerraf became President and CEO of the Dana-Farber Cancer Institute until he retired in 1991. He had been Chair of the Department of Comparative Pathology at Harvard Medical School since 1970.

Moloney's life was much better with Frei as Head of the clinic at the CCRF. Apparently, they collaborated well, and Frei had use for Moloney's knowledge about clinical hematology and cytology. Moloney served at both the Peter Bent Brigham Hospital and the CCRF for many years after his retirement. He was still around when Benacerraf stepped down in 1991 as CEO of the Dana-Farber Cancer Institute, the present name for the enormous establishment that started as the CCRF with Farber as its head.

Benacerraf was succeeded by my colleague David Nathan, who questioned both residents and his boss Frank Gardner during the rounds at Peter Bent Brigham Hospital in the 1960s. He was also Head of Hematology at the Children's Hospital.

The last time I met Moloney was at a congress in Boston in the early 1990s, when he invited me to lunch at the Harvard Faculty Club and we talked about old memories and, of course, the latest tennis events in the world.

Moloney was never nominated for a Nobel Prize. According to Alfred Nobel's will, the Prize was not given for great knowledge or skill, or for educating students. Moloney was one of the most knowledgeable clinicians I ever met. Although I never was his student, I learned a lot about diseases and hematology from him. In addition, I liked him for his kindness, friendship, and integrity. And, of course, because of his interest in tennis!

It is no secret that Frei was nominated for the Nobel Prize on several occasions, but he never received it. Frei received a number of other awards, including the 1972 Albert Lasker Award for clinical medical research, now the Lasker-DeBakey Clinical Medical Research Award. However, in contrast to the Nobel Prize, there was no limit to the number of awardees who could receive the Lasker Prize for a specific year. In 1972, the Lasker prize was also given to Emil Freireich, Vincent DeVita, James Holland, Gordon Zubrod, who was Frei's mentor, and many others. All these clinical scientists had participated in the research that led to miraculous improvements in the treatment of cancer patients. Although I tend to believe that Frei, and perhaps DeVita, were the main innovators of combination cancer chemotherapy, it is difficult to know. The Nobel Prize can only be given to a maximum of three winners in any specific year.

24 Louis Sullivan and William Castle

I got to know hematologist Louis Sullivan through Einar Perman in 1963. Since 1961 he had been working at Thorndyke Memorial Laboratories, which was founded in 1923 and was a unit of Harvard Medical School at Boston City Hospital. Sullivan had worked under the supervision of the world famous William Castle (1897–1990), known for the discovery of intrinsic factor, which was involved in the pathogenesis of pernicious anemia[56].

In 1925, Castle was invited to join the Thorndyke Memorial Laboratories, by its first director Francis B Peabody (1881–1927). Peabody was interested in pernicious anemia, which was a deadly disease at that time. Castle knew that two hematologists had treated patients with pernicious anemia with raw liver. They were George R Minot (1885–1950), Physician-in-Chief of the Collis P Huntington Memorial Hospital at Harvard University, and member of the staff of the Peter Bent Brigham Hospital, and his colleague William P Murphy (1892–1987). Minot had been influenced by the results of George H Whipple (1878–1976), who had seen the effects that this liver treatment had on anemia in dogs.

Castle approached Minot with the idea that patients with pernicious anemia lacked something in the stomach that was associated with achlorhydria, as this was a constant finding in these patients. He tested the idea on a 60-year-old woman with pernicious anemia. First, she was fed with raw hamburger meat, which did not increase her reticulocytes. Then, he stimulated his own stomach with similar hamburger meat, recovered the stomach contents after one hour and gave it back to the patient via a nasogastric tube. After a few days her reticulocytes rose, proving improvements could be obtained if achlorhydria was ameliorated. This later led to the isolation of the intrinsic factor that is important for absorbing the vitamin B12 that is lacking in patients with pernicious anemia. Today, patients with pernicious anemia are treated with vitamin B12, which circumvents the need for intrinsic factor.

Castle was appointed director of the Thorndyke Memorial Laboratories in 1948 and stayed in this position until 1963. However, he was still around and worked with patients at the Thorndyke Memorial Laboratories and Boston City Hospital after his retirement. Perman, who worked with Dr Charles S Davidson, Head of the Division for Liver Disease and Nutrition at Thorndyke Memorial Laboratories, saw him frequently and said he was an excellent clinician, great researcher and a very kind person.

When Whipple, Minot and Murphy received the Nobel Prize in 1934, Castle was not included as a winner. One reason was probably that the importance of his intrinsic factor discovery had not been fully recognized at that point. Another was that there could be only three awardees, according to Nobel's will. However, Castle was nominated four times after that, twice in the 1930s (1935 and 1938), and twice in the 1960s (1963 and 1967), but by then it was too late.

Louis Sullivan left his research fellowship at Thorndyke Memorial Laboratories in 1963. He turned to Boston University and in 1965 he became a co-director of Hematology at Boston University Medical Center. He eventually advanced to Professor of Medicine at Boston University and founded the Boston University Hematology Service at Boston City Hospital.

I first met Louis at Boston City Hospital in November 1963. He told me that he planned to participate in the Congress of the International Society of Hematology in Stockholm in the early fall of 1964. At that time the President of the Society was Professor Jan Waldenström and the Secretary was Lars Erik Böttiger, Associate Professor at the Serafimer Hospital. Louis had not arranged any accommodation and I invited him to stay in our apartment in Stockholm, which he gladly accepted. I returned to Stockholm with my family before Louis arrived for the Congress. We both participated and presented our own research. If I remember correctly, Louis presented his studies on the impact of alcohol on blood cell production[57] and I talked about my microspectro-photometric studies on neutrophils leukocytes. When I returned to the CCRF in 1968 for another year, Louis had joined Boston University as an assistant professor and the University wanted him to build a hematology unit at Boston City Hospital. This resulted in the Boston University Hematology Service, and Louis was its Chief.

Louis was black and so was his wife, Ginger. Both had partic-ipated in the March on Washington in 1963 when Martin Luther King delivered his famous *"I have a dream"* speech. According to Louis, black people were still widely discriminated against in the USA, although the Government had tried to stop it. Louis was an example of both discrimination and how attempts were being made to get rid of it. He said that if you had as little as 5% black genes, then you were black. Many generations of white input were necessary to be recognized as white, if, of course, that was somebody's wish. He had now moved with his family to Lexington, which was a *"white"* neighborhood of Boston. When the neigh-bors found out, through the broker, there were protests, because they thought that house prices would fall. Louis did not hesitate and bought the house. He then visited his neighbors, introduced himself and talked about what he was doing. In the end he became friends with most of them and the house prices remained stable.

One evening my wife and I were invited to his home for dinner, along with his colleagues and friends. There were about 30 guests and only one other couple was white. It seemed that more needed to be done to eradicate discrimination, despite the progress that had been made.

In 1975, Louis was invited to build a medical school at Morehouse College in Atlanta, Georgia. I visited him a few months later. He had great plans. He took me for a drive in Atlanta and parked on an enormous, untidy plot, that was partly being used as a parking lot. *"Here, I will build the Morehouse School of Medicine"* he declared. The idea was to build a medical school for *"under-privileged students"*, in other words mainly the black ones. I thought that this was a great, but difficult, plan. In 1987 I got an invitation from Louis to give a lecture at the Morehouse School of Medicine. He had used the plot I had seen in 1975 to build a wonderful medical school, just as he had promised. He was now its Dean and President. A four-year program had been launched so that students could take their final examinations and become qualified doctors. I was impressed. I was taken around to visit the administrators and teachers. The students and the administrators were all black, but the medical teachers were all white. *"It is about competence"* Louis explained. He said that it was difficult to find competent teachers among the black population and that is why he mainly employed white ones. His argument was that if he was able to provide the best teachers to educate his black students, then eventually he would be able to recruit more black teachers. That was the wisdom of Louis Sullivan. In the future it would be different. Getting rid of discrimination would be based on improving the quality of education for black students. He was totally against fixed proportions of black and white employees, irrespective of competence.

Louis was the best example for how competence could be obtained. He graduated with great distinction from Morehouse College in 1954 and then achieved the same distinction when he received his medical degree from Boston University Medical School. He then advanced his research education at Thorndyke Memorial Laboratories.

Louis remained the President at Morehouse School of Medicine until his retirement in 2002, with a four-year gap from 1989–1993, when President George H W Bush asked him to be Secretary of Health and Human Services. He thinks that the president's wife Barbara Bush may have suggested him for the role, as he and his wife Ginger had met her at a reception and the First Lady had been very interested in his work in Atlanta and at the Morehouse School of Medicine.

Louis served for the full period of President Bush's presidency and he claimed, with some humor, that *"I am responsible for the largest federal budget, larger than the budget for defense"*. The reason for the size of the budget was that it included all the federal pensions. His big headache was how healthcare should be financed. He wanted better financial cover for sickness, but he believed in private insurance rather than in federal or state protection. Louis was a Republican, and his wife was a Democrat. This may have had something to do with Abraham Lindquist, Ragnhild abolishing slavery, as many black people voted for the Republicans after his death. However, this seemed to have changed after the middle of the 20th century and most black people, like Ginger, voted for the Democrats.

I visited Louis in 1991 when he was halfway through his role as Secretary of Health and Human Services. I was impressed by the security precautions. He had a private elevator from the parking garage to his office. He had invited me and a few other people for lunch, together with the chief of the National Institutes of Health (NIH), Bernadine Healy (1944–2011)[58]. Louis had recently appointed her to become the first woman in the USA to hold that position. He explained to me that it was very important to have someone from the medical profession in this important position, as it was undoubtedly the most important research establishment and funding institution in the world. He placed her next to me at the lunch table.

Healy was very open about her plans for the NIH and research funding in the USA. She had graduated from Harvard Medical School and trained as a cardiologist. She was considered to be both an excellent scientist and administrator and had enjoyed an extraordinary career at the Cleveland Clinic Lerner Research Institute before she was appointed as chief of the NIH. She had also been an advisor to President Ronald Reagan. Unfortunately, there was a considerable debate about her appointment, and she had to leave that post after about two years. However, during her short period in office she built the world-famous laboratory for human genomics and shaped the steering group of world-famous researchers in the Human Genome Project. She was a feminist and she decided that the NIH should only finance clinical therapy projects that included both men and women, if the conditions that were being studied affected both sexes.

I asked Louis if he would consider coming to the Huddinge Hospital and the Karolinska Institutet in Stockholm to give a lecture about the American health and medical care system and his views on how to organize it in the future. To my great pleasure he accepted. He came over to Sweden with Ginger, who had devoted herself to a project to try and establish mammograms for women. I asked her to give a lecture to the Department of Oncology at the Karolinska Hospital on 15 November 1991. I was now Head of the Department of Medicine at the Karolinska Institutet at Huddinge Hospital, south of central Stockholm. I travelled back and prepared my Institution and the President of the Karolinska Institutet, the Nobel Prize winner Bengt Samuelsson, and the hospital's Director, Lars-Åke Flood, for the arrival of one of the most important people in global medical research. However, I had forgotten one important player in the game and that was the American Embassy. It did not take long before I had a phone call from an official at the Embassy. From that moment on I was contacted almost every day for a couple of months by staff members working for the Ambassador, Charles E Redman. Every step Louis was going to take needed to be planned in detail. He would stay at the Embassy. Two American security officials appeared two days before the Sullivans arrived. We walked the path from where the car would arrive to the lecture hall, with me acting as Louis and discussed any corner that could be considered a risk for terrorism. My naive idea that I would meet Louis and Ginger alone at the airport was thwarted by the Ambassador. He and his chauffeur arrived before me in the Embassy's armored car. The Ambassador told me to wait in the VIP room, while he and his wife met the couple at the aircraft stairs. My ignorance about security regulations at the airport made me obey. After a while, they all appeared in the VIP room, and I embraced Louis and Ginger to the great amazement of Redman and his wife. I noticed how unhappy Louis was with the Ambassador when he realized how I had been treated.

Redman's attitude changed and we were left in peace to plan the lectures, dinner at my house, dinner with the President (Rector) of the Karolinska Institutet and a sight-seeing trip around Stockholm. Then the Ambassador took Louis and Ginger in the armored car to the Embassy, which would be their home during their visit to Stockholm. Redman and his staff improved their attitude to me, as I had extended the invitation to the Sullivans.

Louis delivered an acclaimed lecture and there were many important people in the audience, including the President (Rector) of the Karolinska Institutet. The Swedish Public Service and press were amazingly uninterested, and we realized that we had probably not publicized the lecture well enough. But Louis did not seem that bothered, as he was more interested in talking with the medical professionals.

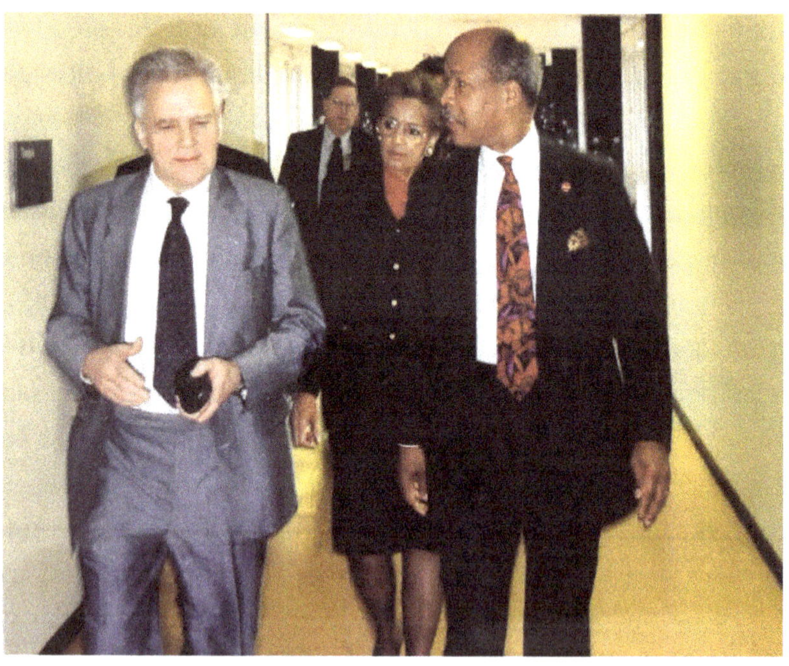

Louis Sullivan was Secretary of Health and Human Services during the Presidency of George H.W.Bush. He visited me at the Huddinge Hospital in Stockholm to give a lecture. Here he is seen with his wife Ginger and the author after arrival at the hospital.

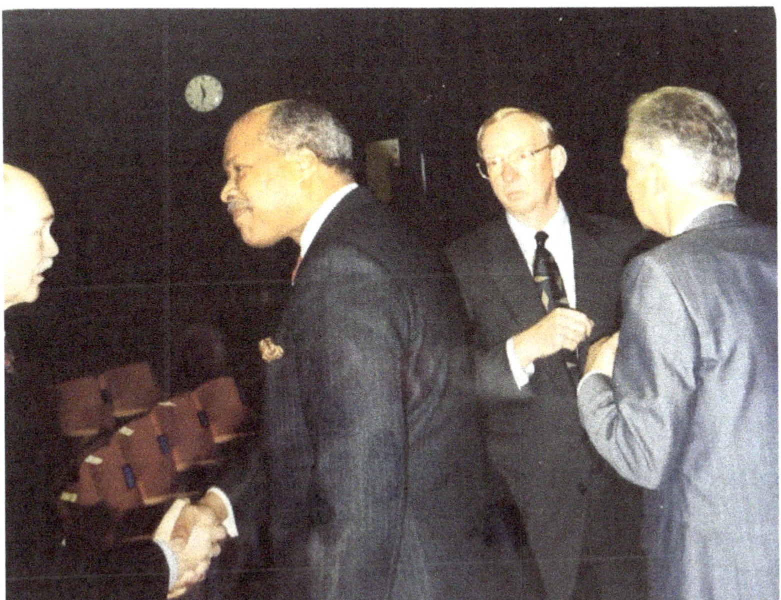

Sullivan before the lecture, greeting chief physician Anders Persson with the President (Rector) of the Karolinska Institutet and Nobel Laureate Bengt Samuelsson in the background talking to me.

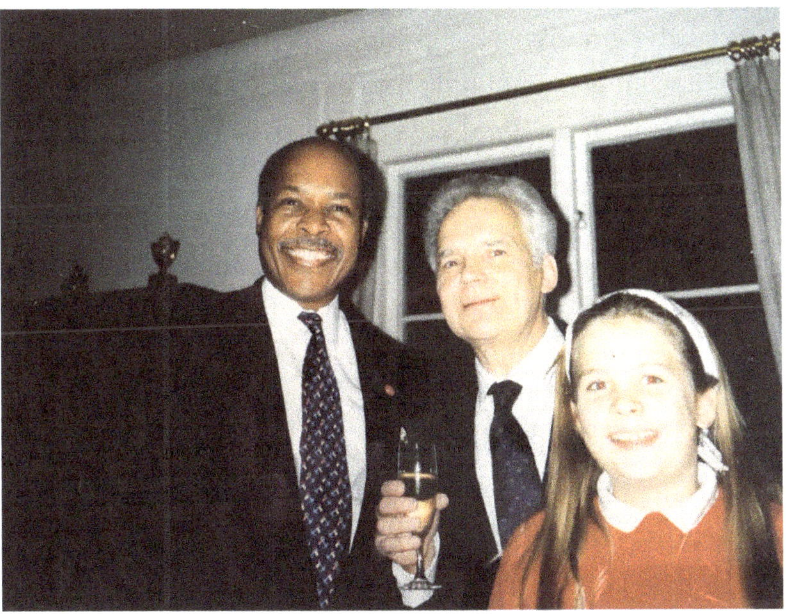

Louis Sullivan with me and my daughter Elisabeth.

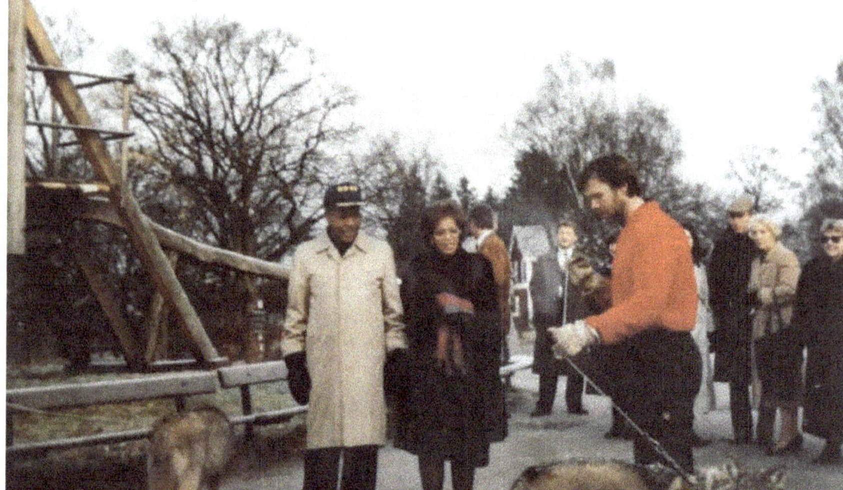

The astonishing meeting between the Sullivans and the wolves during a tour to Skansen.

Security guards accompanied the Sullivans everywhere. During the dinner at our home for some 20 people, security guards were stationed in armored cars outside our house, to the great amazement of our neighbors.

Louis resigned from his position when President Bush lost the election for a second term in 1993. He continued as the President of the Morehouse School of Medicine and expanded the facilities, with new laboratories and education space.

I met Louis Sullivan again a few years ago. He had retired as President of the Morehouse School of Medicine, but not completely, as he was now the Honorary President. He took me for a trip round the school. It was an amazing expansion. One building was called the Louis and Ginger Sullivan Building and their names were in large letters at the entrance. Louis had the right to be proud. His journey from a black middle-class family to Professor in Hematology, builder and president of a medical school and a member of the Government of the richest country in the world was outstanding. If there had been a Nobel Prize for *"the most outstanding achievement in counteracting discrimination due to color or ethnic origin"* he would have been a candidate. However, that was not specified in Alfred Nobel's will.

25 To the Karolinska University Hospital and the Creation of the Leukemia Group of Middle Sweden

"Platelets…?" I had picked up my telephone in my laboratory at the Cell Research Institute. I asked who was speaking and the voice continued to ask me *"What do you know about platelets?"* After a while, I realized it was the Head of the Department of Medicine at the Karolinska Hospital, Professor Henrik Lagerlöf (1907–1999). He had called me because I had contacted his associate, Peter Reizenstein, who was responsible for hematology, to ask him if they would consider admitting me to the department. This was in 1966, when I had just defended my thesis with the highest grade, and wanted to continue my career as a clinician. Lagerlöf wanted to check whether I was interested in working with him and his new interest, which was platelets, rather than work with his associate Reizenstein. Lagerlöf was an innovative, but somewhat eccentric person, who had made some interesting scientific discoveries about gastroenterology and cardiovascular diseases. Now he had some ideas about the impact of platelets on cardiovascular disease. My thesis dealt with leukemia and not platelets, and I answered honestly: *"Not much. My thesis*[36]*dealt with leukemia and my intention is not to focus my research on platelets".* In fact, I had defended my thesis in the great auditorium of the

Karolinska Hospital, and Lagerlöf was probably not there. He was disappointed when I reported my main interest. He had a collaborator in his department, Stig Arne Johansson, who had passed his thesis about the importance of platelets in cardiovascular diseases. I guess Lagerlöf wanted me to join him in his team.

Although I didn't want to participate in the project that was being run by the head of the department, I still secured a position as a resident in the Department of Medicine. Lagerlöf was an understanding and good-hearted person. Although I became attached to Reizenstein's group, I worked in Lagerlöf's private ward during my first six months in 1967, but my research continued to focus on hematology.

After five years of full-time experimental research, my clinical skills had declined. However, it did not take very long until I felt that my clinical education in Lund with teachers like Inge Edler, Arne Gustafsson and Åke Nordén gave me something to build on. Furthermore, during my time as a theoretical doctor I had seen and treated patients when I participated in the emergency service in Stockholm City at nights and weekends.

I was allowed to combine my clinical service at the Department of Medicine with research at my laboratory at the Cell Research Institute, which was located just on the other site of Solna Street, which separated the Karolinska Institutet from the Karolinska Hospital. I obtained my clinical material, mainly blood and bone marrow, from the Hospital and was able to use it immediately for my studies, helped by one and, later, two technicians. My studies were translational clinical studies and eventually they could be included in the concept of personalized clinical medicine.

After my second term in the USA from 1968–1969, I decided to change my research direction.

Firstly, I decided to switch from microspectrophotometry to chromosome analysis, as my goal was to define the importance of chromosomal aberrations in hematologic malignancies. The discovery of the banding method by Torbjörn Caspersson and Lore Zech had enormous potential and we were ahead of other research groups. My technicians had been trained by Zech and I also started to collaborate with her.

Secondly, I decided to devote myself to randomized clinical trials and start with a new approach to acute myeloblastic leukemia. Farber had started using new drugs, like vincristine and cytosine arabinoside relatively late, because he believed that methotrexate was the right drug for acute leukemia. However, when I visited Jim Holland at the Roswell Park Memorial Institute in Buffalo, New York, he was at the forefront of randomized studies to compare new drugs. He started the first clinical trial in acute leukemia while he was already at the National Cancer Institute (NCI) in 1953, but he moved to Roswell Park the following year while the study was still running. It was continued by the new Head of Oncology at the NCI, Gordon Zubrod, who was accompanied by Emile (Tom) Frei (Chapter 23). Frei now started to design a protocol for acute leukemia involving the NCI, Roswell Park and the Children's Hospital in Buffalo. This Group became known as the Acute Leukemia Group B and was later renamed as the Cancer and Leukemia Group B. It was the master model for multicenter collaborating groups for clinical cancer trials that needed large numbers of patients.

I started working with my friend from the Cell Research Institute, Dick Killander, who like me had returned to clinical medicine. I designed a study that compared cyclophosphamide plus cytosine arabinoside (ARA-C) plus prednisolone, with or without the addition of l-asparaginase for treating acute leukemia in adults. L-asparaginase had been shown to be efficient in treating acute lymphoblastic leukemia in children and now we decided to try it in adults. However, we needed many more patients than those we could enroll at the Karolinska Hospital. I therefore managed to bring together the responsible hematologists from Karolinska with four other academic hospitals: the South Hospital and Serafimer Hospital in Stockholm, the Academic Hospital in Uppsala and the Regional Hospital in Örebro (now the University Hospital), to form the Leukemia Group of Middle Sweden (LGMS) trial group. Killander performed several studies on l-asparaginase metabolism, as well as concentrations studies. Although l-asparaginase did not turn out to be a very good drug for acute leukemia in adults, it is still used in children. The results of the study were published in the prestigious scientific journal, *Cancer*, and everybody was happy[29]. It was the first time a randomized study had been performed in cancer patients in Sweden, and it had been blessed by our famous professor, Jan Waldenström (Chapter 18).

The LGMS had to be structured and I asked the Head of Medicine at the South Hospital, Lars Engstedt, if he would consider being the first chairman of the group, with myself as secretary. I would write the protocols and he only had to run our meetings and help to reach agreements within the group. The people involved were Peter Reizenstein and me from the Karolinska Hospital, Lars Engstedt, Jan Palmblad and Ann-Marie Udén from the South Hospital, Göran Holm from the Serafimer Hospital, Andreas Killander (Dick Killander's brother) and Bengt Simonsson from Uppsala and Bengt Wadman from Örebro Hospital. Other clinicians from these hospitals could be brought in by the lead clinicians at the respective hospitals. Scientific journals now had to accept larger numbers of authors on scientific papers and there were 15 co-authors on the l-asparaginase trial.

The LGMS was not just important for running studies, it was also used to bring ideas to the table and as a learning group. We followed what was ongoing in the USA and Europe and this provided useful input. Over the years, I think that the two most interesting projects were based on ideas from the Nobel Laureate, Christian de Duve from Louvain, Belgium, and someone who many people thought should have been a Nobel Laureate, Georges Mathé from Paris.

26 Georges Mathé and Immunotherapy of Cancer

The controversial hematologist and cancer scientist Georges Mathé had used the BCG (Bacillus Calmette-Guérin) vaccine against tuberculosis to treat children with ALL[59]. He had published a study in 1969 that had compared the outcomes for children with ALL who had received conventional chemotherapy, with or without subsequent BCG treatment. My boss Peter Reizenstein was very interested in the approach and thought that this could be something that the LGMS could look at. I contacted Mathé and was invited to study the journals of the children he had treated. This was an opportunity I did not want to miss, so I went to Paris.

Mathé (1922–2010)[60] was a French hematologist and cancer researcher who graduated in Paris. He spent some time at the Sloan Kettering Institute of Cancer Research in New York City and then joined the famous hematologist Jean Bernhard at St Louis Hospital in Paris. Mathé soon outshone his boss and moved to Villejuif outside Paris in 1961. There he became the Head of the Department of Hematology at the Gustave Roussy Institute and built the Institut de Cancérologie et d'Immunogénétique.

In the early 1950s, Mathé had tried to infuse bone marrow cells into animals that had received deadly irradiation. He claimed it was successful, but he also induced a disease that he called secondary disease. This was later called graft versus host disease

(GVHD). Mathé was probably the first researcher to describe this important disease that hampered successful allogeneic stem cell transplants.

In 1958, Mathé used the knowledge gained from the experimental transfer of bone marrow to animals in an attempt to save six Yugoslavian workers who had been exposed to high-dose irradiation from a nuclear plant accident[60,61]. One of the workers died before he got the bone marrow and one received very low dose of irradiation and a transplant was not felt to be useful. Thus, only four workers received the bone marrow, which had been donated by volunteers. They all survived and, furthermore, it was possible to show that the donated bone marrow gave rise to the production of blood cells. Although the bone marrow transplant might have helped the workers to survive, later investigations showed that none of them had persistent transplanted bone marrow cells[62]. All returned to their own original bone marrow and Mathé did not manage to prove that bone marrow transplants could be a permanent cure for bone marrow failure.

However, Mathé continued his trials with bone marrow transplants and, in 1963, he managed to cure the first patient with acute leukemia in the world[63]. The donated bone marrow had taken over the production of the patient's blood cells and Mathé considered that the disappearance of the leukemic cells was partly due to the immunological effect of the donor bone marrow.

Mathé's belief that immunological mechanisms could be used to treat malignancies, in particularly leukemia, encouraged him design a project for the immunological treatment of children with ALL. Based on experimental data, 30 children with ALL received BCG, which was an immune stimulant used to vaccinate against tuberculosis. They also received irradiated leukemic cells that had been donated by other patients after treatment with conventional chemotherapy. Mathé claimed that he had randomized 10 children to be treated with just chemotherapy and 20 with chemotherapy followed by a BCG, with or without leukemic cells. The results of the study were published in the *Lancet*[59]. Mathé claimed that all 10 of the patients who had not received immunotherapy had short remissions of less than 130 days. In contrast, eight of the 20 who were treated with immunotherapy were still in remission 295 to 1150 days after the start of their treatment.

It was now 1971 and I was going to study the patients' original medical records. Mathé understood that I was interested, but was skeptical about the results. But when I arrived, I was given full access to the patient records. I worked hard for about a week but could find nothing wrong with the results. The patients who had received immunotherapy had the best outcomes, as claimed in the published report.

Mathé was an extraordinary person, who was overflowing with initiatives and activity. During my visit I followed him like a shadow when he held his outpatient clinics. He made the most of the necessary investigations while the patient was still there. He took bone marrow samples by puncturing the sternal bone, prepared them on glass slides and had them stained immediately for him to analyze the bone marrow cells through the microscope within minutes. Where I worked it usually took days before you had a written reply from the cytology laboratory, telling you if the patient was in remission or if their leukemia had recurred.

Mathé performed most of the processes himself. If he had a cancer patient that needed an X-ray, the X-ray pictures were ready to be analyzed while the patient was still in the room. Mathé analyzed the pictures himself and decided on the spot about treatment or additional necessary investigations. No time was lost waiting for a written opinion by an X-ray specialist.

Despite my youth and the fact that I was still a resident, Mathé treated me as if I was an important scientist from abroad. I felt like a king!

Mathé had a joint lunch meeting with his group of physicians and scientists every day. About 40 people gathered around him. Foreign guests frequently participated, either as visitors or lecturers. During my visit I was the guest of the day and sat next to Mathé. After the lunch he was often interviewed by journalists.

My visit did not result in any formal collaboration with LGMS. However, Reizenstein was impressed by my report and started a prospective study using immunotherapy that was copied from Mathé's model. Our study was on adults with acute myeloblastic leukemia, not children. There were other differences as well. We used the patient's own (autologous) irradiated leukemic cells for immunization instead of the cells from voluntary donors (allogeneic) that Mathé used. After a few years, there seemed to be an additional effect from the immunotherapy.

During that period in 1977, I received another invitation from Mathé, and this time it was to present our preliminary results. When I arrived at Villejuif, I was met by large posters *"Le Docteur Gösta Gahrton (Karolinska Institutet, Huddinge, Suède) donnera, Lundi, 4 Avril, 1977, á 13 heures, au Paedagogium de l'Institute de Cancérologie et d'Immunogénétique, Hopital Paul-Brousse, un séminaire sur Chimio-Immunothérapie des leucémies aigues myeloides"*.

This was typical of Mathé. Everyone he invited to visit him was important and treated with dignity. My presentation was appreciated, and the discussion was extensive, although the results were very preliminary. A later follow-up study was an anticlimax. We could not see any advantage of the immunotherapy and the study was stopped prematurely.

However, in 1977, I was somewhat optimistic when I was lecturing at one of the most important institutions in Europe and presenting facts in favor of immunotherapy. Mathé had invited me to have dinner with him at the prestigious Automobile Club at Place de la Concorde. He was, of course a member, and the club was one of his favorite places for dinner. It was just him and me. We started the conversation in French, but soon I realized that I did not meet my own expectations. My French was much poorer than his English and we continued in English, although it was alien for both of us.

Mathé was a controversial person in the scientific community and his lectures were frequently provocative. Maintenance therapy meant that patients with leukemia, who had been treated intensively and were in remission, were then treated continuously or at regular intervals. The drug companies loved maintenance therapy as their drug consumption increased dramatically. Mathé did not believe in maintenance therapy and thought that the documentation for its efficacy was poor. During his excellent lectures he frequently claimed that: *"maintenance therapy maintains the disease"*. The value of maintenance therapy is still debated, but there is no doubt that it is effective and prolongs survival for some malignancies. However, its value may be overestimated for others.

Many important researchers have claimed that Mathé should have been awarded the Nobel Prize in 1990, together with Donnall Thomas, because he was the first to describe what he called secondary disease following bone marrow transplants. This was the immune reaction exerted by the graft against the patient and was later named GVHD. Mathé, in parallel with Donnall Thomas, performed the first bone marrow transplants in humans. In Mathé's case this was in 1958 and the patients were Yugoslavian workers with bone marrow failure due to exposure to irradiation. He also cured the first patients with acute leukemia with bone marrow transplants in 1963. Mathé's importance in how immunotherapy was advanced in cancer patients is not disputable. He created the concept of adoptive immunotherapy but did not manage to prove its importance. The breakthrough in that field came much later. Today, numerous registered drugs provide antibodies that have high efficacy against cancer. Part of the effect of bone marrow transplants is the immune effect that donor cells have on the patient's cancer cells. Today, bone marrow is usually substituted for hematopoietic stem cells recovered from peripheral blood. These are as effective for engraftment and for the production of immunoactive cells, e.g., so-called T-cells.

Although nominated once in 1960, Mathé did not receive the Nobel Prize, despite all these important contributions, but he did receive numerous other awards and he became a Commandeur de la Légion d'honneur, which is the most important honor in France. The reasons why he was not awarded the Nobel Prize together with Murray and Thomas in 1990 (Chapter 30) cannot be revealed until 2040, when the investigations by the Nobel Committee members and the discussions in the Nobel Committee can be opened.

Mathé was active until he died in 2010 at 88 years of age in the hospital where he treated his leukemia patients, l'Hôpital Paul-Brousse in Villejuif.

27 To the Huddinge Hospital

Huddinge Hospital, which is now the Karolinska University Hospital, Huddinge, opened in 1972 and it is located about 20 kilometers south of the Karolinska Institutet in Stockholm. It immediately became more of a competitor than a complement to the old Karolinska Hospital, located next to the Karolinska Institutet. Many of the new professors who were appointed came from the Karolinska Hospital. Young doctors could enhance their career by moving 20 kilometers from north to south.

In 1972, I was asked by the newly appointed Professor of Medicine and Head of the Department of Medicine, Gunnar Birke, to apply for one of the associate professor positions, namely a clinical teacher at the Karolinska Institutet. This would be combined with the position as Head of Hematology, a division within the Department of Medicine at the Huddinge Hospital. I hesitated because I had just secured a full-time clinical research position at the Karolinska Institutet that came without any clinical obligations.

In 1971, when I visited Mathé and saw his investment in immunological treatment methods and bone marrow transplants, I was convinced that this was the way to go. The next year I went back to Boston for a couple of weeks to finish up some of my ongoing projects at the CCRF. I had the chance to visit Seattle, the Mecca of bone marrow transplants, and Donnall (Don) Thomas at the Fred Hutchinson Cancer Institute. I made contact with

Thomas in advance, and he invited me to spend a couple of days with him and his team. I was impressed by what they had done and were doing. Bone marrow transplants had to be the way to go to cure leukemia and other disorders of the bone marrow, like aplastic anemia. I learned what was required and made up my mind to start a bone marrow transplant program.

I understood that the Karolinska Hospital was not the place for such a program. Firstly, I worked under the Head of Hematology, and our relationship was tense. Secondly, the organ transplant unit was going to be established under surgery at the Huddinge Hospital and a transplant immunology laboratory, led by Professor Erna Möller, was going to be established at the Hospital.

Eventually, I decided to apply for the position at the Karolinska Institutet and the Department of Medicine at the Huddinge Hospital. I got the position and started my new job on 1 January 1974.

Inspired by the developments in the USA, and my meetings with the pioneers in hematological malignancy treatments, Donnall Thomas, Tom Frei, Jim Holland and others, I was eager to develop a unit that followed the direction that I had seen during my visits to them. However, as head of a division, and not of a department, I did not have a budget and depended on the Professor of Medicine, Gunnar Birke (1920–2004), who was also Head of the Department of Medicine. This department was huge and included three other divisions, in addition to hematology, namely cardiology, metabolic disorders and allergology/lung disorders. Birke, like most of us, had come from a head position at the Karolinska Hospital. He had been Chief of the King Gustaf V's Research Institute, which belonged to the Karolinska Hospital. He had formed collaborative groups at this Institute that were focused on metabolic disorders and endocrinology. Birke was particularly interested in the metabolic changes that occurred in association with severe burns. He was educated in the school launched by the first woman Professor of Medicine in Sweden, Nanna Swartz (1890–1986). She worked with the pharmaceutical drug company Pharmacia AB to discover and develop the first effective drug against ulcerous colitis. That drug, Salazopyrin (sulfasalazine) is still used. Birke had a reputation for being tough and outspoken, but honest. He was better known as a good organizer and friend of the most important local politicians, who were responsible for health care in the Stockholm region, than for great scientific successes. He was an old soccer and ice-hockey player in the greater Stockholm area, and he had friends in every corner.

Birke had taken part in planning the Huddinge Hospital at a relatively early stage and was appointed Head of Medicine from its inception. He was a good friend of the first Hospital Director, Nils Otto Witting, who was a non-medical administrator, but had a good reputation for his collaborative skills. He had appointed Birke as the Chief Physician at the hospital, in addition to his position as Head of Medicine.

Despite holding all these powerful positions, Birke was mainly unknown to the media, and he did not seem too bothered about it. He obtained results directly by negotiation with politicians and did not seem to need the media.

After my first meeting with Birke, I felt that I could trust him. He expected me to build a strong hematology division. He claimed that he did not know anything about hematology. My previous boss, Peter Reizenstein, had warned me that Birke had not worked in clinics for many years and I should not refer to him when I had questions about patients. This seemed to be true, but

I was not concerned about this because the hematology clinic was my own baby. I only wanted financial resources for a potentially expensive division.

The relationship between me and my boss was good most of the time, although we were very different personalities. I started to introduce combination chemotherapy for acute leukemia and built on the programs I had already started at the Leukemia Group of Middle Sweden, where I was initially the Secretary, but later the Chairman (Chapter 25). Birke was very positive in the beginning, but soon realized that my division was much more expensive than the other divisions. He asked me why that was the case. I had to explain that the drugs for leukemia treatment were more expensive than most of the drugs used by the other divisions. However, it was worth the cost, because now we were able to cure a significant number of patients. My division slowly started to show both clinical and scientific results and these were reported in the international scientific press. Birke agreed to let me expand my division, but repeatedly complained about the costs.

Birke was not a Nobel Prize candidate, but he was an important old-style leader. Although his way of leading a department of medicine would seem old fashioned and impossible today, I learned a lot from him.

Birke did not like formal meetings or long discussions. He was both Head of the Institution of Medicine, a section of Karolinska Institutet, and of the Department of Medicine at the hospital with patient responsibilities. So was I when I much later occupied the same posts. The Institution of Medicine should have had a formally elected board. Birke tried to make sure that it did not meet. He took all decisions himself anyway. However, one day there was a problem and he sent out his secretary, Anita Johansson, to gather the board. I had been there for a year, and this was the first time I realized that I was a member of the board. The problem that Birke wanted to discuss concerned the Head of the Department of Rheumatology, which did not belong to the Department of Medicine, but was part of the Karolinska Institutet Institution of Medicine. She had denied more than two students access to her ward, and she had also asked these young students to perform knee joint punctures on patients. There were other issues as well. Birke wanted to relocate her, but he did not have the authority to do this. Of course, the board members came to his aid, and she was relocated after some time. As far as I remember this was the only board meeting that was held when I was a division head.

The hospital had a ward for night admissions of non-surgical patients from the emergency department. Every morning there were about 20 patients that had to be distributed to ordinary wards, usually within the Department of Medicine. Birke led his rounds at 8am every morning to empty this ward. It was his way of making sure he had an overview of the admissions to his department. Birke also went on the rounds of one of his divisions after his emergency admission ward round. He visited a different division each day and came to my division once a week. Birke just needed a report, and he did not interfere with the patient treatment plan. These visits took about half an hour to one hour at the most. It was his way of seeing what we were doing. Then we carried out our own rounds to plan how to treat the patients.

Birke had his own outpatient clinic. I was not involved in it for many years. It was mainly patients that he had seen for a long time and brought with him to the Huddinge Hospital from the Karolinska Hospital. He did not see new ones. If there were problems with a patient, he just admitted them to a specialist ward for investigation and treatment. When he went on vacation, first in line as his deputy was the Head of the Metabolic Ward, a specialist in diabetes called Jan Östman. Second in line was the Head of Cardiology, Erik Orinius, who was also a very competent physician. Third in line was Dieter Lockner, who was responsible for educating students and was also an experienced hematologist with a focus on coagulation disorders. We collaborated very well, and he was as well an able member of the Leukemia Group of Middle Sweden.

I was last on the list. Obviously, Birke trusted his more established colleagues more than me. Another reason may have been that the order had already been established before I arrived at the Huddinge Hospital a year later. It is also possible that he felt that the patients that I specialized in were rarely admitted from the emergency department.

I only remember one time when I was deputy head and responsible for the whole department. It was for a few weeks in the summer when all the others were on vacation. I also had to take care of Birke's outpatient clinic. To my great amazement, his secretary brought me a box of cards, that were as small as post cards. The patient's name was hand-written on the card and there were about one to three lines for each patient. I do not remember the number of patients that I saw. I talked with them, listened to their hearts, took their blood pressure and checked that the medication they were on was OK. They all felt very well and were very satisfied with their treatment and there was no reason to change it, because they were going to see their professor very soon. I might have exaggerated the lack of need for interventions, but it was not a hard job. Most of the patients had previously been admitted for extensive investigations, usually to the metabolic ward and sometimes to the cardiology ward. They had received excellent care. Birke handled it his way. I wrote on his card the same as he had done. One line noting the same medication.

Birke was a heavy smoker and he had at least 40 unfiltered Camel cigarettes a day. This was not without its problems, for him and his surroundings. Every morning all the doctors from the Department of Medicine gathered in the X-ray department so that a radiologist could present the X-ray pictures from the previous 24 hours. This meeting, in the demonstration room, was an old tradition and a way for the boss to see his doctors every day. Birke sat in the middle in front of the X-ray pictures and started his third or fourth cigarette of the day. The crowded demonstration room was cloaked by an impervious fog.

Towards the end of Birke's reign, a no smoking rule was introduced at the hospital. A big no smoking sign was posted on the door to the demonstration room. Birke stopped, looked at the sign in stunned silence, then entered, sat down and started and finished his cigarette as if nothing had happened.

Birke had an ashtray on the top of the picture cabinet that he used to grab every morning when he entered the demonstration room. The radiologists decided that they had to stop Birke smoking during the demonstrations, so they filled the ashtray with water. The next morning Birke grabbed the ashtray as usual and was covered in water. He muttered something, sat down, and started to smoke as usual. However, the radiologists did not give up. The next morning, they glued the ashtray to the cabinet in the usual place. When Birke grabbed it, it did not give away and cut his hand, making it bleed slightly. Birke sat down. No cigarette. This was the end of Birke's smoking during the X-ray demonstration rounds.

Although I knew that I was not Birke's favorite, I felt he supported me developing the Hematology Division. For some time, he did not interfere. However, I had not yet revealed my plan to develop bone marrow transplants. I was hesitant to start it only in my own division. I had to find another way and that meant I had to find a partner.

28 Bone Marrow Transplants at the Huddinge Hospital

After my visits to Paris and Seattle, I understood that bone marrow transplants were not easy. You needed a hematology laboratory, a transplant immunology laboratory and a blood transfusion unit. I had slowly started to build a hematology research laboratory in my division. The hospital had an excellent laboratory for all kinds of routine hematology work. A blood transfusion unit was available and the transplant immunology laboratory that had been established at the Huddinge Hospital when it opened, was the best in the country. The reason for that was that it had been decided that all the organ transplants in the county of Stockholm should be performed at the Huddinge Hospital when it was being planned. The Head of Surgery, Professor Curt Franksson (1916–2007), had been recruited from the old, now discontinued, Serafimer Hospital, which was the oldest hospital associated with the Karolinska Institutet. He had earlier spent two years in the Department of Urology at the University of Washington in Seattle, where he had learnt about renal transplants. In 1964, while he was still at the Serafimer Hospital, he performed the first renal transplant in Sweden. When he moved to the Huddinge Hospital, he continued the transplant program and managed to convince his previous apprentice, Carl Gustav Groth (1933–2014), to come back to Sweden from the University of Colorado in Denver. In 1963, Franksson had met the most celebrated transplant surgeon in USA,

Thomas Starzl (1926–2017), and arranged for Groth to spend a year in Denver. Groth started as an associate to Starzl in 1965 and was obviously highly appreciated by the famous surgeon. After a short spell back in Sweden, Groth became Starzl's closest collaborator in Denver in 1970.

Thomas Starzl was born in 1926 in Le Mars, Iowa, and he was the son of a publisher and science fiction writer. He embarked on his career as a surgeon after his studies at Northwestern University Medical School in Chicago and an internship at Johns Hopkins Hospital in Baltimore. He became interested in the idea of liver replacements and started experimental studies on dogs after he moved to the University of Miami Medical School and the Jackson Memorial Hospital. He returned to Chicago and Northwestern in 1958 and continued his experimental dog liver transplants. In 1962, Starzl was recruited by the University of Colorado School of Medicine in Denver as an associate professor, and he was promoted to Professor of Surgery in 1964. By that time, he had already built a renal transplant program, inspired by the successful transplants performed at the Peter Bent Brigham Hospital by Joseph Murray (Chapter 30) and his team. However, liver transplants were his main interest, and, after a few unsuccessful attempts in 1962 and 1963, he managed to successfully perform the world's first liver transplant in 1967. He had learned how to use the new drug azathioprine, which was invented by the later Nobel Prize winners George Hitchings and Trudy Elion and marketed under the brand name Imuran. He combined it with prednisone to suppress the immunological response and thereby prevent rejection. The University of Colorado, and its two associated hospitals, Colorado General Hospital and Veterans Administration Hospital, became world famous. Starzl, who later became Head of Surgery in 1972, was the star. Patients arrived from everywhere.

Despite his enormous success in Denver, Starzl left in 1981 to take up the post as head of the surgery and transplantation program at the University of Pittsburgh School of Medicine, where he enjoyed similar success. The liver transplant program expanded at three hospitals that were associated with the medical school: the Presbyterian University Hospital, the Children's Hospital of Pittsburgh and Oakland Veterans Affairs Medical Center. They eventually joined forces to become the University of Pittsburgh Transplantation Institute, which was renamed the Thomas E Starzl Transplantation Institute in 1996. Starzl was now the head of the largest transplant center in the world, and he improved the techniques and used new drugs, like cyclosporin and tacrolimus, to prevent graft rejections.

Although he was head of the center until 1998, Starzl decided to end his career as a transplant surgeon in 1990, when he was 64 years old. He said he felt tired and when he wrote *The Puzzle People: Memoirs of a Transplant Surgeon*[64], he admitted that every transplant he had carried out during his career had caused him psychological stress. He decided to devote himself to experimental transplants and focused on such areas as xenotransplantation, which involves transplants between different species, and multi-organ transplants. However, his research did not provide any new real breakthroughs.

Starzl received many awards, including the Lasker-DeBakey award, and he was sometimes a runner-up for the Nobel Prize. History will tell if he was considered worthy of the Nobel Prize for performing the first successful liver transplant. He did not receive it in 1990, when his forerunner in renal transplants, Joseph Murray, received it with Donnall Thomas (Chapter 30).

My friend, the young transplant surgeon Carl Gustav Groth, met Starzl in Stockholm in 1965 when he arrived with his wife for a series of conference lectures. Starzl had been invited by Franksson, but Groth was assigned to be their host during the visit. Two years earlier Franksson had recommended Groth to Starzl and he was probably happy to have the chance to meet the person who later joined him in Denver.

Groth (1933–2014) was born in Helsinki and was six years old when Finland was invaded by the Russians in 1939, at the beginning of World War Two. In 1944, his family emigrated to Sweden, like many other Finnish families, and Groth went to Swedish schools. He chose to pursue his further education in medicine and graduated from the Karolinska Institutet. He soon joined Franksson at the Department of Surgery at the Serafimer Hospital and started a PhD project, which concerned the impact that trauma had on blood flow and erythrocyte aggregation.

When Groth met Starzl for the first time in 1965, he had not yet passed his thesis, and that was one reason he hadn't moved to Denver, which Franksson had arranged during his meeting with Starzl in 1963. However, he joined Starzl in the fall of 1966, just in time to be part of the great transplant surgeon's second attempt to perform liver transplants in humans. When he first moved to Denver, Groth mainly dealt with experimental transplants in dogs, but it seems that he also played an active part in early liver transplants in humans. One of them was performed in 1967 and was said to be the first successful one worldwide. Groth returned to Sweden in 1968, as planned, but Starzl invited him back to Denver in 1971 and he became his closest associate. Groth was highly appreciated by Starzl, but Groth returned home again in 1972 to rejoin Franksson and followed him to the Huddinge Hospital when the Serafimer Hospital was closed down in 1973. Groth worked under Franksson at the Department of Surgery, but headed up transplant surgery.

I decided that I needed to team up with Groth at the Huddinge to start a bone marrow transplant program.

Up to that point I had only known Groth through other colleagues. One afternoon in 1975 I met Groth in the hospital elevator. I asked him: *"Would you be interested in starting a bone marrow transplantation program together with us at the hematology division? Bone marrow transplantation is not surgery, but the immunological problems are, in many respects, the same or like those of organ transplantation."* His immediate and positive response was the start of a long and productive collaboration.

We discussed how it would work in practice. I had to agree not to use the beds in the hematology division for bone marrow transplant patients during the transplant procedure and the immediate posttransplant period. This would avoid all discussions with my head, Birke, about costs. The work-ups before the transplant, and the posttransplant care and follow-up of the patients, would be carried out in the hematology division. The handling of the donor would also be the responsibility of the hematology division. The bone marrow would be harvested in the operating theater by one doctor from the hematology division and one from the transplant division. One of my research technicians would be in the operating theater to make sure that the donor marrow contained enough cells. An interesting point in the deal was that neither of us was a head of department with budget responsibility. However, Groth had been recruited as head of the transplant program and was less restricted by his boss with regard to costs than I was. Also, at that time transplants and surgery were, in general, much more costly than internal medicine, which meant that the cost for the new transplant cases at the Department of Surgery was not a problem for the administration.

If I decided to keep the bone marrow transplant patients in the hematology division, I would have had to fight my corner with Birke. He was already complaining about the rising costs of the expensive drugs that I used for the intensive treatment of other patients with hematological malignancies.

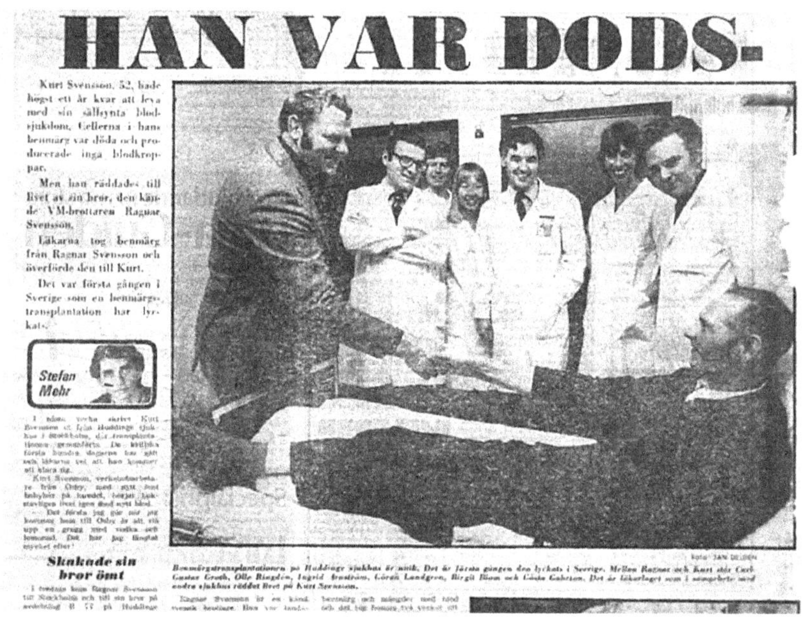

In 1977, we performed the first successful bone marrow transplant in Sweden. The patient, Kurt Svensson, had severe aplastic anemia that was cured with marrow from his brother Ragnar. This picture shows Ragnar congratulating Kurt as the transplant team looked on. From left to right: The donor brother Ragnar Svensson, Carl Gustav Groth, Dr Olle Ringdén, nurse Ingrid, Dr Göran Lundgren, nurse Birgit Blom, the author Gösta Gahrton and the patient Kurt Svensson.

The brothers were happy to talk with the press and this coverage reported that Kurt had been sentenced to death because of his medical condition but was saved by his brother.

Erna Möller was born in 1940. She was an MD and PhD and was educated by George and Eva Klein at the Department of Tumor Biology at the Karolinska Institutet, where she had passed her thesis. Möller had joined Franksson in 1964 before his transfer to Huddinge and had built a transplant immunology laboratory at the Serafimer Hospital. She and her laboratory staff moved together with Franksson to Huddinge where she build a new advanced transplant immunology laboratory.

Möller's sister Ulla Persson was also an MD and was extremely experienced in tissue typing, which had been considered important at the beginning of the organ transplant era. It turned out that this process was much more important and crucial for bone marrow transplantation. Persson became responsible for collaborating with us and for human leukocyte antigen (HLA) typing.

I thought that we were ready to start in the fall of 1975. We agreed to perform the first transplant in a patient with aplastic anemia that had not responded to any other treatment. Aplastic anemia was a deadly disease because the bone marrow could not produce normal blood cells. Eventually, the patients became dependent on blood transfusions. But it didn't just affect red blood cells. Eventually platelets and leukocytes were not produced in sufficient numbers and the patients died of anemia, bleeding and/or infections.

Our first patient was a 17-year-old boy that had received more than 100 blood transfusions. He was in a poor condition and the chance of saving him with the drugs and transfusions that were available at that time was zero. After we had informed his parents about the situation, we discussed the new bone marrow transplant method that had proved successful for a few patients with aplastic anemia in other parts of the world. We offered to try it. His parents agreed and then so did he. He had an HLA-matched sibling who was ready to serve as a donor. After we had carried out all the necessary work-up, we performed the transplant on 12 November 1975. Groth and I drew the marrow from the donor by introducing a needle with a syringe into the iliac crest and drawing the marrow out using repeated punctures. About one liter of marrow mixed with blood was infused into one of the patient's veins. Groth's close collaborator Göran Lundgren was at the patient's side and oversaw the infusion.

After a few days there were signs that the patient was producing red and white blood cells, but unfortunately, we soon realized that the graft had been rejected. This was probably because the patient had undergone so many previous transfusions that his body had induced antibodies that had caused the rejection. The only chance of saving the boy's life was to try a new transplant. Although there was only a small chance of success, his sibling allowed us to try again. So, we did. We tried to increase the number of cells compared to the number infused at the first transplant. Amazingly, it worked. This time there was no rejection. The graft was perfect, there was no graft versus host reaction and the boy was ready to leave the hospital after a couple of months. However, just as we planned to release him, he got a pneumonia due to the cytomegalovirus. This was the most serious one of its kind and was not treatable at this time. The patient died a few months later.

The tragic outcome of this first transplant at the Huddinge Hospital made us revisit our strategy. We had to find another patient with a life-threatening aplastic anemia, but one who was in a better condition than our first patient and had not received as many blood transfusions. The risk of complications would then probably be reduced, and the chances of success would be better. It took nearly two years until we found the right patient in 1977.

His name was Kurt Svensson, he was 52 years old, and he had severe aplastic anemia that did not respond to the normal hormone treatment used for the disease at this time. He had received a limited number of transfusions and was physically well.

Kurt had several brothers and two were international wrestling champions. The most famous one was Pelle Svensson, who had been a world champion, but the most suitable one, according to the HLA patterns, was Ragnar Svensson. Ragnar was therefore used as donor, heavily supported by his more famous brother when they both appeared repeatedly in the media after the transplant. The transplant took perfectly, and the family was happy to take part in media coverage about the successful transplant (Chapter 52). Kurt had limited acute graft versus host disease at first, but then developed a chronic form that mainly affected his skin and caused him some trouble. The red blood cells, leukocytes and platelets produced by the transplanted marrow were soon normal, both in terms of numbers and function. Kurt lived happily and in a good condition, except for some trouble with the chronic graft versus host disease, for more than 15 years after the transplant. Unfortunately, he eventually died, partly due to this complication.

The bone marrow transplant program at Huddinge Hospital was now running. I worked hard to fine-tune the organization, mainly based on the agreement I had made with Groth. A patient that was considered a transplant candidate was admitted to the Division of Hematology. A search for a family donor started. If the patient only had one sibling, then there was a 25% chance that he or she would be HLA compatible. The chances increased if there were more siblings. During the early years we only used sibling donors, which was a severe limitation. We frequently found that no compatible siblings were available, which meant that the transplant could not be performed. As time passed, unrelated donors, found in international registries of HLA typed voluntary donors, were used (Chapter 42).

When all the necessary investigations had been performed and a suitable donor had been found, we were ready for the transplant. The patient was transferred to the transplant unit, where Groth was responsible for the patient. The donor stayed in the Division of Hematology. The unique situation now was that a physician from the Department of Medicine entered the operation theater and worked with a healthy donor on the operation table. It took some time for the nurses to fully accept this situation, probably because there was a transplant surgeon on the other side of the table. During the first 10–15 transplants Groth and myself drew the marrow, but then he obviously got tired of it and some of his residents took over. After all, he was a surgeon. After we had treated another 10–15 patients, I decided that my residents could do it as well and I let my closest collaborator in the transplant program, Berit Lönnqvist, assume this responsibility. We always drew the marrow from the iliac crest. My technician Nita Dahlberg took care of all the necessary cell counts, to ensure that enough marrow had been drawn. This was usually about one liter of marrow mixed with blood. It normally took about 3–4 hours to draw the marrow. When enough marrow had been drawn and collected in blood bags, it was immediately transferred to the patient. They were cared for by Göran Lundgren, who soon became the anchor in the bone marrow transplant unit. The technique was not technically difficult, as the marrow was infused for 20–30 minutes, just like a blood transfusion. In some cases, this happened after we had withdrawn some blood from the patient. No knives were used. The fluid balance was more important, and Lundgren was the expert.

Very soon, another surgeon became interested in bone marrow transplants and that was Olle Ringdén, who much later became the medical Head of the Centre for Allogeneic Stem Cell Transplantation (CAST). He eventually took over most of the work originally carried out by Lundgren.

Berit Lönnqvist was taking over more and more of the routines that I had run in the beginning, and eventually Per Ljungman teamed up with her (much later, when I had retired, he took over from me as Head of the Department of Hematology and even later as Head of CAST when Ringdén retired).

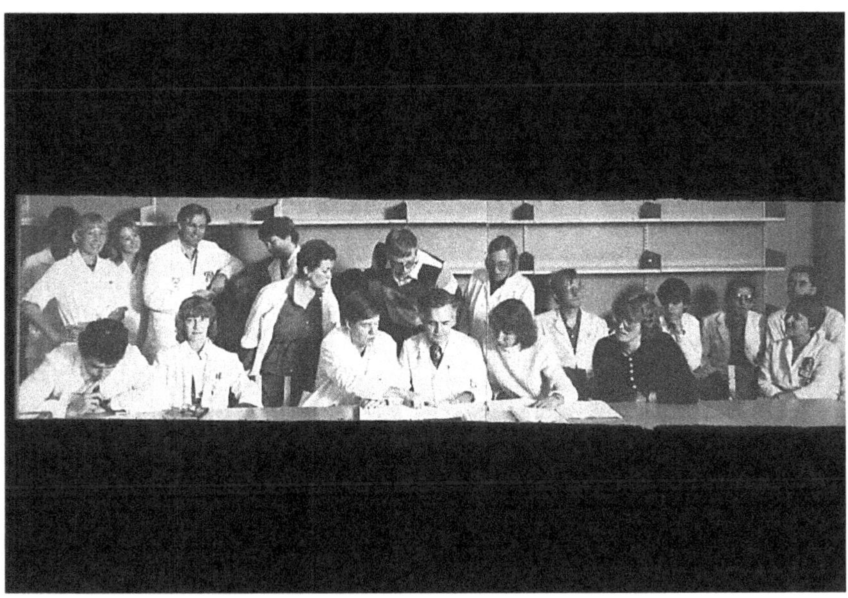

The transplant team met once a week, with all involved specialties and laboratory representatives, for updates and planning. Standing in the middle are from left to right: Berit Lönnqvist, Per Ljungman and Else Svensson. Sitting in the middle from left to right are Olle Ringdén, the author Gösta Gahrton and head nurse Birgit Blom.

After two to three weeks in the transplant division the patient was usually moved to the Division of Hematology and the responsibility was ours. If the patient had to be readmitted to the hospital due to complications, or for a second transplant after they were discharged, the Division of Hematology was responsible.

It did not take long until we were well known both nationally and internationally for our transplant program. We started to have a waiting list. In the beginning I had one secretary, who together with Lönnqvist and later Ljungman, were responsible for the waiting list, which contained the necessary information about the patients and if there were any potential donors. Every week we had a conference with representatives from both units and people from the laboratories. A short report was presented about patients that had been admitted to any of the divisions. Then Lönnqvist, and later Ljungman, reported how the waiting list looked and decisions were taken about the schedule for future transplants. In the beginning I chaired these meetings, together with Groth, but it did not take long before he gave it up. His focus turned to liver transplants and his team performed the first one in Sweden in 1984. So I chaired the bone marrow and stem cell transplant meetings for more than 20 years from 1975 to the end of 1997, when I retired from all my lead positions at the hospital.

Very soon Per Bolme from the Department of Pediatrics became an important collaborator. Many patients were children, and it was logical to have the same arrangements between the Department of Pediatrics and the Division of Transplantation as we had. However, all potential transplant candidates were put on the same waiting list. The weekly conferences expanded to about 20 people, including representatives from the three clinical units, the transplant immunology unit and from other laboratories and research laboratories as necessary. The participants changed over the years, but I was in charge for most of the time and Lönnqvist, Ljungman, Ringdén, Bolme and Persson were present, together with nurses and other collaborators. The organization is almost the same today (2024), under the leadership of Professor Stefan Mielke, Head of CAST.

I was dependent on Birke, from the late 1970s until I succeeded him as Professor of Medicine at the Karolinska Institutet and Head of the Department of Medicine at Huddinge in 1985. He was not just my boss; he was also the Physician in Chief of the entire hospital. He worked in close collaboration with the Hospital Director Nils Otto Witting and later with his successor Lars-Åke Flood. Although his role was to give advice to the Hospital Director, his influence on what happened in the hospital was greater than it should have been. That is why I had not entirely succeeded in circumventing his power by teaming up with Groth. The cost of the whole bone marrow transplant program became an issue for the Hospital Director. I had to justify the cost by demonstrating the great success we had achieved in curing patients, not only with aplastic anemia, but also with acute leukemia and eventually chronic myelocytic leukemia. The strength was that I now had support of both Groth and from Bolme at the Department of Pediatrics. At the same time, Birke was disappointed with the location of the program. He said: *"Groth wants more resources for the bone marrow transplant program. Why is part of the bone marrow transplantation activity located in the surgery department? It is not surgery."* This time he was right, but he did not understand that he was the reason I had made the arrangement with Groth.

Birke arranged a meeting with the Hospital Director so that I could explain what the new development meant in terms of organization and cost. In turn, the Hospital Director had to explain the benefits of my work to the Stockholm County politicians and administrators who had to pay the bills with the taxpayers' money.

I defended both the costs and the organization. I also pointed out that the Division of Hematology was heavily underfinanced with regards to the new developments in diagnostic methods, new effective drugs and transplant techniques that could cure patients who would have previously died due to lack of effective treatment methods.

I had realized that the more departments I could get involved in the program the greater chances we would have of receiving adequate finance. Eventually national politicians, as well as those involved at the local Stockholm County level, reacted. I was called to a hearing with the Socialutskottet government committee, which was responsible for social welfare and health affairs in Sweden. Birke was not invited.

I provided an overview of the rapid developments that had taken place in the treatment of hematological malignancies and of the new bone marrow transplant treatment method. Then I pointed out that we were the first department in the country, and one of the first in Europe, to use this method to cure previously uncurable patients. I ended by concluding that this development was costly and heavily underfinanced. One of the members of the committee, Ulla Leissner, who was previously a Hospital Director at the university hospital in Lund, South Sweden, asked a relevant question: *"What do you do if you do not have the money for a transplant that you consider the only way to save a patient?"* I answered: *"I do it anyway"*. The interesting comment from her was: *"I am happy about that"*.

When I succeeded Birke in 1985, I continued for a while with this do it anyway policy, which was, of course, not sustainable. It led to an argument with the Hospital Director, Lars-Åke Flood, that almost cost me my head position. I solved the funding issue with the help of my associate head Olle Edhag, who I had made responsible for the departmental budgets. But it took many years until Flood and I eventually became friends again.

The main parts of the original organization that I shaped in the late 1970s still prevail, despite numerous hospital reorganizations. These have included new principles for cost counting, changes in transplant methods, such as using peripheral blood stem cells, unrelated donors, cord blood stem cells and, recently, so-called haploidentical donors. More than 3,000 patients had received stem cell transplant at Huddinge Hospital by 2023 and most of them have been cured of an otherwise uncurable disease.

29 Stem Cell Transplants — The Patient in the Center

Jan Waldenström (Chapter 18) always pointed out that it was a doctor's responsibility *"to help patients and not to harm them"* At first glance this seems obvious, but methods like bone marrow transplants showed that this goal could be difficult to reach. The earliest example was the discovery of cytotoxic drugs for cancer treatment. So-called high-dose treatment was shown to cure a fraction of the patients that could not be cured by other means. However, the toxicity was significant, and some patients died because of the treatment, instead of being cured. Patients that have deadly cancers are prepared to endure a lot of side effects without complaining if they know they will be cured. However, if there is a very high risk that the treatment will kill them, they may well abstain from treatment. Bone marrow transplants, or peripheral blood stem cell transplants, are perhaps the best example of such a dilemma. It is not possible to know if the transplant will be successful or if the patient will die from the transplant, often after severe suffering.

Many research attempts have tried to find so-called prognostic factors that can predict if a patient can be successfully transplanted or if the outcome will be poor. The problem is that these factors are very unreliable. It all boils down to statistics. If a prognostic factor indicates that there is a 50% chance of surviving with a bone marrow transplant it also means that there is also a 50% risk of not being cured or dying as a result of the procedure. A patient with a deadly cancer must be informed of the chances of a cure with a bone marrow transplant, and the risks, and then decide what to do. It is not an easy task. Most of the time the patient will ask their doctors for their opinion and advice. It can be a long discussion and Waldenström's view of not harming the patient may, at the end of the day, not come true in many cases. Some patients will die from severe complications, without having had any benefit from the attempted treatment. Thus, the information that is provided to the patient is crucial. At the end they need to make the decision themselves.

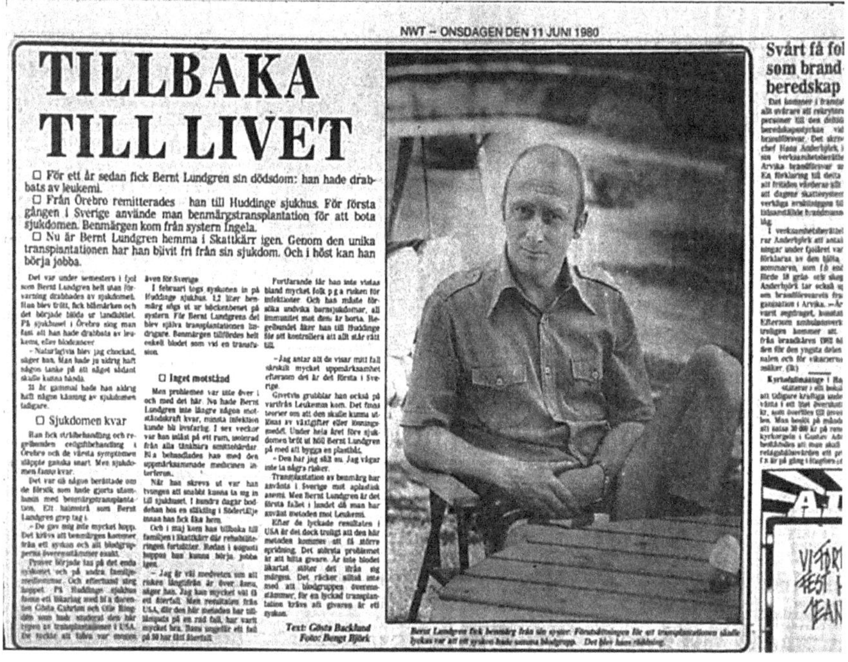

TILLBAKA TILL LIVET

□ För ett år sedan fick Bernt Lundgren sin dödsdom: han hade drabbats av leukemi.

□ Från Örebro remitterades han till Huddinge sjukhus. För första gången i Sverige använde man benmärgstransplantation för att bota sjukdomen. Benmärgen kom från systern Ingela.

□ Nu är Bernt Lundgren hemma i Skattkärr igen. Genom den unika transplantationen har han blivit fri från sin sjukdom. Och i höst kan han börja jobba.

Text: Gösta Bäcklund
Foto: Bengt Björk

In 1980, we performed the first successful bone marrow transplant on a patient with acute myeloblastic leukemia. In 2022, I talked with the patient who was then in good condition at 73 years of age, 42 years after the transplant. He had had no signs of the disease during that time and was obviously cured. He died from other causes in 2023. The headline in this news article, one year after the transplant, was "Back to life".

It is important that the patient's closest relatives take part in the discussion and understand the risks. My experience is that most of the time they understand that there are no promises that the procedure will be successful. If the patient does not survive, then the relatives understand that this was a possible outcome. If the attempt had not been made, the patient would have died anyway, although perhaps later. An attempt had been made to save the patient but unfortunately it had been unsuccessful.

All doctors that deal with similar types of difficult and risky treatments have experienced the contrary. When the patient dies, the doctor is accused by the relatives of having given the wrong advice or even of having killed the patient. It is almost as bad if the patient, having survived, must live with serious side effects due to the treatment. The doctor then can be accused of maltreatment.

CML is a malignant blood disorder that always led to death before we started to perform bone marrow transplants (Chapter 19). The median time from diagnosis to death was about three years. A cytotoxic drug called busulfan led to temporary remission, but occasionally patients could live for many years without symptoms and could then often work full time. I once had a patient who lived and was in an excellent condition for 15 years. Death was usually foreshadowed by signs in the bone marrow. The previous mature looking cells changed to immature so-called blast cells that resembled those seen in acute myeloblastic leukemia. This was called blast transformation of CML. The patients would be dead a few months later.

In 1977, Donnall Thomas and his coworkers in Seattle showed that 13% of patients who had relapsed after they had been treated for acute myeloblastic leukemia could be cured by a bone marrow transplant. This encouraged them to try to treat patients with CML during the blast phase. The results were very poor, but patients were occasionally cured. Therefore, attempts were made to treat

CML patients earlier, during the chronic phase. About 50% of the patients were cured, but the problem was that 30–40% of patients who could have lived for some years before blast transformation succumbed to transplant-related early deaths. Many patients who were still in the chronic phase wanted to take the chance, despite knowing the risks. Others preferred to wait until they showed signs of blast transformation, even though they knew that there was only a small chance that a transplant would be successful once they got to that stage.

A well-known colleague and friend of mine at the South Hospital in Stockholm had a patient, a 40-year-old man with CML, who had been in excellent condition with busulfan for many years. Then a check-up showed minor early signs of blast transformation. His only chance, although small, was a bone marrow transplant. I saw him at my outpatient clinic. I explained the risks and told him that there was a small chance of somewhat better than 10% that he would survive with a bone marrow transplant, as he was not yet displaying clinical symptoms of the coming blast transformation. He understood the situation and wanted to go ahead with the transplant. I wanted his closest relatives to be involved in our discussions, so that they could understand how serious the situation was. He refused to accept that advice. I tried to convince him that it was necessary for his wife to be prepared for the worst. He refused. My efforts were in vain. I asked myself whether I should perform the transplant. Eventually, I gave up trying to persuade him to involve his loved ones and we performed the transplant. Everything went wrong. Severe infections caused complications during the early posttransplant period, and he died within two weeks of the procedure.

About a month after his death, I received a handwritten letter from his 10-year-old daughter, who I had never met. She asked me how it could be that her dad, who was completely healthy when he was admitted to the hospital, got worse during the treatment and died two weeks later. Why had we killed her father? She did not reply to my lengthy response, and I felt sure she would never understand. How could she?

After this unfortunate outcome I made sure that the patient's closest relative was present at some of the most important discussions and that they were fully informed of the risks and the chance of survival. Most of the time, the closest relatives understood that an unfortunate outcome was just that, unfortunate, but that it was a possibility due to the risk assessment that we had discussed before the transplant.

However, in a very few cases the relatives still did not understand, and the team and the doctors were accused of maltreatment. However, this was extremely rare. In general, patients, who had to live with severe complications, like chronic graft versus host disease, were remarkably understanding. So were the relatives who had lost their loved ones. That is why providing accurate information before any transplant is crucial.

30 Donnall Thomas and the 1990 Nobel Prize

In my opinion, the most important person involved in the development of bone marrow transplants as a useful clinical treatment method was Donnall Thomas. Others shared my view, including the Nobel Committee.

Donnall (Don) Thomas[65,66] was born in 1920. He graduated from Harvard Medical School and spent his first years as a physician in the 1940s at the Peter Bent Brigham Hospital. This was the hospital that I visited during my postgraduate time at CCRF in the 1960s. It was there that I attended rounds with Frank Gardner and David Nathan, Sidney Farber's successor at the CCRF (Chapter 21).

Thomas met Farber during his time at the Peter Bent Brigham. Farber obviously appreciated his work because Thomas was given a laboratory at the nearby CCRF. As a young doctor, Thomas participated in the treatment of the first leukemia patient who received the folic acid antagonist amethopterin in 1948 under the leadership of Farber (Chapter 21)[44]. He saw the first patient to go into remission, but he also saw that all the patients eventually had a recurrence of the disease.

When Thomas was at CCRF, he became interested in transfer of bone marrow between individuals and its potential for treatment. He was fascinated by the pioneering experiments published in the early 1950s by Leon Jacobsen[67] (nominated in 1961 and 1963 for the Nobel Prize) and Egon Lorenz[68]. They showed that mice that had received deadly total body irradiation could be saved by their own bone marrow, which had been harvested before the irradiation. At the start of the 1950s he was invited by Dr Joe Ferrebee to the Mary Imogene Bassett Hospital in Cooperstown. They started bone marrow transplant experiments in dogs and eventually achieved the first bone marrow transfer in humans. They were able to show, for the first time, that donor bone marrow cells could create red and white blood cells in the peripheral blood if they were infused into human beings after total body irradiation. The bone marrow was infused into the veins of six terminally ill cancer patients and all of them died from their cancer. However, specific markers made it possible to identify the newly produced cells from the donor bone marrow in the blood of two patients. One had an advanced stage uncurable bone marrow disorder, multiple myeloma, and the other had chronic lymphocytic leukemia. This was the first evidence that donor bone marrow could grow in the bone marrow environment of the new host and start to produce vital, mature red and white blood cells. The results were published in 1957 in the prestigious *New England Journal of Medicine*[69].

Those early transplants led to an international debate about the future prospects for bone marrow transplants, but few believed its value for treating patients. However, Thomas did not give up. In 1959, his group performed transplants from identical twins to two patients with acute leukemia, who were considered uncurable despite the cytotoxic drugs that were already available[70]. The transplants were performed after total body irradiation. Both patients were saved by the bone marrow, as their leukemia disappeared. However, the success was short lived. After a few months, both patients died of their disease.

Thomas moved from Cooperstown to Seattle in 1963, where he became Head of Oncology at the University of Washington School of Medicine. Shortly afterwards, he established his research activities at the Fred Hutchinson Cancer Research Center. For some years he focused on experimental transplants in dogs and his methods improved. The discovery of the human leukocyte antigens (HLA) system by the later Nobel Prize Awardee Jean Dausset (Chapter 42) made it possible to select donors that were compatible with the recipient for these antigen markers. In 1977, Thomas's group had performed 100 transplants on patients with relapsed or chemotherapy-resistant acute leukemia. Of these, 13 were apparently cured, due to the improved therapeutic approach, total body irradiation with lung shielding and the use of HLA-compatible sibling donors[71]. However, the real breakthrough came when transplants were performed earlier in the course of the disease and after an induction period with drugs before the transplant to reduce the tumor burden. If the transplants were performed when the patients were in clinical remission, 50% could be cured.

Thomas's group in Seattle soon became the world leaders in bone marrow and stem cell transplants. The use of peripheral blood stem cells instead of bone marrow made the procedure technically easier[66]. The technique was continuously improved and the graft versus host reaction and disease was graded and described in detail. New preventive treatments were used and one that was particularly important was the combination of methotrexate and cyclosporin. Healthy HLA-typed unrelated donors and new conditioning methods were used. Results improved drastically. Indications expanded and soon more than 50% of patients with acute myeloblastic and chronic myeloid leukemia were cured.

During the 1970s, the method spread to the most important university hospitals in Europe and the USA. The expansion exploded. About 100,000 transplants are now performed worldwide every year and by 2019 an estimated 1.5 million (about half of them allogeneic and half autologous) had been carried out[72]. Donor registries now include more than 40 million HLA-typed volunteer donors (Chapter 42).

I met Thomas in Seattle for the first time in the early 1970s when I was planning to start a bone marrow transplant program at the Huddinge Hospital in Sweden (Chapter 28). He was a nice, gracious, low-profile person who seemed happy to let his collaborators be more visible. He had a shadow who followed him at the office or wherever we went and that was his wife Dorothy Martin, known as Dottie, who he met during his early studies. She was also his technician and secretary and appeared to be his constant companion.

Thomas generously shared his knowledge with me. The visit was of great value, and when we were building our later program we could always call Thomas and Seattle for advice.

Thomas visited us at the Huddinge Hospital several times. The first time he was invited to give the Huddinge Hospital Transplant Lecture during the yearly Läkarstämman. This was a physicians' meeting that was held at a big congress site called Älvsjömässan, outside Stockholm. It attracted about 25,000 healthcare workers, mainly doctors. However, the most spectacular visit was in 1990, when Thomas arrived to receive the Nobel Prize with his friend Joseph Murray, who had performed the first successful renal transplant. They received the prize *"for their discoveries concerning organ and cell transplantation in the treatment of human disease"*. This interesting wording showed that it was possible to research the will of Alfred Nobel and award the Nobel Prize to clinicians that had made practical clinical *"discoveries"*.

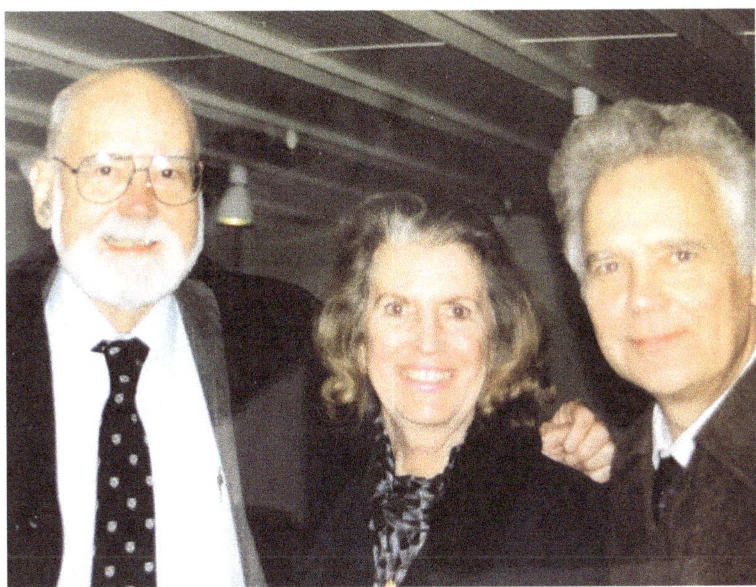

Donnall Thomas was awarded the Nobel Prize in Physiology or Medicine in 1990, together with Joseph Murray. He visited Sweden and the Huddinge Hospital several times. He is seen here on the left with his wife Dorothy (Dotty), who was also his secretary, technician and companion during his frequent travels, and the author Gösta Gahrton.

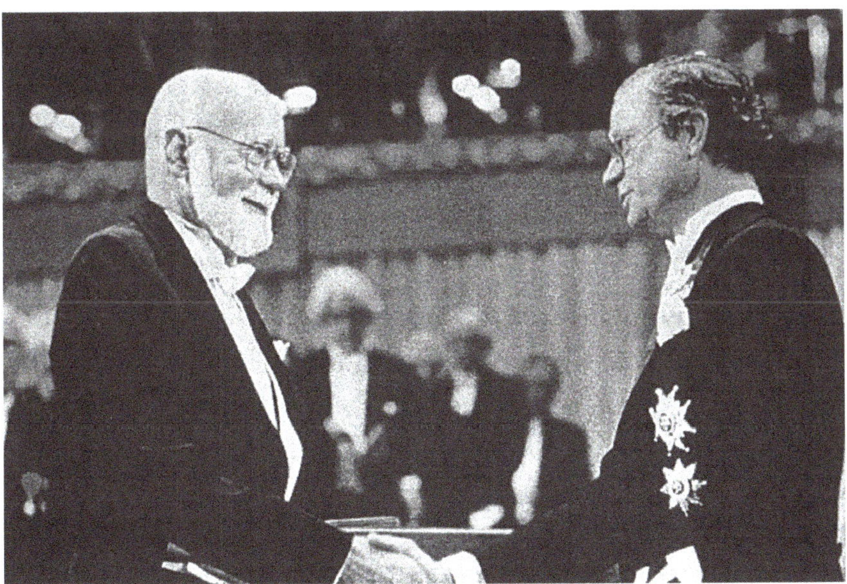

Donnall Thomas receiving the Nobel Prize from His Majesty the King of Sweden on 10 December 1990.

However, these are often more difficult to define than basic scientific discoveries and are therefore awarded less frequently.

A few days before the Nobel Prize award ceremony and banquet, all Laureates must give a Nobel lecture about their research. Thomas gave an excellent historical lecture at the Karolinska Institutet about bone marrow transplants.

The day before the award ceremony there was a general rehearsal at the Concert Hall in Stockholm, directed by the Chief Executive Officer of the Nobel Foundation, Stig Ramel. I was Thomas's official companion for the ceremony. Thomas seemed confused at first and thought that this meant that Dottie would not be able to attend the ceremony the next day. I had to explain to him that she would be seated in one of the front rows among the guests. Because I had the honor to present both him and Joseph Murray to the audience, and to the world, I would accompany him from the back door onto the stage, together with the other Laureates and their companions. I would then sit opposite him, behind the King and Queen of Sweden, until it was time for my presentation. Thomas appeared satisfied with the arrangements. The next evening Thomas received his Nobel Prize. Everything went well and according to protocol.

The selection of the winners for the 1990 Nobel Prize in Physiology or Medicine was the result of considerable work and the Nobel Committee spent a very long time engaged in interesting discussions. This was the case with all the previous winners as well. Unfortunately, the content of these discussions cannot be revealed until 50 years have passed, due to the secrecy rules of the Nobel Foundation. I have, therefore, written a summary of and left those notes in storage at the archives of the Nobel Committee at the Karolinska Institutet. They will be open from 2041.

Chapter 31 · Competing to Become a Professor

When Donald Thomas received the Nobel Prize in 1990, I was a well-established Professor of Medicine at the Karolinska Institutet and a member of the Nobel Committee. However, the path from the time of our first bone marrow transplant in Stockholm in 1975 until my appointment as Professor and Head of Medicine at the Huddinge Hospital had been tough. Although my account of that time falls somewhat outside the scope of this book, no potential or successful Nobel Prize winners were involved so I am free to talk about it. It may be interesting to follow the procedure from being powerless to reaching a top academic and clinical position in Sweden.

In the early 1980s, there were only eight Professors in Medicine (internal medicine) in the whole of Sweden: two each at the University of Lund and the Karolinska Institutet and one each in Gothenburg, Uppsala, Linköping and Umeå. A position as professor became open only if the holder of the position had retired or died and no other positions were available.

Three positions as Professor of Medicine became open in the early 1980s: one in Linköping and two at the Karolinska Institutet. The one in Linköping had been held by Professor Ragnar Berlin, a hematologist. The two in Stockholm were at the Karolinska Hospital and the Huddinge Hospital. The Huddinge Hospital vacancy was held by my predecessor Gunnar Birke and had been predicted for some years, since professors had to retire at 65 years of age. The other position at the Karolinska Institutet had not been predicted. Some years before his formal retirement, Professor Lars Erik Böttiger decided to accept an offer to be the medical chief at the drug company KABI and had left his position at the Karolinska Institutet and the Karolinska Hospital.

With rare exceptions, there were no chairs or head positions in medical subspecialties, such as hematology, cardiology, lung disorders and endocrinology, as the Professor of Medicine was the head of those specialties. They headed both the clinical department and academic department and were responsible for graduate and postgraduate education in all those disciplines.

The reason for having two Professors in Medicine at the University of Lund and the Karolinska Institutet was that two large hospitals with education in medicine were associated with each of them. These were the Malmö General Hospital in Malmö and the University Hospital in Lund associated with the University of Lund, and the Karolinska Hospital and Huddinge Hospital in Stockholm and Huddinge associated with the Karolinska Institutet.

The position in Linköping was thrown open for applications somewhat earlier than the other two and I decided to apply. However, before the reviewers at the Linköping University had come to any conclusion, the two positions at the Karolinska Institutet also became available. I applied for both. After some time, I came to the strategic conclusion that if I withdrew my application to Linköping, then maybe I had a better chance of securing the one that I really wanted at the Karolinska Institutet's Huddinge Hospital. And that is what I did.

Now the usual Swedish circus for professor appointments started. The Karolinska Institutet appointed three specialists and reviewers, all Professors in Medicine, to evaluate each applicant, by focusing on their scientific and educational achievements. To avoid bias, these three advisory positions should not be filled by people with a conflict of interest, such as the professor who had just retired. It meant that only the Professors in Medicine in Lund, Gothenburg, Uppsala and Umeå were eligible to provide advice on the Karolinska Institutet positions. Eventually, Professor Leif Hallberg from Gothenburg, Professor Harry Boström from Uppsala and Professor Per-Olof Wester from Umeå were appointed to review the applicants.

They had the delicate task of reviewing and evaluating the competence of the applicants for the two chairs at the Karolinska Institutet and suggest who should be appointed to the two chairs by ranking their preferences. They had to review 14 highly competent applicants, who each had hundreds of scientific publications and other merits as well.

The reviewers presented their proposal to the Tjänsteförslagsnämnden, which was a body within the Karolinska Institutet that comprised nine professors from the Institutet. Once the majority had reached a consensus, they made their recommendations to the Minister (Secretary) of Education, who at this time was Lennart Bodström, a Social Democrat. He then made the final formal appointment.

Reviewers frequently tried to agree on one candidate, but each would give their own ranking. If they reached a unanimous proposal, then the Tjänsteförslagsnämnden would support them and make that recommendation to the Ministry. This made the appointment easy. However, if they could not agree on the successful candidate, and the Tjänsteförslagsnämnden could not agree, then they would recommend the candidate with the most votes and that would be the name they sent to the Government.

Reviewers are also human beings, and they frequently have to compare apples and pears. This means that their own personal view on a candidate may bias their evaluation. To avoid this, as much as possible, the unwritten rule was not to participate if you were the retiring professor from the position that was being filled. I was particularly happy with this rule, because I knew that the issues I had experienced with my boss Birke could have been detrimental if he had been a reviewer.

And that is exactly what happened. Professor Per Olof Wester from Umeå decided to apply for the two Karolinska posts and that meant he could no longer be a reviewer. To my great astonishment, the Karolinska Institutet appointed Birke to be his substitute. He had a strong position at the Karolinska Institutet and was also a member of the Tjänsteförslagsnämnden. I was sure that his very competent and closest collaborator, docent Jan Östman, was his first choice, as he stood in for him when he was on leave. I was sure that I would not achieve the first two rankings for either role. However, I was wrong. The two strong professors in Gothenburg and Uppsala disagreed with Birke's ranking. They recommended Göran Holm, who was Professor in Clinical Immunology at Karolinska Institutet, for the Karolinska Hospital vacancy and recommended me for the Huddinge Hospital role. Meanwhile, Birke recommended Östman for the position at the Huddinge. Seven of the Tjänsteförslagsnämnden members supported the first proposal by the professors from Gothenburg and Uppsala. Göran Holm and I were recommended to the Ministry for the two positions, and we were both appointed accordingly.

Birke was completely open about his preference. Immediately after the voting by the Tjänsteförslagsnämnden had finished he informed me that *"the voting ended seven to two in your favor, and*

I did not vote for you". I appreciated his honesty, but he should not have been involved in the process to appoint his successor. He came up against two equally strong and honest reviewers and was unable to convince them about his first choice for the role. If I had ever been asked to be a reviewer for my successor, I would have said no. Fortunately that never happened.

32 The First Years as Double Department Head

On the day that my appointment as Professor of Medicine at the Karolinska Institute was officially announced in 1985 the Hospital Director, Lars-Åke Flood, visited my office with flowers and congratulations. As the Professor of Medicine, I automatically became Head of the clinical Department of Medicine at the Huddinge Hospital, which had about 400 employees. The academic institution at the Karolinska Institutet was much smaller and mainly comprised administrators, secretaries, laboratory assistants and researchers. A few physicians, who were also clinical teachers, had dual appointments at the Karolinska Institutet and the Hospital. They were all located within the huge Huddinge Hospital.

My predecessor Birke steered this complicated structure in his own way, running the clinical department with his right hand and the academic institution with his left hand. Formal meetings with the institutional board had mainly been abandoned, as he found it easier to make the necessary decisions by himself. At that time, I was one of the five associate heads of clinical sections and two of us had dual positions at the Karolinska Institutet and the hospital.

We were all treated in the same way and were given great freedom to run our specialist sections. This involved research and clinical practice, if we had grants, our clinics with patients and teaching both graduate and postgraduate students.

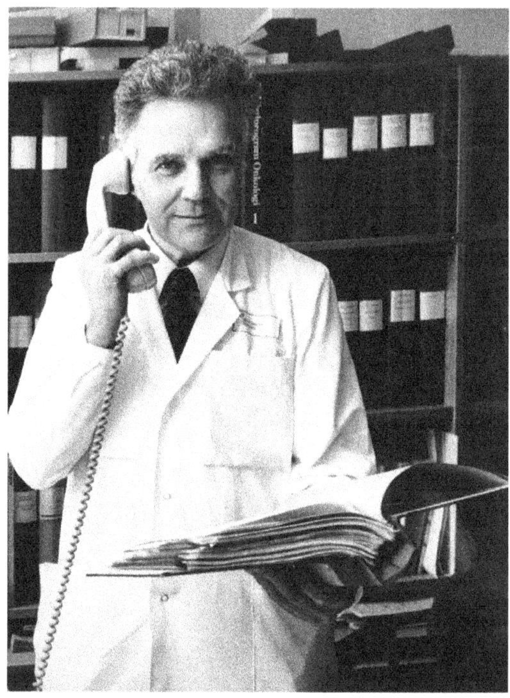

The old telephone was an important tool for running my department and international communications.

Computers and mobile phones had not yet arrived.

I thought that this way of running the dual departments seemed administratively effective but was convinced that there should be a greater focus on clinical research. After I was appointed Professor of Medicine, I gathered the institutional board together. They had not met for months, even years, and I hoped that the members would be happy to be involved with my ideas for the future. There was a deafening silence and I soon realized that something was wrong.

After a few days I was approached by some of the board members, who claimed that the institutional regulations had not been followed. There should have been elections for membership of the board, for example from various groups of teachers, students, and laboratory personnel. This had never been done before, but they still felt it was illegal and not acceptable.

I took this very seriously, followed the regulations and organized elections. Eventually, after about two months we had a new institutional board. It mainly consisted of the same members as before, but now everybody was happy.

Many of my associates were excellent clinicians and researchers, but they were certainly not Nobel Prize candidates. The whole Karolinska Institutet had only one Nobel Prize winner in office and that was Bengt Samuelsson, who was its acting President and Rector. By this time, Ragnar Granit and Sune Bergström had both retired and Ulf von Euler had died in 1983. My primary goal was not to produce Nobel Laureates, but to make the department internationally competitive in research. At the same time, the clinical activities had to be efficient and be able to combine clinical practice with clinical research.

My first associate head was the docent Olle Edhag, an excellent cardiologist and friend. He had succeeded another very able cardiologist, Erik Orinius, as Head of the section of Cardiology, when he decided to move to the other side of the city to the Karolinska Hospital. Edhag was also very good at dealing with our budget. Birke had exceeded this in recent years, and this was probably partly due to my own expensive hematology section (Chapter 27). Edhag had numerous ambitious ideas about how to make the department more effective and he wanted to use part of the budget to promote the wellbeing of the employees. He made a deal with the Hospital Director that if we managed to make a profit by using our budget, we could use it for unspecified measures to support the employees. To our amazement, and particularly to the amazement of the Hospital Director, we managed to make a profit of about 350,000 US dollars that year. Edhag suggested that we should buy a house in the Swedish ski mountains for conferences and that it could also be used by our employees during their leisure. This was a hard nut to crack for the Hospital Director. This was not what he had expected when he had made his promise about what we could do with the profits. The county government lawyers made a series of accusations in the local media about this plan, but I successfully defended the project. We bought the house, which had 10 beds, created an employee association, set up a bookings system and charged the employees the lowest possible fees allowed to avoid taxes, when they used it privately for skiing and recreation. Although the hospital owned the house, my department had priority to use the facility, as it was considered responsible for it. I decided not to use the house myself, in fact I have never seen it. However, it was highly appreciated by the employees and effectively used.

During the following years I copied much of my predecessor's way of running a large clinical department. Once a week I went round to each specialized section. Every morning I visited the emergency department to see patients who had been admitted during the latest 24 hours and were due to be discharged or admitted to the specialized wards. Once a week I had an outpatient clinic. However, I soon realized that this was an impossible and ineffective way spending my time. My focus on hematological research was being hampered. My input in the running of the specialized sections outside hematology was zero. A new organization had to be put in place and that called for new departmental structures. Birke's Department of Medicine had to make way for a more efficient model.

33 The Liquidation of the Clinical Department of Medicine

I was in charge of two different departments of medicine. One reported to the Hospital Director and was responsible for patient care. The other reported to the President and Rector of the Karolinska Institutet and was responsible for research and education in both graduate and postgraduate internal medicine. It wasn't possible to change the structure of the academic Department of Medicine that came under the Karolinska Institutet. However, it was possible to increase the collaboration between the subspecialties within the clinical Departments of Medicine and Surgery, as well as other ones. Those actors now wanted to form new departments, such as gastroenterology, by bringing together the divisions within medicine and surgery and by cardiology teaming up with thoracic surgery. Strong forces within the subspecialties wanted to liquidate the gigantic medicine and surgical departments. I initially hesitated to support this development, but increasing specialization forced the changes. There were considerable weaknesses in lumping hematology and gastroenterology together in one department. Although I had given the division heads full responsibility for their patients, I was still responsible for their budgets. I eventually decided that the idea of forming new departments was good and supported the split of my clinical Department of Medicine. I eventually ended up being Head of the clinical Department of Hematology under the Hospital Director and continued as Head of the academic Department of Medicine under the Rector of the Karolinska Institutet. The process had been started by the dynamic Head of Surgery, docent Göran Hellers, who now took over my division of gastroenterology and established a medical/ surgical gastroenterology department. Just before this transition, I had managed to install the very competent new Professor of Gastroenterology, Curt Einarsson, to my department at the Huddinge Hospital, which is now called the Karolinska University Hospital, Huddinge. I had been in competition with my colleague and Head of Medicine at the Karolinska Hospital, now Karolinska University Hospital, Solna. After the transition, Einarsson was no longer part of my clinical department, but still belonged to the academic Department of Medicine Karolinska Institutet.

The process continued and the clinical Department of Medicine at Huddinge was dismantled and, in addition to gastroenterology and cardiology, allergology, lung and metabolic disorders disappeared from my realm. This reorganization of my department was in line with what had happened in other disciplines and was forced by the increasing need for specialization. I was convinced that it was the right approach and that it would benefit the patients.

I was relieved as it meant that I could focus on hematology, but still oversee the graduate and postgraduate education in medicine. The scientific developments in my academic department bloomed, not only in hematology, but also in other disciplines. During my 12 years as head, 63 dissertations were approved and the number of highly cited scientific papers that were produced exploded. The heads of the clinical departments still belonged to the academic Department of Medicine and their colleagues should have the full credit. A growing number of strong scientists became independent in hematology and that is how it should be.

Some people may think that I am bragging, and some may think that closing the clinical Department of Medicine was the wrong way to go. My previous boss Birke, who was now retired, disagreed with the closure. One day, when I arrived at a reception for the Nobel Laureates at the reception hall in the Karolinska Institutet he shouted loudly at me, so that everyone could hear: *"Here comes the guy who liquidated the Department of Medicine at the Huddinge Hospital"*. In some ways I understood his view. He was the one who had seen the first patient when the hospital opened in 1972, and he did it as the Head of the new Department of Medicine that he had created. His weakness was that he had difficulties accepting that increasing specialization called for change. I saluted him and we were still friends.

Some unforeseen things happened on the road to the new organization. When I was still head of the two Departments of Medicine, a new Hospital Director, Birgitta Böhlin, was appointed. She was a strong lady and at her first meeting with all the heads of departments she stated that her primary goal was to cut the budgets for all of the departments. Although she had nothing to do with the departments belonging to the Karolinska Institutet, she decided that no one was allowed to have a head position at the Huddinge if they were head of an academic department at the Karolinska Institutet. In her view, that involved competing loyalties. This was totally against my own view on coordinating patient care and clinical and translational research involving patients. Böhlin colluded with my friend Anders Persson, who was the Physician-in-Chief at the Huddinge and decided that nobody was allowed to sit on both chairs. I was asked to choose if I wanted to continue as head of the hospital department and leave the academic department or vice versa. I refused to accept the offer and went to the Rector of the Karolinska Institutet, Bengt Samuelsson. He seemed like a shy person, but he was actually very strong and firm. He advised me to stay on and not to agree to leave any of my positions. He was sure that I would not be fired from my head position at the hospital. He shared my opinion that the two positions worked together effectively and were advantageous for both the patients and for research. However, he was wrong. I was fired as the Head of the hospital's Department of Medicine. The strange thing was that I had a very good relationship with both Böhlin and Persson. I was asked to choose who I wanted to replace me as head of the department and was told that I would be allowed to stay on as the associate head. I decided that I could not choose a hematologist, as this would suggest that I would try to govern the department through a dependent colleague. Instead, I chose my associate head, Hans Vallin, who until then had been responsible for the departmental budget. I agreed to be the associate head. Hans was an excellent head and much better than me in handling money matters. This arrangement lasted until the dissolution of the department. Then there was a new organization, a new Hospital Director and a new organizational level between the heads of departments and the Hospital Director. The so-called division head, who sat above the department heads was Lars Collste, who was a friend of mine and lived opposite our house. He thought that it was OK to be both Head of Hematology and Head of the academic Department of Medicine in the new organization.

Although Böhlin and I had very different opinions about whether it was feasible to occupy the head positions in both the academic and clinical departments, we became very good friends. The day before she moved to a quite different head position at the

Försvarets Materielverk, the Defense Material Administration, she approved an application for five million crowns, about 600,000 US dollars, from me and my collaborator and friend Edvard (Ted) Smith. The money was to support a Gene Therapy Research Center at the Hospital (Chapter 46). It was a happy end to our *"collaboration"*.

34   Tutor and Teacher

"You were not a particularly good tutor". This claim was made by Per Hörnsten, the first student who passed his thesis under my supervision at the Huddinge Hospital. It was many years later and by that time he had become a colleague. I was not upset by what he said.

It is important to be a formal tutor in the Swedish system. That means that you initiate, and follow up, projects carried out by PhD students until their thesis is approved. A thesis usually consists of four or more scientific papers and at least half of them have to be published in international scientific journals. The candidate produces a book that contains a printed summary of their thesis, and the contents are officially defended during a session that lasts for about two hours. A recognized senior scientist is usually invited to oppose their thesis and they are frequently invited from abroad. They then recommend whether the students pass their thesis to a central committee appointed by the respective university.

In the 1970s, when Hörnsten was working on his thesis, the role of the supervisor was less formal than it is today. Despite my failure, he produced a very good thesis and defended it properly. He did not continue with a scientific career but became a doctor who was appreciated in the north of Sweden. He was a dedicated moose hunter and invited me to join him several times.

In the 1960s, when I worked on my thesis, there were even fewer formalities, but the requirements were tougher. The supervisor was the soul of the thesis and they needed to approve of what you intended to do. They were also expected to help with resources and be available for help when needed and for testing ideas.

Torbjörn Caspersson was automatically my formal supervisor, or tutor, at the Nobel Institute, as he was the supervisor for every PhD student working there. This, in turn, meant that his engineers educated me on the machinery, the microspectrophotometers and microinterferometers, that had been specifically built for single cell measurements. I also had laboratory space. Then it was up to me to carry out my project. Some of Caspersson's students were working more directly on his projects and saw him nearly every day. Other students, like me, arrived with their own projects and did not see him for several weeks. During the time I worked at the Nobel Institute, from 1961–1966, Dick Killander, Anders Zetterberg, Rudolf (Rulle) Rigler, Lore Zech and an overseas scientist belonged to the group with regular contact, while I, Britta Wahren and Lars Sörén spent less time with Caspersson. At many other of Karolinska Institutet institutions, the heads were rarely formal supervisors. Young docents, namely associate professors, with research groups wanted to supervise as many students as possible. It was an important step in their own career and it meant being the senior author on many publications. Thus, the Head of the Institution could abstain from being the formal supervisor in order to satisfy their docents.

It was not easy to be a supervisor at Caspersson's institution. When I arrived in 1961, he had two docents, Nils (Nisse) Ringertz and Gunnar Blom. They had both been supervised by Caspersson, but now they were docents and had their own PhD students. Both of them later became Caspersson's enemies. This resulted in Blom's departure to the University of Umeå in the northern part of Sweden. Meanwhile, Ringertz held on until Caspersson had retired and then succeeded him (Chapter 19). Caspersson's later docents, including me, had all planned to move to other institutions or clinical departments after we passed our dissertations. Then it would be no problem to start a career as supervisor.

I passed my dissertation in 1966, after I had eight papers published in well-known scientific journals and one summary. I immediately became a docent in medical cell research and genetics. This meant that I could recruit PhD students for my own projects, but I decided not to challenge Caspersson. Instead, I started collaborating with young students who suited my research profile and who agreed with Caspersson's ideas. The intention was not to produce a complete thesis, but to participate in a project for one or two years, hopefully leading to one or two scientific publications. One of them, Xenophon Yataganas, was Greek. He returned to his homeland after a one-year stay, having published three scientific papers on the content and distribution of hemoglobin in single cells in thalassemia, which is a genetic disorder that was common in his country.

Yataganas and I became very good friends. I visited him later in Greece, when he had married a charming, beautiful and rich relative of the famous shipowner Aristotle Onassis. After spending some time as a clinician and clinical scientist at the University of Athens, he changed his career to pursue philanthropic healthcare activities in Africa.

Another young student was Wolfgang Habicht, who spent one year investigating the changes in DNA, RNA and proteins in single cells during the development of leukemia in a mouse model. It resulted in one publication in the scientific journal *Experimental Cell Research*. I lost track of him after he left.

Caspersson said I could keep my laboratory and technicians at the Nobel Institute after I moved to the Department of Medicine at the Karolinska Hospital on the other side of Solna Street, which separated the Karolinska Institutet from the Karolinska Hospital. This was an ideal situation. I could continue my basic research and successively switch to translational research using clinical patient material from the Hospital. But what about supervising PhD students?

When I was in the Department of Medicine, I wanted to continue working in the Division of Hematology, led by docent Peter Reizenstein. Non-dissertation-ready physicians, namely PhD students, seemed to be under his supervision. As I previously explained, it did not seem to be a good idea to supervise PhD students in Caspersson's domain. This meant that I had no PhD students during the whole time I was at the Karolinska Hospital, from 1967–1973. Instead, I started working in collaboration with others. Together we built clinical research on leukemia that focused on new treatment methods and evaluated the prognostic importance of chromosomal aberrations. This was now possible because of the new banding technique that had been developed by Caspersson and his colleagues. It wasn't until I moved to the new Huddinge Hospital, south of the city, that I started to recruit PhD students. My first student was Hörnsten, who I mentioned above. However, I soon realized that I did not have enough time to be a good tutor. So, I teamed up with Britta Wahren, who had now left Caspersson for the Institute of Infectious Disease Control. From then on, Wahren was as much a tutor to Hörnsten as I was, perhaps more.

As mentioned, Hörnsten received his PhD for his excellent thesis about stem cell culturing and how the results could be used in the clinic[73]. So, although Hörnsten thought I was a lousy tutor, his dissertation was excellent.

My poor contributions as a supervisor only improved modestly during my time at the Huddinge Hospital. After I was appointed Professor of Medicine at the Karolinska Institutet and Head of the clinical Department of Medicine at the Huddinge I had little time to spare. I had not foreseen all the other engagements that followed my new roles. For example, I was member of the Board of the Medical Research Council and chairman and member of various committees, and I joined many foundations and editorial boards of journals. Sometimes I was the main supervisor and sometimes I was the associate supervisor, by teaming up with somebody else. This was frequently Britta Wahren, but others included the Head of the Transplant Immunology laboratory, Professor Erna Möller. Most of those that I supervised went on to have excellent careers. I was not able to break Caspersson's record, which was that 13 of the PhD students that he supervised went on to become full professors. However, I am not far from this figure if I count those that passed their dissertations in hematology while they were working at my department.

Karl-Henrik (Kalle) Robert was a shining star who passed his dissertation during his time in my department. He was a close associate and had a full-time position in the Department of Hematology, but Möller was his main supervisor. His main contribution was in succeeding to stimulate malignant cells from peripheral blood of patients with chronic lymphocytic leukemia (CLL) to divide in a culture. The trick was to use a virus, the Epstein-Barr virus, which caused Burkitt's lymphoma, as the stimulating agent.

I saw the possibility of using the same method to study Q-banded chromosomes. At this time, chromosome studies required that cells divided and formed metaphases. The mature cells in CLL did not divide and this meant that chromosomes could not be studied unless the cells were externally stimulated to divide. Robert's success in stimulating the cells was the key. Together with Zech we managed to discover the first specific chromosomal aberrations in this disease, which was the most common leukemia in elderly patients. It was a breathtaking discovery that opened up discoveries of prognostic subgroups of this disease and the possibility of adapting the therapy to chromosomal patterns[40,41]. The discovery aroused great international interest in analogy, with the discovery of the Philadelphia chromosome and the 9;22 chromosome translocation (Chapter 19) in chronic myelocytic leukemia (CML). Robert wanted to name the extra chromosome 12 that we discovered *"the Huddinge chromosome"*, because many years earlier Nowell and Hungerford had named the Philadelphia chromosome in CML after the city where it was discovered. I thought that was too much and it ended up being called trisomy 12, which indicated that the cells had one extra chromosome 12.

Roberts ended his career at the Karolinska Institutet and Huddinge because he wanted to save the world from being destroyed by man. His early understanding of the devastating way that humans treated the environment was admirable. His medicine was, in my opinion, excellent. He wanted to convince industrial leaders that they could make more money by changing to sustainable environmental methods. I did not want to lose him, but my efforts were in vain. After his two-year leave of absence from the department, he had to make up his mind. He chose to leave and created The Natural Step, a non-profit organization that promotes a sustainable society and world. He never became full professor at the Karolinska Institutet, but he eventually became Professor of Strategic Sustainable Development at Blekinge Technical College in Ronneby, southern Sweden.

The Natural Step is now an international organization that operates in 12 countries. In 2000, Robert received the Blue Planet Prize *"for scientifically formulating the principles and theoretical framework required to establish a sustainable society and for enhancing the environmental awareness of business, municipalities and others"*. The Blue Planet Prize *"goes to the outstanding individuals or organizations whose work have contributed and continue to contribute significantly to the improvement of the global environment"*. It was created by the Asahi Glass Foundation in 1992 and is awarded to two people every year. The Asahi Glass Foundation is affiliated with, and was founded by, the Japanese company AGC Inc., (previously the Asahi Glass Co. Ltd), the largest glass manufacturing company in the world. The Blue Planet Prize is sometimes referred to as the Nobel Prize for ecological sustainability, although it has nothing to do with the Nobel Prizes. Robert received many other rewards, and he was worthy of all of them.

Per Ljungman wanted to be a hematologist. He was, and still is, a brilliant clinician, who is particularly interested in the infectious disorders associated with hematopoietic stem cell transplants. I called upon Wahren to be the main supervisor for his dissertation work and Ljungman wrote an excellent thesis on this subject[74]. I soon recruited him to be my associate head of the clinical department and he stayed on in this role until my retirement. He turned out to be a talented administrator and, on my recommendation, he was appointed as my successor as Head of the Department of

Hematology in 1997. Ljungman eventually became an adjunct professor at the Karolinska Institutet.

Gunnar Juliusson was interested in hematology and was working as an intern at Danderyd Hospital a few kilometers north of the Karolinska Hospital when he made contact with me. He asked if I would consider him for a position in my department and I recruited him after his interview, when he showed a great interest in research in hematology. Robert, who had passed his dissertation, became his main tutor. Juliusson produced an excellent thesis[75] and continued to produce research of the highest international level in the field that was my main interest at the time. This was determining the prognostic impact of chromosomal aberrations in hematologic malignancies. He continued the work on chronic lymphocytic leukemia (CLL) that was started by me and Robert, and eventually had his work published in the highly esteemed *New England Journal of Medicine*.[76] It was one of the first comprehensive papers about the prognostic impact of this disease of chromosomal aberrations, as determined by the Q-banding pattern. However, Juliusson was ambitious and didn't just want to be a resident. He wanted to become a head of department and professor and successfully applied to become the Head of the Department of Hematology at the University Hospital in Linköping, south of Stockholm. Juliusson continued to produce important research, particularly in CLL, and soon became Professor in Hematology at the University of Lund in southern Sweden. It was a loss for the Karolinska Institutet and for my department. However, after some years our paths crossed again. When I retired, I asked him to be co-editor of the third edition of a textbook in hematology that I had previously published with my friend and colleague, Bengt Lundh. He was former Head of the Department of Medicine at Helsingborg Hospital, also in southern Sweden, but had died. We ended up producing a totally new hematology textbook. It was a bestseller in its field in Sweden and this was mainly due to Juliusson's efforts.

Christer Paul joined the Huddinge Hospital when it opened in 1972, as an inexperienced, newly qualified doctor. This meant that he was already there when I moved to the hospital. Paul was interested in hematology and became an important member of the Leukemia Group of Middle Sweden (LGMS) that I had established in 1971. I became his supervisor, together with two very able scientists, i.e., Dieter Lockner, a senior physician, who was responsible for the education of undergraduate students in internal medicine, and Curt Peterson, a pharmacologist, who later went on to become Professor in Clinical Pharmacology at the University of Linköping, south of Stockholm (Chapter 25). Paul's dissertation was about the production and use of a DNA-anthracycline complex for treating acute leukemia. Doxorubicin, an anthracycline, was bound to DNA and the resulting complex was used by the LGMS for a prospective study on the treatment of acute myeloblastic leukemia[77].

The idea of using a cytotoxic drug-DNA complex came from the 1974 Nobel Prize winner Christian de Duve[78]. He had shown that drug DNA complexes could be *"eaten"* by the leukemic cells through the lysosome, a cell organelle that he had discovered. As soon as the complex reached the lysosome it was dissolved, and the drug could then attack the leukemic cell from the inside and kill it. In the 1940s, de Duve had been working in the biochemistry section of the Medical Nobel Institutes at the Karolinska Institutet, headed by the 1955 Nobel Prize winner Hugo Theorell.

Curt Peterson and the American pharmacologist William (Bill) Plunkett were responsible for producing the complex. Then the LGMS, with Paul as the main researcher, embarked on a prospective study of patients with acute myeloblastic leukemia. This compared treatments with drug combinations that included either doxorubicin (DOX) bound to DNA (DOX-DNA) or DOX alone. The complex combination was better than the non-complex one, as it led to better overall survival and progression free survival and fewer severe side effects[79]. However, other new drugs and drug combinations were available, and this treatment never became generally accepted and stopped being used to treat leukemia.

Paul continued his scientific work and became an adjunct Professor in Hematology at the Karolinska Institutet. He has now retired from full-time work but is still regarded as a coveted specialist when remote Swedish hospitals need a qualified hematologist.

Jan (Janne) Liliemark had many interests in addition to hematology. He believed that the reason that he got the position as an intern in the Department of Medicine at the Huddinge was his record as a mountain climber. I understood that he had climbed much more difficult mountain peaks than I had. I faintly remember telling him about my own success in climbing Mount Blanc, Grossglockner and other peaks in Europe and I probably told him that I believe that mountain climbers are usually ambitious, have goals and try to reach them. Liliemark was just that kind of a person. I appointed him, and I co-supervised his thesis work together with Curt Peterson before I became head of the department.

Peterson and Plunkett had collaborated on another drug, cytosine arabinoside, which was effective for treating acute myeloblastic leukemia. However, the drug had some problems and neurological side effects had been seen in some patients. Liliemark's project was about how the treatment could be made more effective and cause less side effects. He studied how the body, and the leukemic cells, metabolized the treatment during different administration methods. From 1985–1986 he published seven scientific papers on the subject and six of them appeared in *Cancer Research*, one of the most prestigious cancer journals. His dissertation took place in 1986[80]. Cytosine arabinoside is still used to treat acute myeloblastic leukemia and Liliemark's work provided important information about how the drug is best administrated for maximal efficiency and what side effects can occur.

Liliemark continued to work on the pharmacokinetics of cytotoxic drugs and collaborated with Juliusson on drug studies on cladribine, which was efficient in chronic lymphocytic leukemia and other lymphoproliferative disorders. Juliusson and Liliemark were on the international frontline during these investigations. Liliemark eventually became a professor at the Swedish Medical Product Agency. One of his daughters married the son of the previous Chief Executive Officer of the Astra pharmaceutical company, Håkan Mogren, who was a good friend of mine, and had followed in her father's footsteps.

Eva Hellström-Lindberg was one of Robert's PhD students. I cannot claim that I had a great impact on her rise to Professor in Hematology, but I did send her on a course that helped young doctors to aspire to become heads of department. Already at that time, I predicted that she would have a great career. After she had defended her thesis on myelodysplastic syndrome, which was a relatively unusual hematological disorder that frequently resulted in leukemia, she continued to devote her scientific life to the disease. She became Professor in Hematology at the Karolinska Institutet and transformed the hematology laboratory into an important scientific unit within the Department of Hematology at Huddinge, the Hematology Center. Hellström-Lindberg was eventually elected to be a member of both the Nobel Assembly and Committee. She remains well known on the international scene and was president of the most important scientific hematology association in Europe, the European Hematology Association (EHA), which attracts more than 10,000 participants to its annual meetings. She has received many awards, including the José Carreras Award, which was established in 1988 by the famous tenor after he had been cured of acute lymphoblastic leukemia by an autologous stem cell transplant. The prize money comes from the José Carreras Leukaemia Foundation, which is based in Barcelona, Spain, and a winner is selected every year by the EHA Board during its yearly congress.

Eva Kimby worked on her thesis on the immunological aspects of chronic lymphocytic leukemia under the supervision of my friend professor Håkan Mellstedt[81]. She worked on this while she was at the Danderyd Hospital, north of the Karolinska Hospital. Although I was very interested in her work, due to our discoveries of the specific chromosomal aberrations in this disease, I had nothing to do with her thesis. After she had defended her thesis, she called me and asked me if she could join my department. Of course, she could. I had known Kimby for a long time, and she was one of the best-known physicians when it came to caring for patients with lymphoproliferative diseases, such as lymphoma, CLL Hodgkin's disease and similar disorders. She secured a position as a specialist and head of the group taking care of patients with these disorders. Kimby participated in numerous international scientific groups running prospective clinical treatment trials, particularly those within the European Leukemia Net and the EHA. She was later promoted to Adjunct Professor in Hematology at the Karolinska Institutet.

Altogether, seven of the docents, namely assistant professors, who I educated and/or worked at my Department of Hematology have been promoted to professors. All of them have done it on their own merits, but I cannot deny that I feel rather proud and happy that most of them made their original scientific contributions when they were working in my department.

I had many other collaborators in my department, including my own PhD students or former collaborators or other PhD students. Many of them have pursued important careers but have not yet become professors.

Bo (Bosse) Björkstrand was one of my foremost collaborators. He started his thesis project under the supervision of Karl-Henrik Robert, but Robert soon focused his main attention on creating The Natural Step. Björkstrand came to me and wanted to change his supervisor. I took over as his main supervisor and arranged for him to start working with the Gene Therapy Group that I had started together with Edward (Ted) Smith. I had already engaged a doctor from Turkey, Sıraç Dilber, who was working on a gene therapy project for his thesis. Because Dilber did not work in the clinic, I thought that he and Björkstrand would form a wonderful team (Chapter 46). Björkstrand became the first clinician in the country to be responsible for a clinical gene therapy project[82,83]. After he passed his dissertation, I convinced him to be the principal investigator for a prospective, multicenter European study that I had initiated within the frame of the European Society for Blood and Marrow Transplantation (EBMT). The study compared outcomes for patients with multiple myeloma that had either been treated with an autologous transplant, the conventional treatment for this disease, or with a new approach that combined autologous and allogeneic transplantations. I had previously been the main investigator for several retrospective EBMT studies on allogeneic transplants for multiple myeloma, but now wanted to run a prospective study to prove the benefit of allogeneic transplants.

We managed to finalize the study and Björkstrand was the main author of the first publication in the high-ranking *Journal of Clinical Oncology*[84]. We were able to prove that combining autologous and allogeneic transplants was superior to just an autologous transplant. Although there have been controversial studies, and new treatment approaches mean that allogeneic treatment has been used less often, some centers still provide this treatment for patients with high-risk disease. Eventually, Björkstrand left the department and the hospital to work in the pharmaceutical industry, first for Roche and then for Novartis. He returned for a short period after 10 years, but then went back to industry as the Global Medical Director of Haematology New Therapies at Swedish Orphan Biovitrum AB.

Dilber came from a university hospital in Istanbul, Turkey. He had been informed about our gene therapy program and wanted to work on a thesis in this field (Chapter 46). Dilber had written to me, enclosing reference letters, and asked if he could visit and, if possible, work with our group. I am not sure how I responded, but one day my secretary announced that a doctor from Turkey had arrived and claimed that I had promised to see him. I was confused, but invited him into my office, listened to him and allowed him to start working in the gene therapy laboratory with two supervisors, my friend Ted Smith and Kleanthis G Xanthopoulos, a Greek doctor who worked with him. I had not made a mistake. Dilber wrote an excellent thesis on experimental gene therapy in mice and how it could be used to treat a tumor that mimicked multiple myelomas[85]. Dilber was an innovative researcher and soon after he completed his dissertation, he became an excellent supervisor. He educated several PhD students who, in turn, passed their dissertations in the field. One of them, Evren Alici, is now an excellent supervisor himself. He has a research group of more than 20 people who are focusing on natural killer (NK) cells and chimeric antigen receptor natural killer (CAR-NK) cell research. This could be seen as an extension of the gene transfer research program that I started with Smith. I try to follow their advanced molecular research projects and they still call me a collaborator. Having friends like these means that the old Swedish disorder of age discrimination does not exist.

Dilber was as well an excellent organizer. When I was asked by the European Society of Gene and Cell Therapy to arrange its congress in Stockholm in 2000, and be its President, I asked Dilber to be the Congress Secretary. He carried out the task excellently.

Unfortunately, Dilber was working on too many tasks at the same time. While he was employed by the Karolinska Institutet, he was also a counsellor to the Ministry of Health in Turkey. The administration of the Karolinska Institutet was not happy about the practicalities of his dual role and Dilber left our group for good. Long after my retirement, I supervised one of his doctoral students, Alexandra Treschow. She passed an excellent dissertation on experimental gene therapy, but then left the group for a job in industry.

Ragnhild Lindquist was one of the patients' favorite doctors. Her empathy had no borders, and she was always available for her patients. She enthusiastically started an ambitious PhD project that aimed to find a correlation between exposure to organic solvents and the development of acute leukemia. Long before she finalized her thesis[86], she had preliminary data that supported the hypothesis that patients with acute leukemia had been exposed to organic solvents more frequently than the general population. Painters were particularly at risk, probably because the paints that were used at the time contained benzene. Lindquist's discoveries were considered sensational, and she was interviewed by Swedish television. Her fame peaked when she was engaged by a US insurance company as an expert, supporting a patient that had developed acute leukemia after a long life as a painter.

She successfully defended her thesis and received her PhD a few years before her retirement, then helped hospitals around the country who needed a qualified hematologist, just like Paul.

Mats Merup was one of Juliusson's doctoral students. He continued the chromosome projects and focused on the molecular aspects, in collaboration with Professor Stefan Einhorn at the Department of Oncology at the Karolinska Hospital. His thesis was brilliant[87], and, if he had not been recruited by industry, I am sure he would have had a great academic career.

Perhaps the most remarkable scientific contribution was the dissertation made by my most talented technician, Britt Sundman, whose later married name was Engberg[88]. I made her head of the hematology laboratory, but that was predictively not enough after her PhD success. She left for industry, where she still is active.

Today I do not have PhD students. The young, enthusiastic and extremely able collaborators that were supervised by my PhD students have long since stood on their own feet. They include Evren Alici, Hareth Nahi, Tolga Sutlu, Charlotte Gran, Johan Lund and many others. They do not seem to know the phrase age-discrimination. Their time is still to come and, while I have mentioned them, they will not be described in this book on my memories.

Although I cannot brag about, or compare my *"success"*, with Caspersson's, I am very happy about the high number of competent hematologists that were educated in my department and continue to hold important positions, either in academia or industry, to the benefit of research and, not least, to the patients.

35 The Swedish Medical Research Council and Nobel Prize Winner Arvid Carlsson

The Swedish Medical Research Council was founded in 1945 by a number of Swedish professors, in particular George Kahlson, Professor in Physiology at the University of Lund in southern Sweden. The Swedish Government appointed a board that decided on funding for scientific medical projects at Swedish universities. Board members were appointed for a period of three years, with the possibility for one additional three-year term. The Council had a great influence on Swedish medical science, as it was its main supporter and had the largest budget. It was as important for Swedish medical research as the National Institutes of Health were for such research in USA. It was also of great importance for Swedish Nobel Prize winners. These included Sune Bergström, Bengt Samuelsson, Ragnar Granit and later Arvid Carlsson. Other internationally well-known Swedish scientists who were maybe worthy of a Nobel Prize also benefitted, and they included the likes of Torbjörn Caspersson, Clarence Crafoord, Herbert Olivecrona, Jan Waldenström, Inge Edler and Nils Alwall.

Shortly after my appointment as Professor of Medicine in 1985, I was approached by the very powerful and dynamic general secretary of the Council, Professor Henry Danielsson. He told me I had been proposed for several important positions within the Council and he invited me to be a member of the board, which was chaired by the Governor of Malmöhus county, Bertil Göransson. I was invited to be Chairman of the Priority Committee for Medicine, which covered all aspects of clinical internal medicine and Chairman of the Board for Ethical Affairs. Finally, I was asked to be a member of two international organizations, the Nordic Co-operation Committee and the collaborative European Medical Research Council. It was a prestigious proposal and I accepted without considering the amount of work it would involve. A proposal by Danielsson was equivalent to an appointment and I took up all these positions. After a three-year term I was reappointed to all these roles for another three-year term, which meant that I held them from 1986–1992. These were in addition to my work as Professor and Head of the clinical Department of Medicine and later the Department of Hematology at the Huddinge Hospital and the academic Department of Medicine at the Karolinska Institutet Huddinge.

The work at the Medical Research Council was hard but rewarding. There was a risk for bias, because many of the members of the priority committees had substantial funding from the Council. If somebody on a committee was involved in an application for funding, that person, including me, had to leave the meeting room. I had the impression that we all handled the task well. There were no complaints during the first five years of my appointment. However, others did not agree with this view during my last year, and afterwards I left.

Danielsson retired in 1990 and his successor was the Professor of Surgery at Gothenburg, Tore Scherstén. I had known him since our summer vacations in Åhus during, and shortly after, World War Two, when we both were teenagers. He and his brother Bengt Scherstén, later Professor of Medicine at the University of Lund, both belonged to our gang of six or seven youngsters who took advantage of the summer season for swimming, dancing and love affairs. Tore Scherstén was a very strong and able gymnast. He walked on his hands on the seashore, in contrast to his brother, who was less aggressive and in love with my sister Anita. Looking back, I did not see any signs that could have predicted how successful his career would be. However, after he completed his PhD in 1967, and his studies in the USA, he became Professor of Surgery at the University of Gothenburg in 1981 and Dean of the Faculty of Medicine in 1984. He started a successful liver transplant program in Gothenburg and carried out the first transplant there in early 1985. He was disappointed that this was some months after the first transplant in Sweden at the Huddinge Hospital by Carl-Gustav Groth and his team. I lost contact with him for many years, and when I met him again at our first joint Medical Research Council board meeting, it was a friendly encounter. I was looking forward to a great collaboration with him.

Scherstén wanted to make the Council even more important than it had been under the rein of Danielsson. However, he ended up killing the Council and sent it to the graveyard, with the help of the future Nobel Prize winner, Arvid Carlsson.

The Minister of Education, Per Unckel, asked the Council to put together a proposal for the Government about the most important research areas in experimental and clinical medicine in Sweden. He also wanted the Council to point out the fields that had the most competent researchers. The Minister had also approached the councils responsible for other research areas and asked them the same questions. The Royal Swedish Academy of Sciences, who was responsible for awarding the Nobel Prizes in Physics and Chemistry, and in Economics, were also given the same task for their own fields. The reason was that the moderate, Conservative government that was now in power had decided to dissolve the enormous so-called employee funds that had been created by the Social Democrats. These funds were owned by the Government but controlled by the trade unions. Companies had been forced to allocate a certain amount of money to these funds and the new Government wanted to use the funds to support innovative research.

The Minister wanted a rapid response from the Council after it was approached at the end of March 1992 and an extra meeting of the board was called on 6 April. The General Secretary, Scherstén, proposed that the priority committees should identify strong researchers and research groups in Sweden, within eight areas of medicine, and that they should each produce a four-page document of about 1,200 words by 22 May. Then Scherstén would use the documents to produce a final proposal that would be sent to the Minister, Per Unckel. The board agreed. The different priority committees had to team up. I wrote one proposal on gene therapy with Professor Erna Möller and one on diabetes research with Professor Ulf Smith. We described the areas and provided the names of the researchers and research groups. Scherstén summarized all the documents under four titles, trying to include most of what we had written. The final documents described growth research, glycobiology and biosurfaces, metabolic syndrome and knowledge refinement and transfer[89]. It described both the areas and the researchers active within those areas. I was confused that we could not find what we had described in our submissions. However, Scherstén explained that, for example, hematology was covered by the heading growth research and so on. There was no time to amend his proposal. It was sent to the Ministry of Education on 12 June 1992. It was a mistake, as the document had been hastily produced and had not considered the consequences. It covered the equivalent of several hundred million US dollars in Swedish medical research. The Royal Swedish Academy of Sciences had refused to respond, claiming it had not been given enough time. We should have done the same.

The documents soon became official and the research community outside the Medical Research Council was furious. Some research groups noticed that their areas were not included and, in particular, that their names could not be found among the important research groups. They claimed that the universities should have been asked to participate. Worst of all, neuroscience research, which was very strong in those days, could not be found in the prioritized areas and none of the research groups in this field were mentioned. It nearly caused a revolution, led by no less than the future Nobel Prize winner Arvid Carlsson, who was now a semi-retired Professor Emeritus in Gothenburg.

Carlsson was an internationally well-known researcher in neurobiology. He had not yet received the Nobel Prize when the Council submitted its proposal to the Government. Carlsson was born in 1923 and been forced to retire in 1988 at 65 years of age, as that was the Swedish system. I had met Carlsson in 1952 when he was a teacher on the medical chemistry course I attended in Lund (Chapter 12). He had switched from the Institution of Pharmacology to the Institution of Medical Chemistry. I did not know anything about his research at the time. He later revealed in his autobiography, which can be found on nobelprize.org[90], that he was inspired by Torsten Thunberg, Professor in Physiology in Lund, who was nominated for the Nobel Prize 15 times. Thunberg discovered a group of enzymes called dehydrogenases, which are necessary so that the body's cells can breathe. He made the discoveries independent of similar ones made by a German scientist, Otto Warburg, at about the same time. Carlsson dryly made the comment that Warburg received the Nobel Prize, but Thunberg did not. My father's sister Hilma worked as Thunberg's personal technician for 25 years and, according to my father, she was the one who had performed all his pioneering experiments (Chapter 4).

Although Carlsson admired Thunberg, he never worked at his Institution of Physiology for obvious reasons. Thunberg was born in 1873 and retired in 1938, long before Carlsson started his career. Soon after he had graduated, Carlsson started to work as an amanuensis, which was an unpaid assistant, at the Institution of Pharmacology. It was headed by one of Thunberg's favorite students, Professor Gunnar Ahlgren. He inspired Carlsson to study the metabolism of calcium, which led to his dissertation. Ahlgren was still the Head of the Institution of Pharmacology when I was a student and took the pharmacology course in 1953. The students arranged the time of their examinations with him. When I called to make my appointment, he was a patient in the Department of Skin Disorders, which did not hinder him from examining me one day in 1953. When I arrived, he was in bed. His foot was stretched out and his big toe had gone brown. He asked me what I saw. Fortunately, I knew that potassium permanganate was used for some skin disorders, and it turned brown after some hours when it was oxidized by the oxygen in the air. It was the correct answer. After about 45 minutes of further questioning, I was awarded the very good grade in pharmacology med beröm godkänd, which means approved with praise. Then he talked to me about my father, who he had met during their early careers in the 1920s. I hoped that I had not got the high grade due to this connection.

After his dissertation on the metabolism of calcium, Carlsson spent a few more years with Ahlgren. However, in 1955 he turned to the influential and later Nobel Laureate Sune Bergström, Head of the Institution for Medical Chemistry, for advice about how to work in an important pharmacological institution in the USA. Bergström provided him with some contacts, which eventually led to a collaboration with Dr Bernhard B Brodie, Head of the Laboratory of Chemical Pharmacology at the National Heart Institute in Bethesda. This was where his interest for chemical pathways in the brain awakened. After having spent five months in USA, he went back to Lund and teamed up with the innovative Professor Nils Åke Hillarp at the Institution for Histology (Chapter 12). Carlsson went on to make pioneering discoveries and the most important one was the discovery of the neurotransmitter dopamine and the role it plays in how humans move. It was shown that a lack of dopamine caused Parkinson's disease, which then led to discoveries of drugs that could help patients with this traumatizing disorder.

Carlsson was appointed Professor of Pharmacology at the University of Gothenburg in 1959, but had been retired for three years by the time the 1992 Swedish Medical Research Council proposal about the important research areas in Sweden was submitted to the Government. However, he was still active as an emeritus professor and involved with a number of drug companies. He was a combative person, and he was furious that the proposal had neglected the important area of neurobiology. He turned to two of his fellow emeritus professors, who had little to lose in a battle with the powerful Council, Björn Folkow and Anders Lundberg. Both were previous Professors in Physiology. They wrote a couple of protest letters to the Council, but more importantly they drafted a protest and asked all the researchers that represented the Swedish universities to sign it. The protest contained three main points. First, that the proposal should be withdrawn due to the conflicts of interest among those who had produced it. Second, that the researchers in the Council that had produced the proposal were overrepresented among the proposed areas of research and were mentioned by name together with those proposed areas. Third, that the General Secretary, namely Scherstén, the Assistant Secretary Professor Håkan Eriksson and the representatives elected by the universities should resign from the Council. They received 700 responses, including many from professors. About 500 sympathized with the protest, while just under 200 supported the Council's proposal. One problem that the protesters faced was that three of the seven elected board members, including myself, had already resigned shortly after they had produced their sections of the proposal, as they had served on the board for the maximum six-year term. I had resigned less than a month after the production of my part of what Carlsson considered a *"conflict of interest document"*. This meant that only four members of the board who were involved in the proposal would be called on to resign and that the newly appointed ones would be asked to resign despite having had no involvement in the process. The Council and Scherstén did not give in and the proposal that he had written was not withdrawn.

Carlsson did not directly name me, even though he probably knew that I was the author of two of the original eight pre-proposals that were reduced to four by Scherstén. Instead, his target was my co-author of the gene therapy proposal, Professor Möller, who was a deputy board member until I left and was then promoted to a regular one. Möller was a good friend of mine. She was Professor of Transplantation Immunology and Head of the Transplantation Immunology Laboratory at the Huddinge Hospital. Möller was also one of the leading professors at the Karolinska Institutet, having been educated at the Institute of Tumor Biology by George Klein, a member of the Nobel Assembly.

I spoke to her later about her feelings at the time and she claimed that she did not take it very seriously. She was elected to the board without problems and did not leave the board until the next crisis years later, when all board members were substituted for new ones. I discuss this incident later.

My old friend Nils (Nisse) Ringertz (1932–2002) (Chapters 1 and 19) was one of the most aggressive critics of the Swedish Medical Research Council's proposal. He thought, like many others, that the universities, and not the members of Council, should have proposed the key areas and important scientists in Sweden. Ringertz was an important person at the time. He had succeeded Professor Torbjörn Caspersson as Professor of Cell Research and Genetics in 1978, had been a member of the Nobel Assembly since then and had joined the Nobel Committee in 1981. In 1992, when the struggle with the Government was going on, he became the Secretary of both the Assembly and Committee, which put him in a very powerful position. Despite our opposing views about the Council's proposal, we stayed good friends, which was important because of the work we had to do together on the Nobel Committee. I had been a member since 1988, became Deputy Chairman in 1995 and was Chairman, with Ringertz as the Secretary, in 1997. We had to do a good job, and, in my opinion, we did. When Ringertz died in 2002, before his 70th birthday, his successor, Professor Hans Jörnvall, stated that he had participated in deciding about Nobel Prizes in Physiology or Medicine for about one-third of all Laureates since the first Nobel Prize in 1901. Not a bad record.

When I look back on the Swedish Medical Research Council's proposal, I can retrospectively agree with the critics. However, I think that the Minister of Education was the villain in the drama. His requirement for us to deliver a comprehensive proposal in less than two months was unrealistic. Maybe we should have refused to do it, like the Royal Swedish Academy of Sciences had done.

So, what happened to our proposal? The truth is not much. The Government had probably listened to the critics. Although Scherstén remained as General Secretary, and the proposal reached the Ministry of Education, it probably ended up in the bottom of a drawer. The Government, under Prime Minister Carl Bildt, mentioned in the Bill (1992/93:171) that the Swedish Medical Council had delivered some interesting thoughts about the issue, but the Government had decided to use the employee funds for the creation of three new research foundations. Medical research came under the new Strategic Research Foundation for Natural Sciences and Technical Research. This meant that the Medical Research Council was not given any share of the money from the employee funds. However, it was some comfort that many important foundations, like the private Wallenberg Foundations, received information about the important research groups in Sweden. Many of the groups later also received funding from the Strategic Research Foundation.

The Council had to endure another crisis before it was closed down. Two female scientists, Agnes Wold and Christine Wennerås from Gothenburg, where Carlsson was a professor, had not received the positions and funding that they felt they were entitled to. They were both clever and important researchers, at least in one respect. They had analyzed how women had been discriminated against when competing for positions and funding. When I went back and read their seemingly excellent scientific analysis of the distribution of research funding to men and women in the prestigious scientific journal *Nature*[91], I was tempted to admit that there was something true about their criticism. However, this was not my own personal experience during my work with the priority committee. I never even thought about whether applications came from a man or a woman. I tried instead to assess the quality and competence of the applicant. Sometimes I preferred an application in my own field, but only if it could favorably compete with another one in a different field. In general, I tried to avoid assessing such applications, to avoid bias, and let others on the priority committee take the lead on decisions in such situations. However, it was sometimes very difficult to compare applications, as it was like comparing apples and pears, and I cannot exclude the possibility that conflict of interests could exist. However, this was never based on whether an applicant was a man or woman, and I don't remember any other members of the priority committee having such thoughts. Today there are those who think that quotas should have been applied, to ensure that more of the few applications from women should have been funded, but back then the committee did not think like that. The goal was always to fund the best applications and the best research groups.

The result of this feminist attack against the Swedish Medical Research Council was that both the general secretary, Scherstén, and the board had to leave in 1995. The new General Secretary, Professor Olle Stendahl was also a good friend of mine and was a very qualified microbiologist. His job was not easy, as he had to restore trust in the Council.

I had to retire at the end of 1997, as I had reached 65 years of age. However, there was an unwritten rule at the Karolinska

Institutet that emeritus professors had the right to office space and that they could continue working, without a salary, if they managed to secure research funding. I intended to use this privilege, as I had ongoing stem cell transplant projects. Some of them were in collaboration with EBMT, the European Group for Blood and Marrow Transplantation (now the European Society for Blood and Marrow Transplantation), and had been highly rated by the Swedish Medical Research Council. I applied for continued funding from the Council in good faith. However, I received a *"nice"* letter from Stendahl telling me that because I had now retired from my position as a full professor, I no longer had the right to receive funding from the Council. Period. My application was not passed to the priority committee. The decision was taken on some formal grounds that I did not recognize from my own time at the Council, which ended in 1992. This was age discrimination and against the agreement Sweden had signed with the European Union (EU). It was more than a year before I was ready to fight my corner. I had to do the groundwork and to find other professors who had also experienced this discrimination, including some who were approaching retirement and some younger ones who could be co-authors on a debate article. I soon found the perfect person. Professor Emeritus Peter Reichard was a top ranked biochemist and occasionally my antagonist in the Nobel Committee. He had been ranked number two out of 40 applicants for the priority committee for biochemistry before the General Secretary discovered that he had retired. He was denied funding for the same reason as me. He agreed to co-author the debate article. Who else would be interested in participating? Carlsson of course. He had fought against the Council before, as described earlier, and then when he had retired, he had been denied research grants from the Council. In early October 2000, he received the Nobel Prize in Physiology or Medicine. What timing! I approached him and described the issue to him. He enthusiastically agreed to participate. Either he had forgotten that I had been his antagonist during the Council struggle many years ago or he just thought that this was an excellent opportunity for another fight with the organization. I worked on the debate article for some weeks and 15 professors put their names to it, including Carlsson and Reichard. It was published in the largest Swedish daily newspaper *Dagens Nyheter* on 30 December 2000 and there was an immediate reaction[92]. The Minister of Education was now Thomas Östros, who was a Social Democrat. He contacted the Rector and President of the Karolinska Institutet, Professor Hans Wigzell, and asked about age discrimination during the allocation of research funding. Wigzell denied all knowledge of the Council discriminating against retired researchers, as described in our debate article. It had to be stopped. Since the EU directive concerning age discrimination was already in writing and supported by Sweden, no further formal action had to be taken. Age discrimination disappeared quickly among all the research funding organizations in Sweden, at least on paper.

Although I cannot recall that age discrimination was an issue during my own time at the Swedish Medical Research Council, either at board level or in the priority committee for medicine, I am not totally sure whether members thought about the age issue. Neither Danielsson nor Scherstén had indicated that they thought that age should be considered when judging the research applications. The quality of the project was the key factor for funding.

The fact that the Council had been accused of so much discrimination may have been too much for the Government. First it was accused of not letting the universities participate in the allocation of funding, then of discriminating against women and finally of defying the EU rules on age discrimination. The fact that the Council had been instrumental in promoting and been primarily responsible for the fabulous scientific achievements by Swedish scientists until the end of the 20th century could not save it. I admit that I am proud that I participated in this development. But the Council was dissolved and disappeared as an organization on its own. A new body for governmental research money allocation was born and was called the Swedish Research Council. Medical science was just one part of it. The principles of evaluating and distributing funding seemed similar to the Swedish Medical Research Council, but now a new organization was in charge. It was obvious that the Nobel Prize winner Carlsson had at least one finger in the pot of this development.

36 The Work of the Nobel Committee

In early 1988, I was asked to join the Nobel Committee as an adjunct member. It would involve hard work and reviewing nominees for the Nobel Prize. The instructions were clear and that was that everything that was discussed within the Committee, as well as information about nominees or nominators, was secret for the next 50 years. I accepted the offer with pleasure. The following year I was elected to the Nobel Assembly, a position that I kept until my retirement at the end of 1997. I was repeatedly elected as an adjunct member of the Nobel Committee, until I was elected to be one of the five ordinary members. In 1995, I became vice chairman of the Committee, and in 1997 I became the chairman.

Without revealing any secrets, it is easy to understand why I was elected in 1988. The Nobel Prize was awarded to Sir James W Black, Gertrude (Trudy) B Elion and George H Hitchings *"for their discoveries of important principles for drug treatment"*. Black had discovered certain molecules in the stomach, the H2 receptors, that became the targets for an H2 receptor blocking drug, cimetidine, that could cure ulcers in the stomach. The discovery caused a revolution in treating stomach ulcers, that until then had been treated by surgery. Now it became possible to cure stomach ulcers with a pill. Surgery was no longer needed for this disease, with rare exceptions. Black also discovered another receptor antagonist, propranolol, which was antagonistic to adrenaline receptors in the heart and helped to prevent excitation of the heart

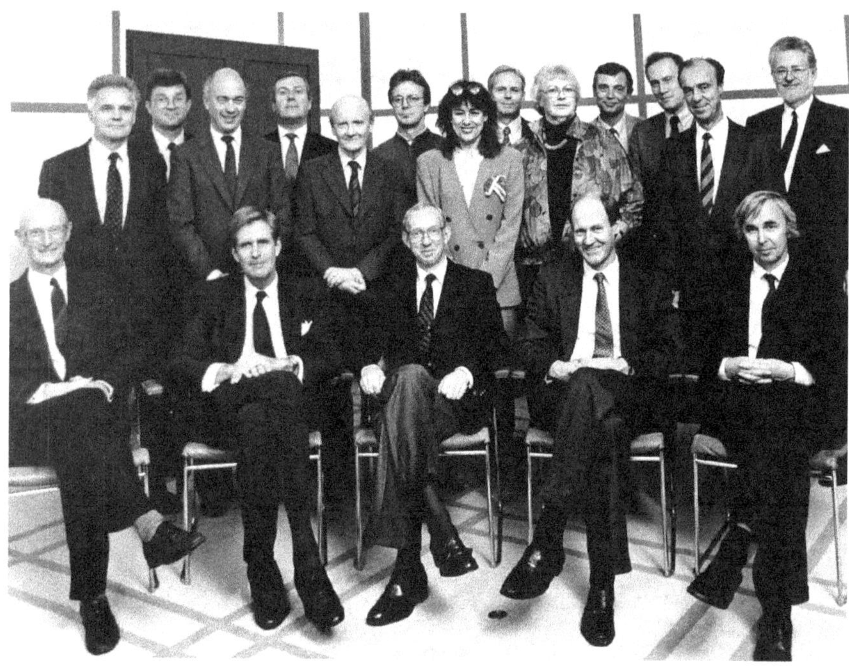

The Nobel Committee in 1988.

Sitting from left to right were the ordinary members: Jan Wersäll, Sten Orrenius, Bengt Samuelsson (Nobel Laureate and President and Rector of the Karolinska Institutet), Tomas Hökfelt, Hans Wigzell (later President and Rector of the Karolinska Institutet).

Standing from left to right were the adjuncts and secretary: Gösta Gahrton (the author), Sten Grillner, Alf Lindberg (later Secretary), Folke Sjöqvist, Viktor Mutt, Göran Akusjärvi, Anita Aperia, Göran Holm, Kerstin Hall, Bertil Fredholm, Nils Ringertz (later Secretary), Erling Norrby (later Secretary of the Swedish Academy of Sciences, responsible for the Nobel Prizes in Physics and Chemistry) and Jan Lindsten (Secretary).

and the risk of atrial fibrillation. This was a new principle for preventing this disorder.

Hitchings and Elion had worked together. Hitchings was the older of the two and considered to be a mentor to Elion. However, Elion was instrumental in developing two mainly new drugs, the cytotoxic drug 6-mercaptopurine that she showed could kill leukemic cells and the first antiviral drug, acyclovir. Both drugs were effective in treating diseases that had not been treatable earlier.

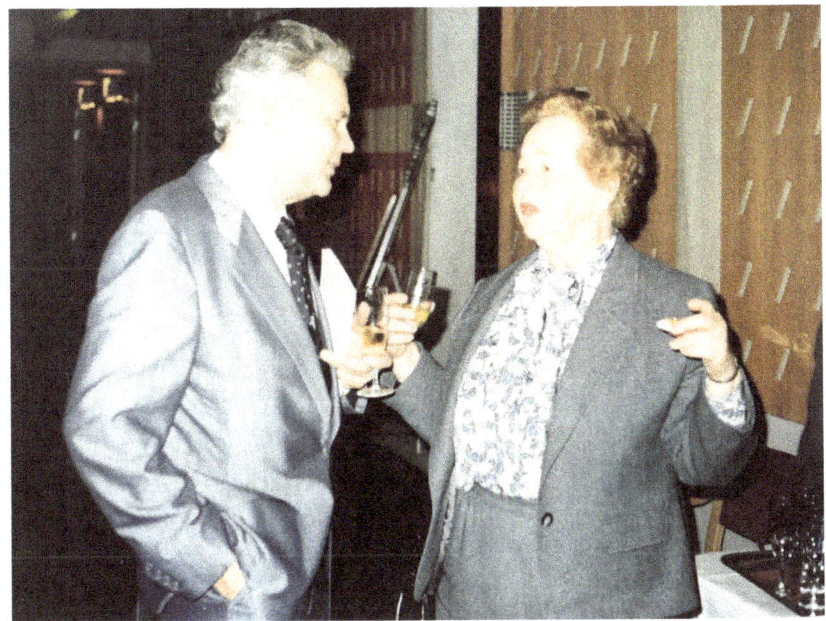

The author in discussions with Nobel Laureate Gertrude (Trudy) Elion, during a reception at the Karolinska Institutet during Nobel Week in December 1988. This picture was taken a few days before the Nobel Prize ceremony in the Concert Hall and the Banquet in the City Hall in Stockholm.

The principles of treatment were new and changed the pessimistic views on cancer and virus disease treatment possibilities. The discussions in the Nobel Committee that led to these prizes can be read in 2039 in an addendum that I will present to the Nobel archives at the Karolinska Institutet.

Of the 21 Nobel Prizes that were awarded during my 10 years on the Committee, I rate the 1990 Prize awarded to Joseph Murray and Donnall Thomas the highest. At last, here was a prize for clinical medicine that related to a very well-defined discovery, i.e. "for their discoveries concerning organ and cell transplantation in the treatment of human disease" (Chapter 30). The Committee's discussions about the other nominees will be made public in 2041.

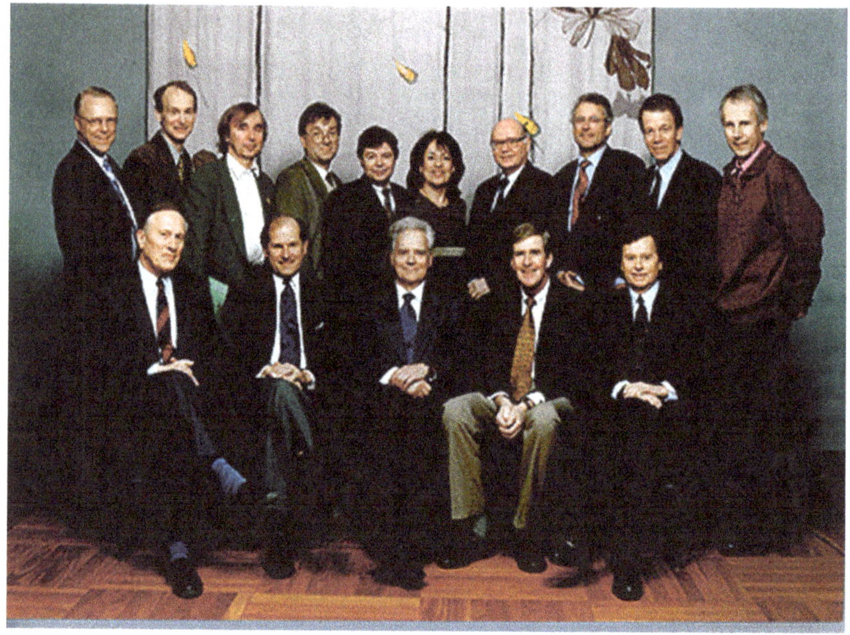

The Nobel Committee in 1997.

Ordinary members sitting from left to right: Nils Ringertz (Secretary), Ralf Pettersson (later Chairman), the author Gösta Gahrton (Chairman), Sten Orrenius and Göran Sedvall.

Adjunct members standing from left to right: Hans Jörnvall (later Secretary), Björn Wennström, Hans Wigzell (President and Rector of the Karolinska Institutet), Sten Grillner, Karl Tryggvason, Anita Aperia, Bertil Daneholt, Bo Angelin, Lars Klareskog and Rune Toftgård.

The last prize during my time on the Committee went to Stanley Prusiner in 1997 *"for his discovery of Prions — a new biological principle of infection"*. Prusiner had studied a group of very unusual disorders that were not caused by bacteria or viruses. He showed that they were caused by some kind of protein particles that were different from both of these organisms, which he called proteinaceous infectious particles or prions[93]. These particles caused a neurological disease in cattle called bovine spongiform encephalopathy (BSE), also known as mad cow disease. Scrapie, which is a similar disease in sheep, was also caused by prions. Creutzfeldt-Jakob disease is a very unusual form of dementia that affects humans and a variant of it is considered to be caused by prions and is known as variant Creutzfeldt-Jakob disease[94]. The disease is considered to be caused by eating meat contaminated with BSE. Cattle that have been fed meat meal are the source of the prions that infect humans, and this is now prohibited in the EU. Prusiner's discovery was controversial at the start. Many research groups in the USA considered prions to be just viruses. In the middle of the night, after the Nobel Prize had been announced, I was woken by the phone. *"Is this Professor Gahrton, Chairman of the Nobel Committee?"* I expected some crazy person at the other end and was ready to hang up. However, after some seconds I said *"Yes, who is calling?"* He continued: *"Are you the Chairman of the Nobel Committee that decided to award Stanley Prusiner the Nobel Prize?"* I repeated *"Yes, who is calling?"* He continued *"I am calling from the journal Newsweek in the USA. Here, most scientists in the field claim that the particles that Prusiner calls prions are just viruses"*.

Although the field related to this Nobel Prize was far away from my own, I had gained valuable information from the specialists on the Committee. This meant that I could inform the journalist about a couple of research groups in the USA that did not believe in Prusiner's discovery, but that after 10 years of debate most scientists in the field had been able to confirm his discoveries about prions. I convinced him that the prize was one of the best documented and original ones in the history of the Nobel Prize. I believed that I had convinced him, and my proof was in the next issue of *Newsweek*, where he had written a short, but positive, comment about the prize. Today, the 1997 Nobel Prize is not considered controversial.

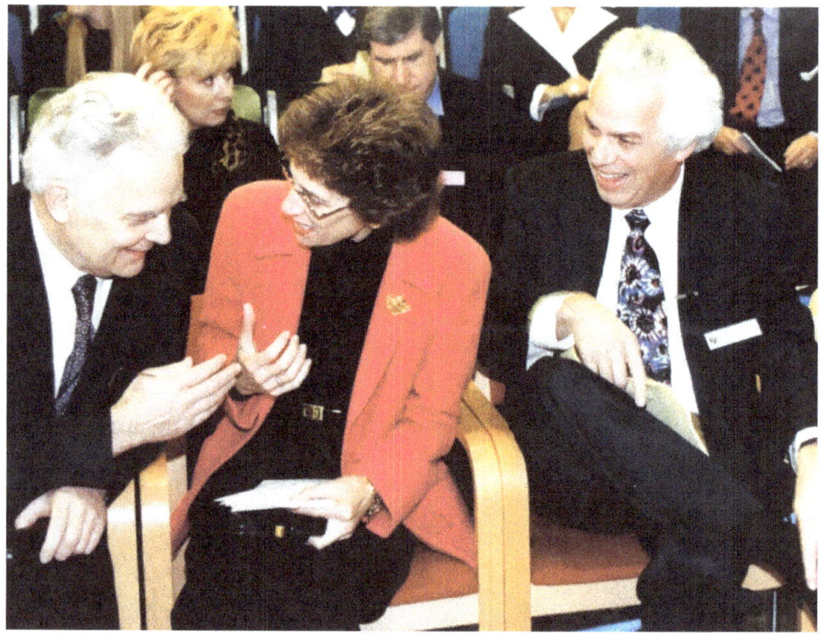

The author with the 1997 Nobel Laureate Stanley Prusiner and his wife before his Nobel lecture at the Karolinska Institutet during Nobel Week in December of that year.

The Nobel Committee has a tradition to invite the Nobel Laureates in Physiology or Medicine to a dinner at the Thielska Galleriet art gallery in Stockholm a couple of days before the award ceremony and the great Nobel Party at Stockholm City Hall on December 10. I had planned to ask Prusiner a tricky question at the end of my dinner speech to him. He had called the proteinaceous infectious particles prions and not proins, which would have been a more logical form. I asked him why he called the particles prions, which according to the English dictionary referred to a genus of sea birds, namely *Pachyptila* in Latin. Prusiner had no answer, maybe for the first time. However, the name is now well established in the scientific community. The discussion in the Nobel Committee about other candidates for the prize in 1997 can be revealed in 2048.

Chapter 37
Researchers Claiming to be Worthy of the Nobel Prize

There are some scientists who claim to be, or at least consider themselves to be, worthy of the Nobel Prize, but never receive it. Sometimes they are right, but sometimes they overestimate their scientific contributions. In addition, individual Committee members are sometimes approached and informed about a scientific discovery that the informer thinks should be worthy of the award. Since all nominations result from invitations, such approaches could come from people who have not been invited or the person that has made the discovery. I was approached a few times because I was a member of the Committee.

On one occasion, the Chief Executive Officer of the Nobel Foundation, Stig Ramel, invited me to a dinner with a few important foreign professors in medicine. It was a few days before the award ceremony and some 20 people attended. I had no idea why those particular dinner guests had been selected. I had been invited because I had been asked to give the speech to celebrate Donnall Thomas's achievement at the award ceremony a couple of days later. I was seated at a table for six people and next to the famous Professor of Medicine, Francesco Balsano, from the Department of Medicine at the University in Rome, La Sapienza. He told me that he was interested in hematology and stem cell transplants and invited me to give a lecture on these topics. I accepted and we agreed that the title of my talk would be *"Bone marrow transplantation today and in the future"*. I did not know him but was later informed by my friends in Italy that he was one of the most powerful Professors in Medicine in Rome and had the nickname *"The Pharaoh"*. It was a very tempting invitation, particularly because the lecture would be given in association with the opening of a new research unit at the hospital called the New Research Center of Fondazione Andrea Cesalpino. It would also be followed by a black-tie dinner. I was disappointed that I would not be able to go, because I was due to be the host for Louis Sullivan and his wife in Stockholm at the same time. However, Professor Balsano insisted that I should come to visit him another time and eventually I went to Rome to give the lecture on 3 December 1991, one year after our first encounter at the dinner party. I gave the lecture to about 100 people, then we took his private elevator from the lecture hall to his enormous and luxurious office. After a short introductory chat, he showed me a couple of electron microscopic pictures showing hepatitis B virus particles and told me about how he had discovered the virus as well as the cell therapy that could kill it. I listened politely and praised his discovery. Nothing was said about the Nobel Prize, although the aim of the conversation was obvious. However, in his defense, I later found out that he had published what he had claimed to me in *Nature* the previous year[95]. Balsano never received the Nobel Prize.

According to my sources, he was accused of abusing his position as a member of the Italian Medicines Agency. In an interview with an Italian newspaper, which was cited in the Swedish press, he denied everything and claimed that he had excellent contacts with the Swedish Nobel Prize Committee at the Karolinska Institutet, which had given him great credit for his discovery of the hepatitis B virus. I felt that a media drive to find the responsible Committee member was not far away, but it never happened.

Another researcher that I knew relatively well was Don Metcalf (1929–2014), who seemed to think that he was worthy of the Nobel Prize. Metcalf was Head of the Cancer Research Unit in Melbourne's Walter and Eliza Hall Institute of Medical Research in Australia at the time. He knew that my research group at the Huddinge Hospital worked with stem cells. We cultured stem cells from leukemia patients in the hope that we would identify important patterns that could lead to treatment options. Per Hörnsten's dissertation dealt with this issue (Chapter 34). We used an ingenious method that Metcalf had published. It demonstrated that individual hematopoietic committed stem cells gave rise to colonies of mature granulocytes in a Petri dish. Later he used the method to show that blood from both normal individuals and patients with leukemia had a soluble factor, namely granulocyte colony stimulating factor (G-CSF), which was a prerequisite for the growth of the colonies and the production of the mature granulocytes. It later led to the commercial production of G-CSF as the drug filgrastim, marketed under the name Neupogen, that can save patients with cyclic neutropenia, which is an unusual disease. In this disease the neutrophil leukocytes, also called granulocytes, cannot be produced in sufficient amounts and this can cause severe, sometimes lethal, infectious diseases. The drug can also save patients with infections caused by neutropenia related to intensive cancer treatment, such as stem cell transplants.

I met Metcalf many times and invited him to Stockholm to give lectures. Once he was very keen to talk about the history of the discovery of the experimental culture system, which was the precondition for identifying the colonies and stimulating factor. He had published the discoveries with Thomas Ray Bradley (1923–2013) but had toned down Bradley's contribution when he described the history. However, the truth was that Bradley had developed the colony assay in the early 1960s after he returned home to the Physiology Department at the University of Melbourne, having spent a couple of years learning cell culture at the National Cancer Institute in Bethesda, USA. Bradley was the first name on the two ground-breaking publications in 1966 and 1967[96]. The 1967 paper was published in the prestigious journal *Nature*. Bradley also seemed to have shown that blood contained a factor that had to be present for the colonies to be formed before they started their collaboration in 1966.

However, it seemed to be true that Metcalf led the work to make it a commercial drug. In fact, his work led to the identification and purification of three additional colony-stimulating factors, the granulocyte-macrophage CSF (GM-CSF), macrophage CSF (M-CSF) and multi-CSF, now known as interleukin-3. His group also cloned the gene for GM-CSF.

Metcalf may well have been worthy of the Nobel Prize, but not without Bradley. His description of the history did not help. Neither of them got the Nobel Prize.

The Nobel Prize in Physiology or Medicine was shared in 2008. One winner was Harald zur Hausen for his discovery of the human papilloma viruses that cause cervical cancer. The other winners were Françoise Barré-Sinoussi and Luc Montagnier for their discovery of the human immunodeficiency virus (HIV). I have reason to believe that at least two people were very disappointed that they were not included in the Nobel Prize for the discovery of the HIV.

Robert (Bob) Gallo was, and still is, an outstanding researcher. By 1982, he had discovered the first retrovirus, the T-cell leukemia virus, which caused an unusual form of acute leukemia in adults[97].

He was also an excellent lecturer and was invited to meetings and congresses to give the most prestigious lectures. I invited him a couple of times to give lectures at meetings that I arranged. The most important was the European Gene Therapy Congress in Stockholm in 2000, when he was the main speaker. At the time we were running the first clinical gene marking study in Sweden (Chapter 46), and I was very interested in clinical gene therapy. Gallo had spent several years researching the cause of AIDS and claimed he had discovered the HIV virus. This was challenged by Luc Montagnier's group at the Institute Pasteur in Paris. The argument between these two research groups about who discovered the HIV virus first was primarily about patents and both had strong backers. Luc Montagnier had Institute Pasteur, which was representing the French Government, and Gallo had the Food and Drug Administration, which was representing the US Government.

The patent struggle seemed to have been resolved when Gallo arrived in Stockholm and I picked him up in my car to drive him to the hotel that the congress organizer, Congrex AB, had chosen. I didn't give their choice much thought. I was too busy driving and listening to Gallo's monologue, in which he described in detail how he had discovered the HIV virus. Knowing about the struggle between the two research groups I decided not to comment. However, I knew that the matter was in arbitration and decided that he must have had another reason to try to convince me about his role in the discovery. Again, as in the case described above, I believe that he thought that my role in the Nobel Committee was still important. He obviously did not know that I had left the Committee three years earlier.

As I approached the hotel, I suddenly realized that this was one of the most basic hotels in Stockholm. On his registration form Gallo, or probably his secretary, had chosen a class three hotel instead of class one, probably thinking that class three would provide the best accommodation. This would not have been a good start to his stay, as he was used to first-class flights and luxury hotels wherever he was invited. Fortunately, his very good friend Professor Peter Biberfeld had, for some reason, realized the error. When we arrived at the hotel, his room had been cancelled and a new reservation had been made by Biberfeld at one of the best hotels in Stockholm. We continued our drive, and everything was in order.

Gallo never received the Nobel Prize, at least he has not received it so far. It was to his credit that when we next met in Mannheim, Germany, we were still good friends and the Nobel Prize was not mentioned. This was at the European Leukemia Net, the year after Luc Montagnier and Francoise Barré Sinoussi received the Prize that Gallo clearly wanted.

A much more direct approach about the 2008 Nobel Prize was made by a friend of mine in the Eurogenethy network, which was financed by the European Commission and led by Professor Odile Cohen-Haguenauer in Paris (Chapter 47). At the European Society of Gene and Cell Therapy Congress in 2009, David Klatzmann presented a 30-minute lecture about the discovery of the HIV virus. He claimed his role in the discovery was as fundamental as, and equivalent to, that of Luc Montagnier. He may have had a point, as his name later appeared on the list of patent owners.

I could not follow his arguments in detail at the lecture, so I asked him to write about his own involvement in the discovery of the HIV virus, which caused AIDS. In 2021, I received a 20-page document. First, I thought that it would be better to publish the full story in his own words, so that anyone who had any insight into the complex matter of collaborative research could reach their own conclusions. However, since that would have been too much for a book like this one, I have included his Summary and Conclusion in his own words:

My contribution to the discovery of a new virus that causes AIDS by David Klatzmann

Summary

"Announcing the 2008 Nobel Prize in Physiology or Medicine, the Nobel Committee wrote in short: "Professor Francoise Barré-Sinoussi and Professor Luc Montagnier discovered human immunodeficiency virus-1 (HIV-1), the first human lentivirus. They characterized the virus based on its morphological, biochemical, and immunological properties and demonstrated the capacity to induce massive virus replication and cell damage to lymphocytes."

In the more detailed account of "The discovery of human immunodeficiency virus (HIV)" made by the Nobel Committee, the awarded discovery is described as covered in only two scientific articles:

- *Barré-Sinoussi et al., (1983) Science: Isolation of a T-lymphotropic retrovirus from a patient at risk for acquired immune deficiency syndrome (AIDS).[98]*
- *Klatzmann et al., (1984) Science: Selective tropism of lymphadenopathy associated virus (LAV) for helper-inducer T lymphocytes.[99]*

In this document, I show that (i) I had a key role in the "discovery of HIV-1" (1st article), although I was omitted as an author and (ii) I was the senior independent scientist who demonstrated

HIV capacity "to induce massive replication and cell damage to T lymphocytes" (2nd article), the property demonstrating that HIV was the cause and not a consequence of AIDS. I also show that this article should have been printed in mid-1983, a year earlier than it has been.

My contribution to these discoveries and articles can be summarized as follows:

- *I was the key person who elaborated the "lymph node hypothesis", THE critical hypothesis licensing the first isolation of HIV, and I contributed to the work reported in the first article.*
- *I conceived, designed, performed, and analysed the experiments demonstrating the HIV tropism and cytopathic effect for CD4 lymphocytes; I am the senior and independent author of this work that was a collaboration with the Pasteur team.*

I made the first integrated presentation of the results of these 2 articles in August 1983 at the International Immunology meeting in Kyoto, even before the presentation by Luc Montagnier at the Cold Spring Harbor meeting of September 1983.

The Nobel Prize Committee did not realize my role in the rewarded work, likely because:

- *they missed the true origin of the "lymph node hypothesis" that they erroneously attributed to the Nobelists, although Montagnier himself repeatedly attributed it to us (i.e., in the Scientific American issue of October 1988).*
- *they could not know that I participated in the HIV isolation process because I was erroneously omitted as an author of the HIV isolation report, as later acknowledged by a government appointed independent committee that reviewed the authorship of the report.*

- *they did not realize that I should have the credit for demonstrating that HIV has the capacity "to induce massive replication and cell damage to T lymphocytes", a work that I conceived, designed, and performed, as acknowledged repeatedly by Luc Montagnier.*
- *they could not know that my article on HIV tropism and cytopathic effect was sent for publication to Nature in June 1983, only a few months after the publication of HIV isolation and had suffered major flaws in its review process, in link with the starting confrontation between the French and US groups for the paternity of HIV discovery.*

Conclusion

The 2008 Nobel Prize in Physiology or Medicine has been attributed for the discovery of a new virus that causes AIDS. As claimed by the Committee, this started with setting up experimental procedures to look for a virus in a lymph node of a patient with generalized lymphadenopathy, the key to the success; it ended with the demonstration that the virus was different from previously known viruses and had a specific tropism for CD4 cells that it killed.

The Nobel Prize was rewarded to Françoise Barré-Sinoussi and Luc Montagnier. It is probable that analysing the history of the discovery, the Nobel Prize Committee did not have access to the following information:

- *the lymph node hypothesis was from the working group on AIDS established at the Pitié-Salpêtrière hospital in Paris, and more specifically from me, and the account of this in a letter to the journal Science and even articles by Montagnier himself unfortunately remained unnoticed.*

- *the article on the tropism should have been published just a few months after the paper relating the discovery of the virus and the review process for this paper was strongly flawed. I was the leading investigator for this work, which was a collaboration with and not a supervision by the Pasteur team.*
- *I should have been an author (likely the 3rd after the 2 virologists) of the initial paper on the discovery of LAV, given the fact that I put up the lymph node hypothesis and analysed the lymph node cells, results included in the paper.*
- *I was never under the supervision of Luc Montagnier or Françoise Barré-Sinoussi.*

Despite my frustration, I continued my work from (i) observing no CD4 T cells in AIDS patients; (ii) showing CD4 tropism and cytopathic effect of the virus and (iii) showing disappearance of the CD4 molecules at the surface of infected cells to formulate the hypothesis that CD4 could be a receptor for the virus. I conceived and performed experiments that proved it and discovered what is the first known retrovirus receptor. The description of a specific virus receptor on a human cell drastically changed the field of receptor biology and opened the doors to a whole new science of virus/host cell interaction.

There are ample documentation available and key witnesses to confirm this account of my contribution.

This document was first elaborated under suggestion from Daniel Cohen, a renowned geneticist who I had known since 1981 when I was collaborating with Jean Dausset (Nobel Prize winner) on suppressor T cells at the Saint Louis hospital. Daniel saw my distress and knew this story long before the prize was awarded.

An important witness is Professor Pierre-André Cazenave, who was the chief of the Immunology Department of the Pasteur

Institute at that time. Pierre André Cazenave is both an outsider (he never collaborated with Luc Montagnier, nor with me) and an insider (he was a Pasteur Institute Professor, my teacher for two courses that I attended at the Pasteur Institute — General Immunology, 1980; Specialized Immunology, 1981 — and the president of the Jury of my "Doctorat d'Etat ès Sciences Naturelles" in 1985, in which jury participated both Luc Montagnier and Jean Claude Chermann, among others).

Another important person, who could confirm my contribution to the initial scientific article relating the first HIV isolation, is Laurent Chambaz, my attorney for the litigation that took place regarding this point.

Finally, Norman Letvin confirmed to me in writing that my first integrated presentation of LAV isolation, tropism and cytopathic effect for CD4 T cells at the International Immunology meeting in Kyoto, August 1983, convinced him that this virus was the cause of AIDS."

I must reiterate that this was David Klatzmann's own version about his role in the discovery of the HIV virus that causes AIDS. However, I believe that he had a point, at least about his contribution to the discovery being important. It also illustrates that there are frequently many contributors to a great discovery. Most of the time, the Nobel Committee has managed very well to award the worthiest ones, which seems to be the reason for the Nobel Prize's reputation.

Perhaps it is unfair to include İhsan Doğramacı under this heading. He invited me to Ankara to present a lecture on stem cell transplants at the famous Hacettepe University. It wasn't until I returned home that it occurred to me that my visit to Ankara might have had something to do with my role as a member of the Nobel Committee.

My collaborator and friend Sıraç Dilber, who I first met in 1992, had many contacts in Turkey, including the Minister of Health. He also had established contact with Murat Tuncer, Professor in Pediatrics at Hacettepe University in Ankara, who was interested in gene therapy and transplants (Chapters 45–46). After Tuncer visited Stockholm in 1997, I was invited to give a lecture about stem cell transplants at the University. This formal invitation came from Ihsan Doğramacı, who was a very rich man, physician and great supporter of medical science[100].

Although I did not know anything about the person who had invited me, I accepted the invitation, as Sıraç had assured me that he was a serious person and a great supporter of medical research. He was not exaggerating. Doğramacı was born in 1915 in Erbil, Iraq, which at that time belonged to the Ottoman Empire. His family had amassed a great fortune from the oil market. Eventually, the Doğramacı family moved to Ankara and invested a large part of their fortune in land around the capital. The rumor was that the family owned the greater part of the city. Doğramacı was a pediatrician and seemed to have spent quite some time in this profession when he was younger. He also spent some time on research but was not a well-known scientist himself. Instead, he devoted his life to financially supporting research. He was appointed Professor of Pediatrics in Ankara in 1955, and partly supported the establishment of the Hacettepe University, which was a well-known Turkish institution. However, after some time he became disappointed with the way the government steered the university. This was why he initiated, and partly financed, the building of a new private university in Ankara. The Bilkent University is now one of the leading ones in Turkey. During my visit, when I was guided by Doğramacı himself, it had just opened and was still scarcely populated. However, this seemed to have changed in later years.

Although Doğramacı was not a famous scientist himself, he was known as an enthusiastic organizer and initiator in many important organizations, such as the World Health Organization, UNICEF and the International Pediatric Association. Doğramacı was a gracious man, who gave me a laudatory introduction, based on my *curriculum vitae*, including the fact that I was a member of the famous Nobel Committee at the Karolinska Institutet. I gave my lecture on stem cell transplants and gene therapy for about a hundred of his colleagues at the Hacettepe University.

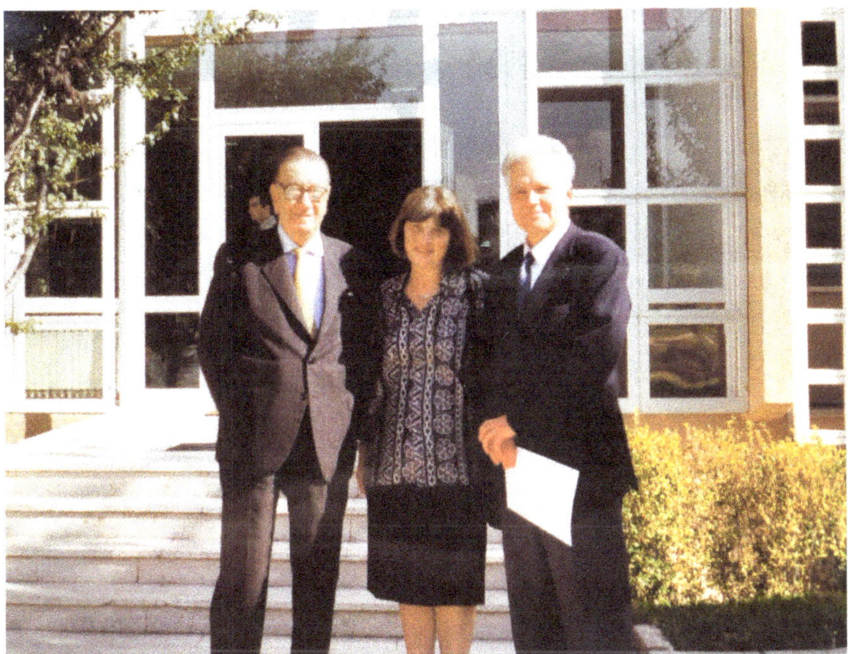

Ihsan Doğramacı, Professor of Pediatrics, initiator, and financier of Bilkent University in Ankara, together with the author and the author's wife Astrid.

An interesting discussion followed the lecture. Doğramacı had invited me and my wife to a party in his home, which was more like a minor palace than an ordinary family residence. An orchestra greeted us with classical music, and we were guided around his home by the host himself. His art collection was impressive, and the paintings included a typical work by Miró, with a dedication to Doğramacı within the artwork. The delicious dinner for some one hundred guests took place in one of the most luxurious dining rooms. At the end of the dinner, I gave a traditional speech of thanks and alluded to an event in Swedish-Turkish history. When the Swedish King Charles XII had lost the battle at Poltava in Russia, he and his closest surviving officers and soldiers fled south to Turkey, where they were treated as important guests by the Turkish Sultan Ahmed III for five years. Being treated as an important guest in Turkey was a great favor.

The question that was ringing in my head was whether Doğramacı had any thoughts of receiving the Nobel Prize for his support for medical research? In that case he had not read the testament of Alfred Nobel, highlighting the need for a *"discovery"*. Without underestimating my own lecture and research, I concluded that I had received a sumptuous reception. It ended with a private guided tour to Cappadocia for a few days.

38 Journal of Internal Medicine and Acta Medica Scandinavica

Scientific journals are the key to documenting new discoveries. Reports at scientific meetings may be important, but it is safer to rely on discoveries that are accepted for publication in important scientific journals. Some journals can publish short communications on important discoveries quickly on their internet pages and this may be enough to prioritize news of a discovery. However, most of the detailed research that is published has to go through a long peer-review process by reviewers who should not have any conflicts of interest with either the subject or the authors. This process may take 4–6 months from submission to publication. If the paper is then rejected, the author has to go through the same process again. David Klatzmann's paper (Chapter 37) illustrates the complications that might occur. Trust in the journal is also important. The impact factor, which measures the number of citations in relation to the number of articles in the journal, is considered to provide a measure of the quality of a journal. A journal with a low impact factor may publish less important discoveries, while a journal with a high impact factor is supposed to publish more important work. The goal of most scientists is to be published in a journal with both a high impact factor and a short publication time, especially if they want a Nobel Prize.

I was the Chairman of a Society that financed a journal that initially focused on Nordic countries, but evolved into an international title, with a high impact factor, that tried to attract potential Nobel Prize winners.

"If I had foreseen that it was to be that excellent, I would not have battled against your action to change its name". That was what my previous boss at the Karolinska Hospital, Henrik Lagerlöf, Emeritus Professor of Medicine at the Karolinska Institutet, said when the first issue of the *Journal of Internal Medicine*, or JIM for short, appeared in 1989. The battle to change the name from *Acta Medica Scandinavica* had lasted a year.

On 18 March 1982, I was asked by my colleague Stephan Rössner if I would consider being a member of the Association for the Publication of *Acta Medica Scandinavica*. Its annual meeting was due to be held the same day at the Karolinska Hospital. I could be elected and be a member of the Association with no membership fee. It was a non-profit association whose sole aim was to publish *Acta Medica Scandinavica*. The Journal was launched in 1863 as the *Medicinskt Arkiv* (Medical Archive) by Axel Key, the former President and Rector of the Karolinska Institutet. In 1869 it became the *Nordiskt Medicinskt Arkiv* (Nordic Medical Archive) and in 1901 it was split into two sections, focusing on internal medicine and surgery. In 1919, the internal medicine section became a journal in its own right, *Acta Medica Scandinavica*. Its long history was attached to the Karolinska Institutet by the statutes of the Association. Any changes had to be approved by the Karolinska Institutet and it would receive any remaining assets if the society and journal was dissolved.

The meeting was attended by a few colleagues that I did not know, together with the Chairman, Leif Hallberg, Professor of Medicine at Gothenburg, and the other board members. The annual report was presented and approved, and the board was re-elected. *Acta Medica Scandinavica* had published good research that year and everybody was happy.

I do not remember participating again in the Association until 27 March 1987, when I agreed to join the Editorial Board and the Board of the Association. The few members that were not on the board had just one task and that was to ensure that the Editor-in-Chief and the board produced the best possible scientific journal within the budget. Interest in being a member was not very high and the yearly meetings were poorly attended. In April 1988, the Association had 62 members, including 31 who were retired, two who were living abroad and 11 who were board members or auditors.

There had been many famous chief editors before I joined the Editorial Board, such as Jan Waldenström (Chapter 18), who had published some of his most important work in the journal. These included the paper on benign monoclonal gammopathy in the 1940s, which made the distinction between monoclonal and polyclonal gamma-protein increases.

The Editor-in-Chief during my first period as a board member was Lars Erik Böttiger. He had been Professor of Medicine at the Karolinska Institutet but had resigned three years earlier to be Head of Medical Research at the KabiVitrum pharmaceutical company. He was an active Editor-in-Chief with ideas about how to improve the journal. There was a lot of competition for the best manuscripts that could receive the highest citations. The journal's publisher, Almqvist & Wiksell, was pessimistic and claimed that the journal could only be published with a financial deficit, which had been the case for many years. Although the journal had good reserves, thanks to clever financial decisions and an important grant from a philanthropist in the 1920s, it could not continue to make a loss.

Together with the Chairman of the Board, Professor Leif Hallberg, Böttiger started to change and improve the journal. In June 1988, he told the editorial staff and the board that he was considering moving to a new publisher, Blackwell Scientific Publications. The board agreed on 1 January 1989, and the Journal was soon making a profit. Böttiger now wanted to make this mainly Scandinavian journal an international publication with an international Editorial Board. We all reached out to our contacts and pulled together a highly competent Editorial Board, including famous scientists from all over the world.

Hallberg and Böttiger arranged mini symposia to generate review publications on current topics and encouraged the submission of better original manuscripts. The aim was to generate more citations and increase the impact factor.

Böttiger told the board that he wanted to change the name of the Journal, as it was too provincial and no longer reflected their international focus. The name change was discussed at a board meeting on 25 April 1988 and Böttiger suggested that *Journal of Internal Medicine* was the best choice. Other names that were discussed were the Scandinavian Journal of Medicine, The New Journal of Medicine, Journal of Clinical and Experimental Medicine and European Journal of Medicine. Three months later, the board unanimously decided to propose Böttiger's suggestion to the Association's members.

The name change had to be approved by two-thirds of the attending members because it involved a change of the statute, and it automatically changed the name of the Association to The Association for the Publication of *Journal of Internal Medicine*.

The Karolinska Institutet had already approved the name change in November 1988, after a letter from Hallberg and Böttiger.

Böttiger wasn't expecting the scale of the opposition that the proposed name change provoked. Lagerlöf, now 81 years old, took the lead, supported by Emeritus Professor Nils (Nisse) Törnblom. Göran Holm and I, both Professors of Medicine at the Karolinska Institutet and chairs of the Departments of Medicine at the two University hospitals, and board members, supported the proposal. Böttiger explained the background to the proposal, including declining sales, increasing competition for the best manuscripts and the declining impact factor. The name change was not the only action that had to be taken. Lagerlöf argued that a name change would not improve the quality of the journal and that *Acta Medica Scandinavica* had worked well since 1919. Nisse Törnblom agreed. Jan Waldenström was not at the meeting, but I had received a letter from him before it took place. He said that he did not *"think it appropriate to break out from the Scandinavian Actas"*. He mentioned *Acta Paediatrica* as an example.

Waldenström had been the Editor-in-Chief for many years. I thought about his paradigm-shifting work on monoclonal and polyclonal gammopathies, which he had published in the journal in the 1940s. I also thought about his later work on macroglobulinemia, which had made him world famous, and, in my opinion, worthy of a Nobel Prize. His words were very important. However, the rest of the letter gave more hope. He said he preferred the name the *European Journal of Medicine*. However, Blackwell had warned us not to use a regional name. Still, this comment indicated that Waldenström might accept a name change.

Our friendship, despite these adversities, was confirmed at the end of the letter, when he said, *"Thanks for the excellent bone marrow symposium*". He was alluding to a symposium on bone marrow transplants that I had organized during the Annual Meeting of the Swedish Medical Association. I replied that I respected his view but would support the proposal at the meeting.

The proposal won with a sufficient majority. Only two members, Henrik Lagerlöf and Stina Björk, voted against the name change. Remarkably, Nisse Törnblom abstained from voting, together with Ed Varnauskas, a cardiologist. Nine members voted in favor. These were the six members of the board, plus Professor Per Björntorp from Gothenburg, Professor Anders G Olsson from Linköping and Torbjörn Lundman, Chief Physician at the Danderyd Hospital and the royal private physician to the King of Sweden.

With the name change agreed, Böttiger wanted to create a national scientific editorial advisory board to complement the international one. This would spread knowledge about the journal across Sweden and encourage clinical researchers to submit their best manuscripts. He asked the members of the Association to help him gather suitable names from all the Swedish universities. Most of the people that were suggested were not members of the Association, and on 7 February 1989 we elected 19 new members. Once again there was a lively debate. Waldenström was present this time. He was somewhat cryptic but appeared mainly positive. Perhaps our correspondence had some influence on his view. Only four opposed the name change and the election of the new members, including Lagerlöf, Törnblom and a former Editor-in-Chief Birger Strandell. Despite some resistance, there was now a national board and the name change had finally been approved. But the battle was not over.

At the next ordinary annual meeting on 10 March 1989, Törnblom led the opposition. Lagerlöf seemed to have given up.

Maybe he had changed his mind when he saw the first issue of the new journal with the new name. The minutes noted that he thought the first issue looked very good. So did Lars Werkö, the well-known Professor of Medicine in Gothenburg and later deputy Chief Executive Officer of the ASTRA pharmaceutical company. When the meeting closed, Henrik approached me and said that he wouldn't have battled against the name change if he had realized how good the name change would be.

Hallberg resigned as Chairman of the Association in 1993, and soon after that Böttiger resigned as Editor-in-Chief. I became Chairman of the Board and Göran Holm became Editor-in-Chief.

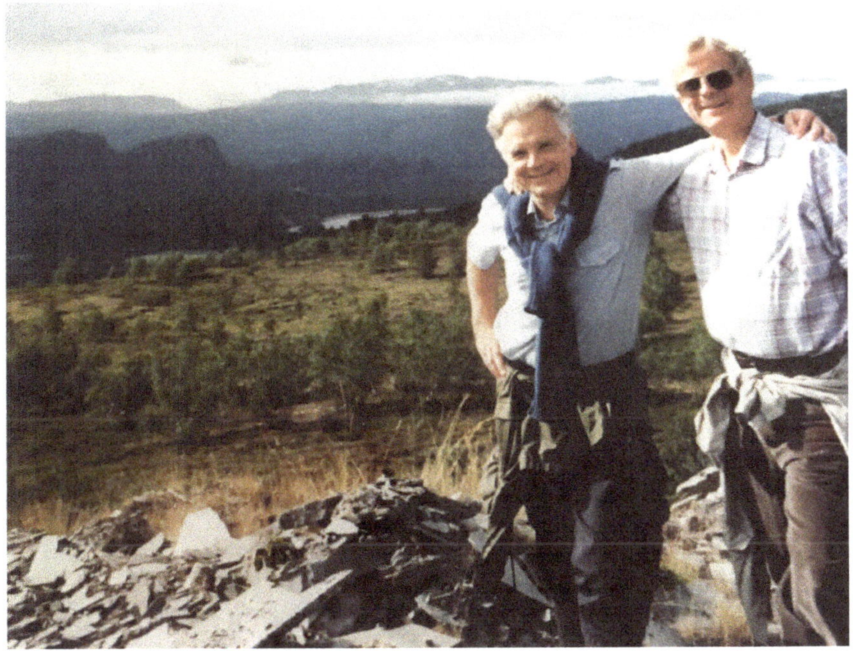

The author together with Göran Holm, Professor of Medicine at the Karolinska Institutet and Head of the Department of Medicine at the Karolinska Hospital. The photo was taken when I was attending a meeting in Tromsö, Norway, when I had succeeded Leif Hallberg as Chairman of the Board of the Association for the Publication of the *Journal of Internal Medicine* and Göran had succeeded Lars Erik (Larsa) Böttiger as its Editor-in-Chief.

He was succeeded by Professor Ulf de Faire in 2006. The journal continued to make spectacular improvements. We attracted review articles from the most important clinical scientists, including Nobel Prize winners, original articles improved, and the impact factor rose continuously. When I resigned in 2009, it had reached 5.942, compared to 1.0 in 1990. de Faire and his deputy editor Bengt Fagrell and later the present Editor-in-Chief Bo Angelin achieved an impact factor of 13.068 in 2023, similar to some of the most important American and European journals in clinical medicine. It is not possible to quantify the importance of the name change, but it probably played some role in the success of the Journal, which started to increase thanks to the aspirations of Larsa Böttiger.

39 Moscow and the All-Union Scientific Centre for Haematology

Only two Nobel Prizes in Physiology or Medicine have been awarded to citizens of Russia or the Soviet Union. Both were awarded during the reign of Tsar Nicholas II. Ivan Petrovich Pavlov was honored in 1904 *"in recognition of his work on the physiology of digestion, through which knowledge on vital aspects of the subject has been transformed and enlarged"*. Ilya Ilyich Mechnikov split the Nobel Prize with Paul Ehrlich from Germany in 1908 *"in recognition of their work on immunity"*. These are both well-known figures in the history of medicine, but without known followers. Looking for potential Nobel Prize winners was not the reason for my professional visit to Moscow.

In the spring of 1990, I was invited to visit the All-Union Scientific Centre for Haematology with docent Sigvard Olsson from Gothenburg. The center was the most important one for the research and treatment of patients with hematological disorders in the Soviet Union. The invitation came from the Deputy Head of the Center, Professor Yuri Nikolajch Tokarev. One reason was that the Head of the Center, Professor Andrey Ivanovich Vorobiev (1928–2020), later the first Minister of Health for the Russian Federation, was disappointed with the agreement on research collaboration between the Soviet Academy of Medical Sciences and the Swedish Academy of Science. The agreement did not include his center, which focused on blood disorders. Vorobiev and

Tokarev thought that we should establish collaboration outside the agreement.

Tokarev, who was born in 1926, was both a scientist and a clinician. He worked in Ghana for many years during the 1960s, where he became interested in tropical medicine, in particular the genetically related hemoglobinopathies thalassemia and sickle cell disease. He collaborated with Susan Holland, a famous hematologist and communist in Budapest, Hungary, who had managed to build an important center of hematology, with support from the country's communist regime.

When he returned to the Soviet Union, Tokarev investigated the frequency of the thalassemia gene among people living in the Soviet republics of Azerbaijan and Georgia[101] and found that it was as high as 10% in certain districts.

I met Tokarev at a hematology congress in Jerusalem and he told me that he wanted to invite me and my friend Sigvard Olsson to give lectures in Moscow. Sigvard had made internationally recognized discoveries about the genetics behind another interesting disease, hemochromatosis[102]. This disorder is characterized by storing too much iron in the body, which damages many organs, particularly the liver, which may shrink and lose function if the treatment is started too late. The plan was for Sigvard to deliver lectures on hemochromatosis and for me to talk about bone marrow transplants.

The situation in Moscow was shaky in 1990. President Mikhail Gorbachev, who had won the Nobel Peace Prize in same year, had introduced the policies of glasnost and perestroika, which mean openness and reconstruction. Free enterprise was allowed to a limited extent. For example, some restaurants were allowed to set their own prices and accept US dollars.

The Baltic states, namely Estonia, Latvia and Lithuania, were trying to liberate themselves from the Soviet Union, but Gorbachev did not like this idea and was not going to give up easily on this point. He accused the Estonians of being ungrateful for the enormous investments by the Soviet Union in factors such as infrastructure.

The situation in the shrinking Soviet Union was not clear to Sigvard or me when we started our journey there. But we travelled with enthusiasm and were eager to experience something new and unexpected and to give our lectures.

When we arrived, we were greeted by Tokarev, who was accompanied by a nice lady who was going to take care of us during our visit. She had been educated in the communist ideals but did not try to indoctrinate us. Instead, she was a good guide who warned us about any problems that could occur.

The visit lasted from 28 March to 3 April 1990. We stayed at a basic hotel a couple of Metro station stops from the hospital and insisted that we travelled back and forth to it every day without our female guide. The Metro stations were far more luxurious than in Sweden, with wonderful crystal chandeliers and the names of the stations written in Cyrillic letters. Sigvard became an expert at interpreting and led our joint travel. This meant that we managed to get around by ourselves, and without the nice politruk (political bureaucrat) lady. We met our host every day at the hospital, and he invited us to join him for breakfast, lunch and dinner in his office. He claimed that the meals in the hospital cafeteria were hardly edible, and he preferred to see us in his office or in the evening at his home. Breakfast and lunch were simple, with some cold cuts, but the dinners at his home were of western quality. Sometimes we were taken by our politruk lady to new, rare private restaurants with excellent food and drink. She told us that these restaurants were only for rich people and visiting foreigners like us, because the prices were extremely high, and you could pay with US dollars. Ordinary people sometimes smashed the windows in protest, but she had been instructed to take us to some of them. We were not impressed. A three course good, but ordinary, dinner for two was about 10–20 dollars, including drinks. One of these restaurants seemed to be in a secret location and was only for upper communist class people. It appears we were part of these select few during our visit.

Tokarev told us that the situation in the country was very bad. People living in the countryside were starving. Gorbachev had destroyed the country. He was as unpopular in the Soviet Union as he was popular in the West. The dissolution of the country was a disaster, the economy was at rock bottom and only a minority with connections to the party bosses and with plenty of money could afford decent food. For most people, bread was the basic food, while meat and vegetables were absent from their tables. We checked a few stores. Bread was extremely cheap. A loaf of bread was about a quarter of a US dollar and could be bought without limits. We also tried a big butcher shop. Numerous sales assistants behind the counters seemed to have nothing to do, while at one corner customers had lined up to get a share of a large sausage, cut into pieces, by the only working sales assistant. We noticed that several hundred small metal jars about 10 cm in diameter covered the shelves. No one seemed to ask for them, so I decided to, to the astonishment of the sales assistant. She brought one down from the shelf and I paid a small fraction of a dollar. I opened it when I got back to Stockholm a few days later, as I needed a can opener. It was just as well, because it contained a disgusting root mash that was not even eaten by the poor Russians. The result of the planned communist economic system was clearly visible.

Our lectures at the hospital were apparently appreciated by the physicians and students, despite the fact that Tokarev had to translate every sentence from English to Russian. This meant that the lectures took about twice as long as normal. After my lecture, I was available for patient consultations. I remember seeing the husband of a patient with chronic myelocytic leukemia (CML) (Chapter 29). He had not brought his wife to the consultation, which meant that I could only tell him about the current results, the possibilities and the risks, and that the only chance for cure was a bone marrow transplant. I also stressed that I did not know about the results at the hospital, or overall, in Russia, but he told me that he already knew that himself. Most of the patients who had received a transplant had died. He had already planned for his wife to have her transplant abroad, either in Germany or in Poland where it was cheaper. Although I tried to stay neutral, I could do nothing but support his decision, because he was clearly one of the few people in the Soviet Union that could afford to go abroad for transplant.

After some discussions with our host, we got permission to participate in a ward round on the transplantation and leukemia treatment unit, together with the responsible hematologist, Dr Valery Savchenko. He was a very knowledgeable physician and very able hematologist and had spent three months in Seattle with Donnall Thomas learning bone marrow transplants and leukemia treatment. This followed the more relaxed relationship between the USA and the Soviet Union following the meeting between Ronald Reagan and Mikhail Gorbachev in Iceland in 1986. Savchenko had returned home from the USA filled with enthusiasm, to find that access to drugs and other resources were extremely limited. He only had six beds to treat all bone marrow transplant patients in the Soviet Union and a few more for those with leukemia that did not need a transplant. Unfortunately, he did not have enough drugs to treat six bone marrow transplant patients at the same time and he did not have enough to treat all the leukemia patients on his ward that did not need a transplant. These were mainly children. I asked him *"How do you cope when you do not have enough drugs to treat all the patients who need effective treatment?"* His response was clear enough: *"I choose the patients with the best chances and who can be effectively treated and hopefully cured. They get all the cytotoxic drugs that I have, while the others get palliative care so that they die without too much suffering. At some hospitals in Moscow the patients only get insufficient dosages of the available drugs so that every patient gets a share. All the patients die, but all have received a small insufficient dose of the drugs. I choose the unfair way, that results in curing at least some patients that would not have been cured with the fair way"*. Of course, he was right.

We had some leisure time in the evenings, and I decided to try to get a ticket to the Bolshoi Theater. At any price. The politruk lady told us that it was impossible. The tickets were always sold out. However, she also confessed that there was a black market, where unscrupulous people sold tickets outside the theater for unaffordable prices, and she advised us not to go down that route. Despite this, I asked her to accompany us to the theater, even though she declared that she would not enter it at any price. But she added that she would not cause trouble for us if we managed to get tickets.

She knew exactly where the black-market guys were positioned. We approached one of them and she checked that the tickets were real ones. She again advised us not to buy them as they cost 20 dollars each and were on the second balcony. We bought two tickets without worrying about the price and Sigvard and I experienced a marvelous performance of Giuseppe Verdi's opera La Traviata. The singers were excellent and so was the solo ballerina who performed on a table in the first act. She was surrounded by performers who were singing ecstatically to the applause of the enchanted audience. Mikhail Gorbachev had not forgotten to support the Bolshoi Ballet and Opera Theater and its actors, and it was the highest world-class performance.

Olsson and I left our hosts Tokarev and Vorobiev with mixed feelings. Despite the difficult situation in their country, they showed some optimism. It could not have been worse than it was. They were anxious to build collaborations with other countries. After all, Vorobiev had managed to handle the medical aftermath of the Chernobyl nuclear plant accident in 1986 fairly well. When he was asked by the Premier Nikolai Ivanovich Ryzhkov if having foreigners in the clinic would compromise the Soviet nuclear program, Vorobiev replied: *"We are ready for openness"* (Chapter 40). Chernobyl may have been the impetus for the glasnost that was declared by Mikhail Gorbachev and Vorobiev may have played a role in it.

40 Chernobyl and Robert (Bob) Peter Gale

On the afternoon of 11 September 2001, I received an email that said *"Will not arrive — no flights from New York. Bob"*. My friend Robert (Bob) Peter Gale was scheduled to participate in a meeting at the Swedish Radiation Protection Institute. A few days earlier, he had sent me a message about his arrival and suggested that we had dinner together. I knew that Bob was a fussy eater and had reserved a table in one of the best restaurants in Stockholm, Ulriksdal's Inn. Bob had become a world celebrity following the Chernobyl nuclear power plant accident in 1986 and he sometimes behaved like a diva. I had learned to be flexible during our long friendship and I was anxious to see him and discuss some issues with him, as he had one of the sharpest brains I knew. Although I was disappointed that he could not visit as planned, I was not totally surprised when I called the Inn to cancel the table. I blamed my friend for the cancellation. *"My American friend was going to arrive from New York and he has either missed the plane, or has found something more attractive to do than to come to Stockholm"* I said, adding *"He is a bit of a diva"*. The head waiter soon put me straight. *"From New York? Haven't you heard that the whole city is on fire and flights are not allowed in or out of New York?"*. He gave me some further information and I checked the media. Bob was excused. The two World Trade Center towers had collapsed after a terrorist attack. I saw the aftermath with my own eyes a year later when I visited New York.

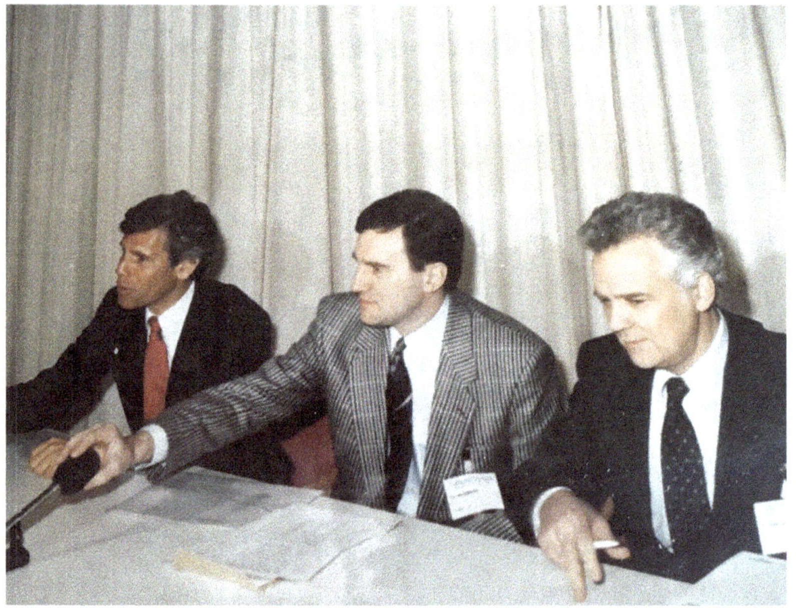

Robert (Bob) Peter Gale (left) and Wolfgang Hinterberger (middle) together with the author (right) at a press conference during the EBMT meeting in Bad Gastein, Austria, in February 1989. Wolfgang was the Congress President and I was the President of the EBMT.

Bob Gale is a super intelligent, but also controversial, hematologist and I met him at international congresses and meetings throughout the world. We have become good friends, mainly due to our joint interest in bone marrow and stem cell transplantation. Bob is much younger than me, as he was born in 1945. He has enjoyed a steep career trajectory and constantly criticizes scientific results that are not well founded. He is extremely sharp and can always put his finger on the weak points in a presentation. Our friendship has not prevented him from being my toughest critic when my presentations have displayed weaknesses. In particular, this happened when I presented our early results on stem cell transplants of patients with multiple myeloma and Bob felt that the transplant-related mortality was too high. Although this issue is still debated by others, the results have improved considerably since those early days.

Some colleagues think that Bob is better in finding weaknesses in others' results than making new discoveries himself. I disagree. In one interview he was asked about his most important discovery, and he mentioned cloning the BCR/ABL gene in CML with Eli Canaani in 1984. I was surprised, as I had no idea that he had been involved in that important discovery. I had to check in PubMed, the virtual database of all medical scientific publications, and found 1,026 of his publications. They included one in the *Proceedings of the National Academy of Sciences*[103], one in the *Lancet*[104] and one in *Nature*[105]. I checked with other colleagues in the field who confirmed his claim. I just wondered why he had never told me that he had been involved in this important discovery in the disease, as

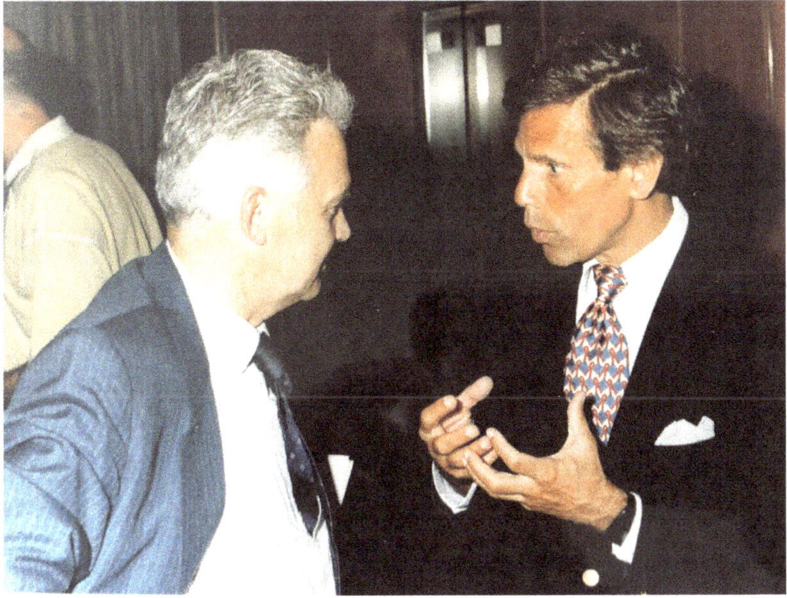

Robert (Bob) Peter Gale (right) in discussions with the author in Vienna in June 1993. We had both been invited by Wolfgang Hinterberger to give lectures at the inauguration of the Ludwig Boltzmann Institute at the Donauspital.

it had been a priority for me when I was a young researcher. I had not been able to identify the translocation between chromosomes 9 and 22, t(9;22) that we had predicted, even though we had the means to discover it as early as 1971.

Interestingly, Bob's discovery had little to do with his international fame. Bone marrow transplants, radiation and Chernobyl were the key elements in this.

From 1973 to 1993 Bob was a faculty member of the University of California Los Angeles School of Medicine. For part of that time, he was Head of the Division of Hematology and Oncology at the Department of Medicine, where he launched a bone marrow transplant program. From 1980–1997 he was Chairman of the Scientific Advisory Committee at the Center for International Blood and Marrow Transplant Research. This was a US-based research organization, whose original aim was mainly to collect reports for retrospective studies of bone marrow transplant data from individual patients transplanted at centers all over the world. This key position was an ideal platform for his efforts to use bone marrow transplants to save patients after the Chernobyl accident in 1986. It was anticipated that the bone marrow of some workers would have been damaged by the radiation leakage during the accident. Bob initiated a rescue operation with the help of billionaire Armand Hammer, who was born in Russia, had contacts with Mikhail Gorbachev and was willing to finance the operation. Bob recruited some of the most competent people in the bone marrow transplant field, including the immunologist Yair Reisner from Israel and Richard Champlin from Houston, and established the team in Moscow. The team worked with Russian hematologists to perform transplants on 13 patients that had received deadly radiation dosages, with allogeneic bone marrow from donors.[106]

Eleven of the patients died, either due to transplant complications or to the radiation damage or a combination of these and other causes. Two patients were still alive three years later, but there are no records that say what happened to them after that.

A poor outcome could have been expected, when I looked back at the results of the bone marrow transplant attempts by Georges Mathé in 1959, following the Yugoslavian atomic plant accident (Chapter 26). This was because radiating particles had probably entered the body and caused continuous radiation damage, even after a transplant. However, Bob still became a world celebrity and an expert in the effects of radiation on the human body. I listened to his presentations on the 13 patients at many congresses without being too impressed. My previous boss, Peter Reizenstein, had also been in contact with the Russians concerning a possible transplant approach. The first impacts of the accident outside the Soviet Union were detected in Sweden due to the cloud of radioactive material that reached the country, particularly around the city of Gävle. When we got information about the extent of the accident, Reizenstein thought we could help. I did not believe in the transplant approach and eventually Bob was ahead of us. No Swedish teams participated in the rescue operations.

Treatment with a new drug called GM-CSF was more important than transplants. It had been produced on an industrial scale after the discovery that the blood contained a protein that stimulated the increased production of white blood cells. The discovery was made by Thomas Ray Bradley and Donald Metcalf in 1967[96] (Chapter 37). The drug seemed to be able to decrease death from dangerous infections, since white blood cells were important in the defense against them. However, GM-CSF was still under investigation and not yet registered for general use. It led to another similar drug called G-CSF (granulocyte colony-stimulating factor) that stimulated the white blood cells better. The Soviet authorities did not give permission for its use, claiming that the side effects were unknown and could be serious. Bob contacted the Head of the Hematology Centre, Andrey Vorobiev, who was also the responsible physician for patients affected by the Chernobyl accident. I later met him, when I visited Russia with Sigvard Olsson in 1990 (Chapter 39). Bob asked Vorobiev to inject the drug into one of his blood vessels to prove that GM-CSF was safe and could increase the number of white blood cells. Vorobiev said he would agree if Bob did the same to him. So that is what they did. They both felt excellent after the injections and agreed to inform the authorities the next day that they had tested the drug and that it was safe. They also agreed to investigate if the number of white blood cells in their blood had increased after a few days.

That evening, Bob went to a dinner at the American Embassy. He had not been there long when he received a message that Vorobiev had been admitted to the emergency unit at the hospital, due to chest pain and suspected heart infarction. Bob took a cab to the hospital and found Vorobiev in bed with chest pain and seemingly miserable. After a thorough investigation, Bob found no signs of heart infarction, but Vorobiev did have a localized pain in the sternum, the bone covering the heart, which is one of the white blood cell producing bones. Vorobiev had completely recovered the next day and both Bob and Vorobiev had increased white blood cells. It is well known that harmless and transient pain may occur in bones that produce white blood cells, including the sternum. Thus, the drug was safe and could now be used to treat patients.

The efforts to save victims of the Chernobyl accident made Bob world famous. He appeared at large international congresses, expert group meetings and radiation conferences, where he presented the results that flooded out of the investigations that he and his team performed after the accident. He appeared on all the important TV channels in the USA and elsewhere as the expert on irradiation damage and disorders. At the height of his fame, he was asked to run for the Senate in California, which he wisely refused. He told me that he had been tempted to accept it, but he had refused for economic reasons. An election campaign for a senator seat was certainly not as expensive as one for the presidency, but it was still difficult to afford.

Instead, Bob continued his scientific career and was eventually headhunted by the successful pharmaceutical company Celgene. It produced one of the most effective drugs for treating multiple myeloma, the cancer disease that was high on my list of interests. Later, I had a fruitful collaboration with this company when we performed trials in Sweden (Chapters 34 and 44). Being an advisor to the company did not prevent Bob from accepting the prestigious position as Chief Editor of the scientific journal *Leukemia*, which he had successfully increased to an impact factor of 12.897 in 2023.

The medical establishment did not rate Bob's transplant efforts to save the victims of the Chernobyl accident very highly and many thought that he exaggerated his importance. However, I am sure that Bob had an altruistic wish to save patients. Maybe his use of GM-CSF was more important than the transplants.

Disregarding the Chernobyl transplant results, Bob became an expert in radiation physics and the radiation damage associated with atomic plant accidents. This included being one of the foremost experts in judging the effects of the Fukushima accident in Japan in 2002. On this occasion there were no attempts to use stem cell transplants. Instead, Bob calculated important estimates of the risk of cancer development due to the radiation. Based on his experiences from Chernobyl, he predicted that the increased incidence of cancer in Japan would not be higher than 0.002%, in other words nearly negligible. The misinformation that the public received in those days was monstrous. For example, children from the Chernobyl area came to Sweden as part of a rescue operation and a TV presenter said that most of the kids would probably get leukemia. The truth is that no increased leukemia incidence was documented after Chernobyl or Fukushima. This in no way underestimates the leukemia-inducing action of high irradiation dosages that were documented after the atomic bombs in Nagasaki and Hiroshima.

Bob wrote an excellent book about irradiation, which focused on the damaging effects on humans[107]. It was, to a great extent, based on his experiences of the two accidents at Chernobyl and Fukushima.

Bob's personal story is more complicated. His ancestors come from both Belarus and the Austrian Empire. During a site visit to the Mecca of stem cell transplants, Seattle, in 1978 he met a friend for life, Wolfgang Hinterberger from Vienna. Like Bob, Hinterberger was learning about transplants at the Fred Hutchinson Institute led by Donnall Thomas. After he returned to Vienna, Hinterberger became responsible for stem cell transplants at the University Hospital and later became Head of Medicine at the Donauspital. Bob made numerous visits to Vienna and Wolfgang Hinterberger and his wife Margareta helped him to find his roots. It was during one of those visits that Bob and I found that we had a common friend in Vienna. Our social encounters in Vienna with the Hinterbergers were highlights in both of our lives and they included visits to the New Year Concert and looking at the fireworks from the roof of the Museum for Natural History.

I did not know whether Bob was married or divorced, until I met his beautiful and wonderful wife Laura. I thought that she was from Israel, and like Bob had a Jewish background, but I was recently informed that Laura's ancestors arrived with the Mayflower and that she was Christian. Although I don't usually have any idea, or bother about, the religion or ethnic background of my friends, I once told her that my great-great grandmother was born into a Jewish family. She then converted to Protestantism, which was her husband's faith. I had heard that Jewish people considered that people were still Jewish if their mother's ancestors were. I thought it was fun to tell her that, despite my long line of Protestant ancestors, we had something in common. She and Bob just laughed at it. They had reason to do so. Like myself, they did not seem bothered about other people's ethnicity or religious background. During my working life I have usually had no idea whether my collaborators were Jewish, Protestants, Catholics or Muslims. My belief is that science can unite people irrespective of the differences that seem so important for many ethnic groups today.

Bob is a great scientist, but to my knowledge he has never rated himself as being worthy of a Nobel Prize. His strength lies in his logic and critical thinking, but perhaps his clear writing style is even stronger. That is perhaps why he has published more than 1,000 scientific papers. I believe that he has written most of them himself, in contrast to many others with similar numbers, who have published papers written by someone else, often by medical writers paid by companies.

Bob has, of course, received many awards, including the Presidential Award by the New York Academy of Science.

41 The European Society for Blood and Marrow Transplantation

In 1985, I was asked whether I would accept becoming President of the European Group for Bone Marrow Transplantation (EBMT), now the European Society for Blood and Marrow Transplantation. I was surprised. The person who asked me was one of the leading hematologists in the world, John Goldman. He was sometimes called Mr CML due to his devotion to scientific work concerning this deadly disease, until a fraction of the patients was cured with bone marrow transplants (Chapters 28–29). I asked him whether he would prefer to adopt the role himself, but I don't remember his answer. During the next annual meeting I was appointed President Elect, which meant that I would succeed the present charming Italian President, Alberto Marmont, when he stepped down in 1988. Marmont was Professor and Head of the Department of Hematology at the San Martino Hospital in Genoa, Italy. He was a brilliant clinician, but a less brilliant organizer. He was the sixth President of the EBMT, which organized annual meetings that were attended by about 100 bone marrow transplant specialists. We usually had our conferences at a pension or hotel in the Alps, in Courmayeur, Courchevel or St Moritz. There were lectures and working parties until lunchtime and then we went skiing until late afternoon. Then we continued working until late into the evening. This meant that we combined working for at least eight hours a day with relaxing skiing. This was an appreciated and effective way of meeting, getting to know each other and exchanging experiences. However, more people wanted to participate. Bone marrow transplants as a cure spread rapidly in Europe and all over the world. The number of centers and the number of transplanters increased drastically. Better organization and more space for the meetings was needed and that meant that the EBMT had to be reformed and reorganized.

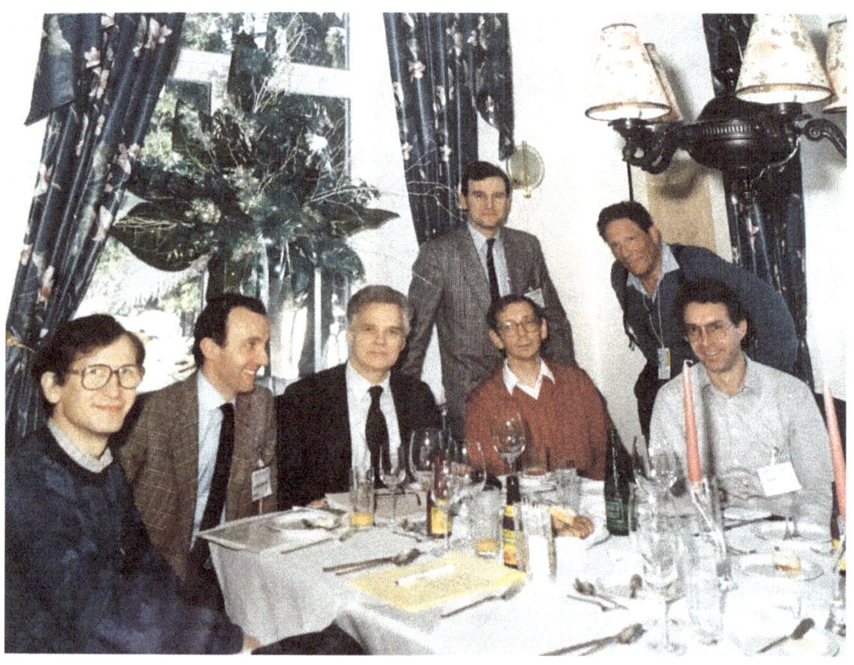

The EBMT board during my presidency 1988–1990.

Sitting from left to right: Alain Fischer (Professor of Immunology at the University of Paris and Head of Pediatric Immunology and Hematology at Hospital Necker in Paris, a pioneer in clinical gene therapy), Andrea Bacigalupo (Head of Hematology at San Martino Hospital in Genoa, Italy), the author, Claude Gorin (Head of Hematology at the Saint Antoine Hospital in Paris) and Alois Gratwohl (Head of Hematology and Stem Cell Transplantation in Basel, Switzerland and later President of the EBMT).

Standing from left: Wolfgang Hinterberger (Secretary of the EBMT and later Head of Medicine at Donauspital Vienna and Jon van Rood (Professor of Immunology at Leiden University Medical Center, co-founder of the EBMT and World Marrow Donor Association and considered by many worthy of the Nobel Prize).

The EBMT was founded in 1975 by the pioneers Bruno Speck, a hematologist from Basel, Jon van Rood, an immunologist from Leiden (Chapter 43) and Eliane Gluckman, a hematologist at the St Louis Hospital in Paris. Gluckman had been a student of one of the most famous hematologists in the world, Jean Bernhard, who was Head of Hematology at the same hospital (Chapter 26). The trio met in 1973–1974 in the Alps to discuss setting up a society to promote bone marrow transplants in Europe. Speck became the first President and a younger colleague, Ferry Zwaan, a hematologist from Leiden, became the Secretary in 1976. Their first project was to establish a database of all the bone marrow transplants performed in Europe. Physicians reported the diagnoses and all possible clinical and laboratory markers on each patient to the database. Follow-up information was reported at regular intervals. The aim of the database was to collate information about the most suitable patients for the treatment, the prognostic parameters and the outcomes in relation to the factors that were investigated. All the transplant centers in Europe were invited to be members. There was only one requirement and that was that they needed to use the report form created by the EBMT Secretary and the board. The first members were the centers led by the founders, namely the transplant and/or hematology centers in Basel, Leiden and the St Louis Hospital in Paris. They were soon joined by the Hammersmith Hospital in London. Carl-Gustav Groth and I decided to apply for membership as soon as possible. We registered for one of the first annual meetings in 1976 in St Moritz in Switzerland. About 70 people had registered and I had submitted an abstract for an oral presentation about how Caspersson's Q-banding technique could be used to identify inherited fluorescent satellites on chromosomes. It covered how these could be used to obtain information about whether the donor cells had taken and started to grow in the patients or if the patient's own cancer cells had taken over and rejected the graft[108,109]. This was important information, but I must admit that it did not receive spectacular attention at the meeting. However, it was the first scientific publication from the bone marrow transplant program at the Huddinge Hospital and it was a starting point for our internationally respected science in the field. Our center joined the EBMT and my right- and left-hand Dr Berit Lönnqvist, a hematologist in my department, became responsible for reporting our transplant patients to the EBMT database.

The EBMT grew rapidly. By the time I was elected president in 1988, more than 100 centers were members. More than 500 delegates attended the 1989 annual meeting in Bad Gastein, Austria, which was organized by my friend and Secretary of the EBMT, Wolfgang Hinterberger, who was also the local President. There were about 350 scientific oral and poster presentations. At the start, the members were centers with any number of individual members. Eventually Stockholm, including the Huddinge Hospital, had five centers registered as members, with more than 40 individual members.

When I became President, Hinterberger was already the Secretary and Peter Ernst, a transplanter and hematologist from Copenhagen, was the Treasurer. We agreed to rewrite the constitution and I also investigated how to get grants from the European Union (EU).

A new constitution was in place when I stepped down as President two years later. The EBMT was now a democratic society with stem cell transplant centers as members and the fee paid by the centers was based on the number of individuals they had as members. I had also managed to secure the first ever EU grant to the Karolinska Institutet. The EU only allowed institutional grants, but it was entirely used to support the EBMT, mainly to continue building the database.

Up to that point I had only secured grants from Swedish sources with reasonable bureaucratic procedures. Although I had managed the relatively difficult EU grant application procedure, I had not foreseen what would happen when the grant was used. After a couple of years, two clerks from the EU grant organization appeared at the hospital and declared that they had come to audit the annual institutional report about how we had used the grant. The administration of my Institution had a good reputation, and I was confident everything was in order. However, I was wrong on one point. It turned out the currency exchange rate from Swedish Krona to Euros and vice versa, had been carried out at the wrong time. I don't remember when it should have been done, when we got the bills or when we paid them, but my secretary, Susanne Barksäter, had got the timing wrong. This meant a small difference, up or down in the currency exchange rate. She had to do it all over again and she did a fantastic job. The auditors were satisfied after about six months.

I once more had to consider that my country, Sweden, was backwards in some respects. Many years after the core states in Europe had formed the EU, we had still not joined them. In 1995, Sweden eventually voted to enter the EU, but only if our 10 million inhabitants could continue to use the Krona instead of the Euro. This silly decision made it difficult for us to receive EU grants and caused problems for all Swedes that travelled or traded with Europe. Interestingly, other countries that became members of the EU around this time had to qualify for being allowed to convert their currency to the Euro, while Sweden that was qualified chose to keep the Krona.

Despite these currency issues, EU grants were important for the development of European stem cell transplant research. The first grant was for three years but was renewed so that we received a total of six years. An American, Donnall Thomas, received the Nobel Prize for his contribution to making cell transplants a valuable clinical treatment method (Chapter 30). However, I think that the transplant research in Europe competed well with the American studies, even though it was slower. The proof was that American transplant researchers came to the annual EBMT meetings, even without a special invitation. This was unusual, because in most other medical disciplines, Europeans went to the meetings in USA, but Americans did not travel to European congresses.

The European bone marrow transplant research expanded and was partly driven by the EBMT. Collaborative initiatives were established with the USA and our group at the Huddinge Hospital was part of the developments. In the beginning, the large retrospective studies that used the EBMT database were the main reason for the successes. Prognostic factors for outcomes were analyzed and the importance of new treatments could be compared to current ones using large numbers of patients. One example was the finding that carrying out transplants with peripheral blood stem cells had similar outcome to transplants with bone marrow cells in most diseases. This was first shown for patients with leukemia and multiple myeloma[75]. My friend Ray Powles and his colleagues at the Royal Marsden Hospital in the UK had shown that the feared graft versus host disease could be diminished by the prophylactic use of a new drug called cyclosporin[110,111]. Large EBMT register studies soon made it possible to show what the treatment meant for the patients[76]. Many received better treatment and fewer succumbed to treatment-related complications.

It took a while before we managed to perform prospective randomized studies within the EBMT. However, I eventually designed a prospective study to determine the importance of using allogeneic (allo) transplantation combined with autologous transplants for multiple myeloma, compared to the current method that only used autologous transplantation. The study started in 2000 and included 23 EBMT centers with my collaborator and previous PhD student docent Bo Björkstrand as the principal investigator. After several years, we were able to show that the auto/allo combination was associated with better overall survival rates than auto or auto/auto methods, despite higher transplant-related mortality[84]. Thus, improved survival was due to a lower relapse rate and death due to the disease. Although this result was later debated and not confirmed by all the similar subsequent studies, it proved that EBMT centers could run large and important prospective studies.

Although I rated the research performed by the EBMT centers as very high, I cannot claim that these discoveries met the standard of the Nobel Committee or Alfred Nobel's will. This does not mean that the individual members of the society could not have carried out such discoveries. The next two chapters are proof of this.

42 Bone Marrow and Stem Cell Donors — The World Marrow Donor Association

A bone marrow or stem cell transplant needs a donor. For some blood and bone marrow disorders the patients can actually be their own donor. In such cases the stem cells are collected, frozen, stored, then thawed when needed and given back to the patient as a rescue operation after intensive bone marrow eradication treatment. This is called autologous transplantation. The name of the concept is questionable since the word transplantation suggests that the organ or cells are transferred to the individual by another individual. Normally when we talk about transplants, we mean that something has been transplanted from one individual to another. This is the one exception.

In the beginning, siblings were used as bone marrow donors for transplants. Before the discovery of the HLA (human leukocyte antigen) system by Jean Dausset in the 1960s (Chapters 27–29, 43), successes were rare unless the sibling was a twin. Each human being has a genetically determined HLA type, which is crucial for the success of a transplant. The HLA type of the donor must be as compatible as possible with the recipient. If the donor is a twin, there is almost 100% compatibility, while one sibling only has a 25% chance of being compatible. An unrelated individual is nearly always non-compatible, but it does happen. This rare possibility has led to establishing registries of unrelated donors who are HLA-typed volunteers. The results of transplants with stem cells from a close to compatible unrelated donor have been shown to be nearly as good as those with HLA-identical sibling donors.

The first national registry of volunteers was established in London. The Anthony Nolan Registry was set up by Shirley Nolan in the hope that it could find a donor for her son. Anthony had a genetic life-threatening disorder, Wiskott-Aldrich syndrome, and his physicians thought that it could be cured with a bone marrow transplant. The registry was the first, and for a long time, the largest one in the world. Slowly, other countries followed and built their own registries. One of my friends and co-founder of EBMT, the immunologist Jon van Rood (Chapter 43), became the driving force and organizer of this activity. He originally created a book, then a database, of most of the HLA-typed volunteers in the world, called Bone Marrow Donors Worldwide (BMDW)[112]. He also created an association for all national registries of volunteer donors, the World Marrow Donor Association (WMDA)[113].

A national registry of HLA-typed volunteer donors was also created in Sweden on the initiative of Marcus Storch, an industry leader and later Chairman of the Nobel Foundation. His son Tobias fell ill with aplastic anemia before the BMDW was established. No donor was found, and his son died from the disease. Marcus and his wife Gunilla became the driving force in building the Swedish Tobias Registry, which now comprises more than 200,000 registered volunteer donors. These can be found in the BMDW database, and the registry is also a member of the WMDA.

It was shown in the 1990s that the umbilical cord had stem cells that could be used for stem cell transplants. Many countries had started to build cord stem cell banks containing frozen

HLA-typed stem cells that had been collected from volunteers after childbirth. They were also registered in the BMDW and could be searched just like any other volunteer bone marrow and stem cell donor.

By 2022, the BMDW had information about the HLA-typed cells of nearly 40 million volunteer donors and more than 800,000 stored cord blood units in 55 countries. The database can be searched on the internet by those with login access.

43 Jon van Rood

"Would you consider being President of WMDA?" Jon van Rood, one of the founders of the association, asked me that question at an EBMT meeting in 1999. I had formally retired in 1998 and quite some time had lapsed since I had stepped down as President of the EBMT. van Rood obviously thought that I had done a good job at the EBMT, but I still hesitated. The members of the WMDA were not usually medical doctors. They tended to be people with a theoretical background in biomedicine and working in laboratories or in blood transfusion units. They had little contact with patients, except during blood sampling activity. On the other hand, they were often knowledgeable about immunology and experts in HLA typing. Many were nurses working in laboratories or transfusion units.

I told van Rood that I did not feel qualified to be the President because I had not dealt with HLA typing or blood transfusions, and I was a poor immunologist. Although I had spent five years in Caspersson's cell biology department in my youth and handled the HLA-typed biological products that were produced in the laboratories during the bone marrow transplant procedure, I was a clinician that worked with transplant patients. van Rood insisted that I was just the kind of person they needed for the job. The WMDA needed a leading clinician that worked with patients as it currently lacked that kind of knowledge. I asked if he thought that the members would accept me as President, and he said he was convinced they would. I accepted.

van Rood was a highly respected immunologist. He had identified antibodies against leukocytes in pregnant women in 1958[114], which was about the same time that Jean Dausset had discovered the leukocyte antibodies that led to the delineation of the HLA system[115]. (See also the forgotten discoveries of leukocyte antibodies in 1952 by my teacher in Zürich, Sven Moeschlin[19] in Chapter 14.) Many scientists in the field felt that van Rood should have been awarded the Nobel Prize in 1980, with Jean Dausset and George Davis Snell. He had shared the prestigious Wolf Prize with them in 1978 *"for his contribution to the understanding of the complexity of the HLA system in man and its implications in transplantation and in disease"*. However, there was no Nobel Prize for van Rood in 1980, although he was nominated six times until 1972 and a special investigation for the Nobel Committee was made by George Klein in 1969. Instead, the third man on the ticket with Dausset and Snell was Baruj Benacerraf. The three men received the Nobel Prize *"for their discoveries concerning genetically determined structures on the cell surface that regulate immunological reactions"*.

Although I felt that van Rood was disappointed, he never mentioned anything about the prize to me. He continued his research career, and his interest in helping clinicians to find donors for stem cell transplants made him create the BMDW and help to establish the WMDA. Although Donnall Thomas and John Goldman were co-founders of WMDA, van Rood was its soul. It was quite clear to me that my role as president of the WMDA would depend on van Rood's support. The plan was for me to be President for two years. John Hansen from the Fred Hutchinson Center in Seattle had been President for the previous two years and he succeeded van Rood himself. He took over from Thomas, who was the first president of the WMDA.

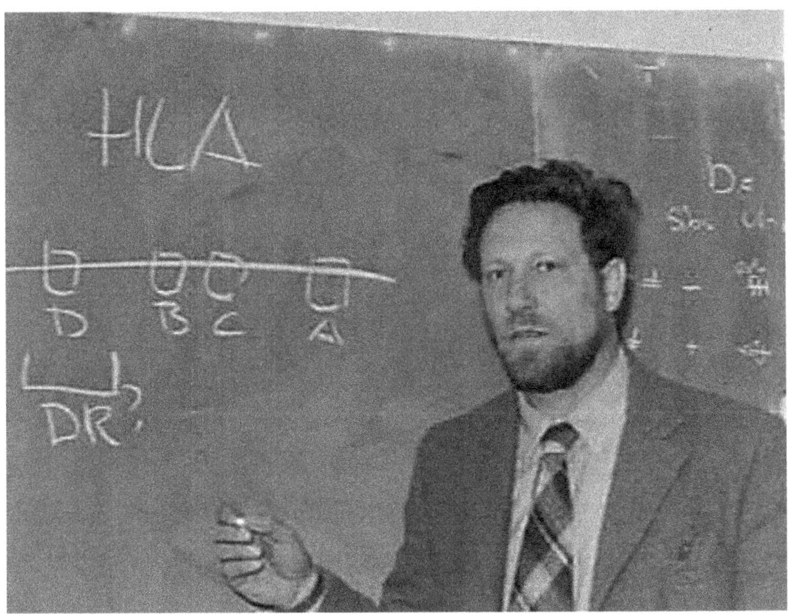

Jon van Rood, Professor of Immunology at the Leiden University, was co-founder of the EBMT and WMDA. He was considered by many to be worthy of the Nobel Prize for the discovery of leukocyte antibodies in pregnant women. He was awarded the Wolf Prize, with Jean Dausset and George Davis Snell in 1978.

Before I became the President, I was President Elect for one year. After my two-year presidency from 2001–2002, I was a member of the board. It was a rewarding experience getting to know the committed people in the WMDA. They were often skilled immunologists and had excellent knowledge of transfusion medicine. One goal was to engage as many transplant centers as possible and increase the number of HLA-typed volunteer donors. The WMDA centers were very successful in this respect. However, the people who worked with the donors were concerned about the lack of feedback from the transplant centers about the outcomes of the transplants with stem cells from the donors that they typed. Ambitious attempts to improve communications with the transplant centers had been largely unsuccessful. This meant that the donor centers concentrated on research around the donors instead, namely their physical and psychological status after their donation and how to handle the donor's wish to get to know the recipient of their donated cells.

I must admit that I was no more successful than my predecessors in establishing effective communication between the transplant centers and donor centers about the outcomes of transplants. The outcome research was driven by the transplant centers, as they had complete information about the donors at the time of transplant, which was the prerequisite for this kind of research.

The typing technique developed rapidly. Certain HLA types were more important for successful transplants than others. Genetic typing provided better results and the number of HLA markers that resulted in optimal transplant outcomes was defined. The results from using unrelated donors soon became about as good as transplants with HLA-identical sibling donors.

As I had predicted, van Rood continued to be the dominating force in the WMDA throughout my presidency. We had an excellent collaboration, and he facilitated my work in all respects. The collaboration with the donor centers also worked well. We also gave a presentation to the EU Parliament that made it easier for stem cells for transplants to cross over country borders. In the past, nurses had sometimes experienced difficulties with officials when they had tried to pass through customs with stem cells for transplants that had come from the USA or Asia. This improved after our visit to the EU.

Even though my presidency went well, thanks to hard work, progress and harmony, I felt that the WMDA was not the place for me. My place was in the hospital with the patients and medical staff. Although I kept my membership after I had stepped down from the presidency and board, my participation in the annual WMDA meetings came to an end.

van Rood continued to be the soul, mentor and grand old man in the organization as long as he lived. He died in 2017, at the age of 91, without having been awarded the Nobel Prize.

44   Multiple Myeloma

My scientific career was about acute and chronic leukemia from the start. The time I spent with Torbjörn Caspersson and Sidney Farber was devoted to leukemia, mainly chronic myelocytic leukemia. After my disappointment when I failed to discover translocation t(9;22), I turned to chromosome studies in chronic lymphocytic leukemia for a while. These were more successful, and in 1979 we discovered the first specific chromosomes associated with this disease, namely t(11;14) and trisomy 12[40,41]. However, I continued my interest in the treatment of acute and chronic myelocytic leukemia with bone marrow transplants. This treatment, together with all kinds of cell therapy, became my focus.

I was not a myeloma guy. I did not have the feeling that I belonged to the scientific myeloma establishment. However, I still entered the field and became fascinated by it due to a single patient.

It happened on a patient round in 1983 with my resident and closest collaborator in the bone marrow transplant activity at the hematology division, Dr Berit Lönnqvist. We were still under the Head of Medicine, Gunnar Birke. Lönnqvist was responsible for investigating and following up most of the transplant patients. She had a brilliant memory, could report all the details about the patients at any time and she was my additional memory. I could call her in the middle of the night for information about a patient and she always had the answer. Lönnqvist also had lots of ideas about science but found it difficult to put them together in a thesis. She was very decisive and if she had an opinion on how to proceed with the treatment it was close to impossible to change her mind. However, she was right most of the time.

During one round, we passed one of her patients, a middle-aged woman with multiple myeloma. She had been treated with melphalan, prednisone and cyclophosphamide, from diagnosis and during repeated relapses. Lönnqvist claimed that there were no more options, except for one, and that was a bone marrow transplant. I recalled that one of the first six terminal cancer patients that had received bone marrow transplants from Thomas in 1959 had multiple myelomas. Like all the other patients, this one died very soon after the transplant, although with identified markers on peripheral blood cells before she died. That proved that they derived from transplanted donor stem cells. I later found out that a couple of twin transplants had been performed in myeloma patients in 1982. Two abstracts from the American Society of Clinical Oncology and American Association for Cancer Research meetings each reported one allogeneic transplant. However, the abstracts, by Alexander Fefer and Elliot F Osserman respectively, did not provide any follow-up that could be evaluated. To my knowledge, the outcomes of these patients have never been reported in any scientific journal.

I listened to Lönnqvist and said that this seemed very experimental to me. She insisted that bone marrow transplants had cured other bone marrow disorders, and this was the last and only chance for the patient. It could be carried out under the patient exemption umbrella, allowed outside a research project. I consented and we made the first successful allogeneic transplant in a patient with multiple myeloma. She went into complete remission, and it was sustained for nearly four years. In the meantime, we started collaborative projects within the EBMT, and we performed further transplants at Huddinge. I became engrossed in the myeloma research field.

The phrase multiple myeloma first appeared several years after Dr William Macintyre described what was said to have been the first case in 1850. However, another case that was described by Dr Samuel Solly in 1844 was most probably myeloma[116]. It is a deadly cancer disorder of the bone marrow and frequently affects other organs as well. The annual incidence is five to six per 100,000 in the western world, and about half of the patients are older than 70 years of age. The outcome without treatment varies but is usually short and can be months or a few years. Treatment has been available since the early 1960s and these short survival times are rarely seen today.

In the second half of the 20th century, multiple myeloma patients were usually taken care of by hematologists or medical oncologists. In Sweden, the disorder was treated by hematologists. Nils Alwall from Lund University carried out initial trials in the 1940s (Chapter 48) to treat myeloma patients with urethane, which later turned out to be ineffective[117]. Melphalan was introduced in 1962 after trials performed by Danny Bergsagel at the MD Anderson Hospital in Houston, Texas[118]. Another cytotoxic drug, cyclophosphamide, was also effective, and both could be combined with prednisone. In the 1970s, some other drugs improved outcome for the patients, namely doxorubicin (Adriamycin) and vincristine and the combination of these drugs, but overall survival was still relatively poor and cures were not seen.

In 1983, Lönnqvist convinced me to perform an allogeneic transplant on the patient that had relapsed after treatment with these available drugs. Allogeneic bone marrow transplants were still risky at this time, but there was a chance that they could provide a cure, as had been shown for other hematologic cancers like leukemia (Chapters 28–29).

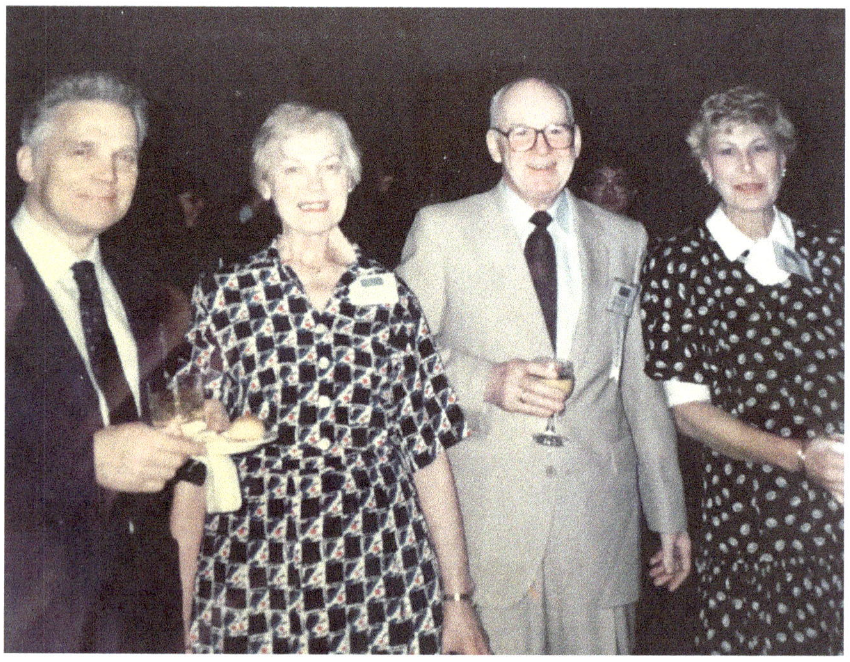

Left to right: the author, next to Joyce and Danny Bergsagel during the International Conference on Multiple Myeloma in Bologna, Italy, in June 1989. Danny discovered that melphalan was the first effective drug for multiple myeloma and it is still in use today.

We reported our success with this and two other patients three years later in 1986[119]. However, we did not claim that they were cured, because the observation time was not long enough. However, other centers started to transplant patients with multiple myeloma, after our group and the group in Bologna, led by Professor Sante Tura, reported encouraging results[120].

Centers that were members of the EBMT slowly started to perform transplants in high-risk patients and reported the outcomes to the EBMT database. I was a member of the Chronic Leukemia Working Party, now the Chronic Malignancy Working Party, and I chaired the Multiple Myeloma Subcommittee for 18 years, which was far too long! We were soon able to report results and describe factors that were important for survival[121]. However, the weakness was that the database did not contain the results of any other treatment apart from transplants. This meant that no comparisons could be made to other treatments, with one exception. This was those patients who had been given an autologous transplant, which started a couple of years later.

I very soon understood that I had to educate myself in the myeloma field and be part of organizations and project groups that had placed their prime focus on multiple myeloma.

I was invited to a workshop at Blenheim Palace in Oxfordshire in the UK in October 1987, where the goal was to form an international group of scientists interested in multiple myeloma. Tim McElwain from the Royal Marsden Hospital in London was behind the initiative. He and his colleague Ray Powles, who had been a good friend of mine since our immunotherapy trials for leukemia (Chapters 25–26), had treated myeloma patients with high-dose melphalan in 1983[122]. Peter Selby, who was also based at the Royal Marsden, later joined this project. They supported the treatment by providing autologous bone marrow cells that were harvested and stored frozen before the treatment. They were then given back to the patient who needed to be rescued from bone marrow aplasia with an autologous bone marrow transplant[123]. The hope was that more myeloma cells would be killed by these high doses and that this would prolong the patients' disease-free survival. A similar approach had been used by Bart Barlogie in Houston, Texas, and the results looked promising[124].

McElwain had asked the most well-known person in myeloma research, Dr Robert A Kyle from the Mayo Clinic in Rochester, New York, USA, to support the meeting and to chair one of the sessions. Another well-known hematologist/oncologist, Professor James Spencer Malpas from the Department of Oncology at St Bartholomew's Hospital, London, was also included in the organizing committee that was mainly run by McElwain and Selby.

There were 34 participants round a square table. The meeting was very informal, and we all stayed at The Bear Hotel in Woodstock, a small inn close to the Palace, from 14–16 October. Each of us presented our approach to multiple myeloma. I presented my results from 24 allogeneic bone marrow transplants that had been reported to the EBMT Registry, including the three performed at the Huddinge Hospital. I claimed that the results were promising, but pointed out that the observation time was too short, at a median of 437 days, to make firm conclusions.

Many important myeloma researchers participated in the meeting, as well as the organizers. The most well-known one was Robert (Bob) Kyle. He was born in 1928 and had spent most of his life at the Mayo Clinic in Minnesota, USA, and would continue to do so after the meeting. His main contribution to the myeloma field was analyzing thousands of electrophoretic spikes in the blood, indicating increases in monoclonal immunoglobulin in the patients he saw at the Mayo Clinic. Many of these were not associated with myeloma. By following their course, he could determine the risk that patients with those spikes would develop myelomas. Jan Waldenström and his students and collaborators had called such a monoclonal spike a benign monoclonal gammopathy if the patient did not have a myeloma. Kyle called this a misnomer, since 40% had developed myelomas after 25 years. He therefore instead called it a monoclonal gammopathy of undetermined significance and that term is still used for this condition[125].

Kyle was an excellent clinician, and he led many other studies that concerned treatment, prognostic factors and staging. During the 1960s, he had spent some years as a young doctor with one of my favorite hematologists, William Dameshek, who I visited during my time in Boston (Chapter 22). But what I did not know was that Kyle had participated in curing a boy with severe aplastic anemia with a bone marrow transplant after contact with Thomas. This was early in the history of bone marrow transplantation. It was the only time Kyle got involved in a bone marrow transplant and he was not a fan of doing it for multiple myelomas.

I met Bob Kyle at many meetings, and we became very good friends. When we attended a small meeting arranged by our colleagues in Poland, we together went to see the death camp at Majdanek, which was used by the Nazis to kill Jewish people. It was not as well-known as Auschwitz but was just as terrible. We were both horrified to see the Mausoleum, where the ashes of murdered Jewish people had been collected and exhibited.

The meeting at Blenheim Palace ended with the formation of the International Myeloma Workshop, which became the International Myeloma Society in 2007. The aim was to arrange scientific meetings about myeloma every other year in the future and hopefully initiate collaborative projects. We decided to have the next meeting in Houston, Texas, under the chairmanship of two leading clinical myeloma researchers, Raymond Alexanian and Bart Barlogie. They had performed many important treatment trials for myelomas and pioneered high dose melphalan treatment, followed by autologous bone marrow transplants, in 1986. This was the same approach that had been used earlier by the Royal

Marsden to treat lymphomas. A couple of years later they also used it for myelomas. Later, when Bart had moved to Little Rock, Arkansas, USA, and built an impressive myeloma research group, he introduced a principally new treatment with thalidomide that was effective and is still used in various combinations[126].

Blenheim Palace was enormous and was the home of the Duke of Marlborough. It had an interesting history that dated back to the 18th century, and it was the birthplace of the legendary Winston Churchill, the former British Prime Minister. He was a descendant of the first Duke of Marlborough, John Churchill (1660–1722). The current occupant of Blenheim was the 11th Duke of Marlborough, John George Spencer-Churchill. He did not need all the space at the Palace for his work and leisure time and he probably needed money to maintain such a huge building. Some of the space was rented out for meetings and probably other income generating activities.

I did not know much about the Palace's history and wanted to spend some of my leisure time exercising in the early evenings. I dressed in my running gear and went outside the Palace, with the intention to run all around it. I went out of the front door on the northern side and started to run in a wide circle in the front park, turning east, then south-east through a forest-like area with some paths. I tried to continue to circle the Palace, left the path and turned south-west. I hesitated when I encountered a run-down steel fence, but managed to climb over it, with some difficulty. This took me out of the forest and into a very nice garden on the western side of the Palace. After a short while, I heard a man shouting at me to stop and he sent out a barking dog, which followed me, biting at my shoes until I stopped. I had strayed into a private area and was interrogated about how I had managed to enter the duke's family area. After some harsh accusations and shouting, he mellowed when I explained that I was part of a group that was working in the Palace, and I was very sorry that I had accidently entered the private area. He showed me the way back to the Palace. I did not see the duke or his family, but I was able to brag about having spent some time in the 11th Duke of Marlborough's private garden.

After a successful meeting I felt sufficiently updated in the field to conclude that both autologous and allogeneic treatment modalities were important and worth continuing.

Although the EBMT provided the main base for my activity in the myeloma treatment field, I started to participate in the International Myeloma Society workshops.

I soon became a member of another working group, the International Myeloma Working Group (IMWG), which was created and funded by the International Myeloma Foundation (IMF). This was, and still is, the most important multiple myeloma funding agency and it has an ambitious educational program and patient-directed activity.

The IMF was founded in 1990 by a myeloma patient, Brian Novis, who later succumbed to the disease. His wife Susie Novis became the driving force in the organization after his death and later married Brian G M Durie, who became the IMF's Chairman and Chief Scientific Officer. He is also a myeloma specialist at Cedars-Sinai Outpatient Cancer Center at the Samuel Oschin Comprehensive Cancer Institute in Los Angeles, USA.

Susie is worth a book of her own or at least a chapter in a book. She is charming, driven and one of the most able persons I have ever met. Numerous projects, prizes and working groups have been established under her leadership. She has managed to raise funds like nobody else and she has involved patients. It seems that everything she touches ends up producing something valuable and good.

Brian Durie, Susie's present husband, had already established himself in the myeloma field well before he got involved with the IMF. Brian proposed the first prognostic myeloma staging system in 1975 based on relatively few, but basic, parameters that could be determined in the laboratory with relative ease[127]. He did this in collaboration with another myeloma star, Sydney Salmon, Founder of the Arizona Cancer Center at the University of Arizona, USA, which he led from 1976–1998. Numerous myeloma studies have used this staging system, which still forms the basis for revised systems.

Thanks to Susie and Brian, the IMF is now an organization that works all over the world with patients and scientists and collaborates with other cancer organizations. For example, it organizes summits alongside the yearly meetings of the European Hematology Association and has financially supported the biennial International Myeloma Workshop (IMW), later International Myeloma Society (IMS) Congresses.

In 1999, twelve years after the first meeting at Blenheim Palace, the IMW met in Stockholm. My friend Professor Håkan Mellstedt, Kenneth Nilsson, Professor in Cellular Pathology at Uppsala University and myself were the organizers, but I must admit that Håkan did most of the work. It occurred two years after my formal retirement and, although I still worked at Huddinge Hospital as emeritus professor, I did not have the same staff and administrative support at my home base as when I was head of both the clinical and academic institutions. We had about 700 participants and the meeting went very well.

In the early 1990s I started working with Brian Durie on a book about multiple myeloma, after I was approached by the Arnold Publishing Company, a member of the Hodder Headline Group in London. They wanted me to be the Chief Editor of the book. I thought about it for a while and only agreed if I could engage a co-editor. At this time, I was not at all well established in the myeloma field. I needed a co-editor who knew the best *"myeloma people"* in the world and nobody had better knowledge than Brian. I approached him and he agreed. We met at an IMW meeting, and he suggested the most able authors in the USA for specific chapters. I took care of the European ones. We approached the potential writers, and, after some months, the author group had been finalized. The book appeared in 1996[128].

Textbooks are short lived and there were special reasons why a book about multiple myeloma published in 1996 would not to be up-to-date for very long. Developments in drug treatment exploded and so did the diagnostic tools. In the year 2000, I was once again approached by the Arnold Publishing Company.

This time they wanted an extended book, including myeloma-related disorders, like amyloidosis and Waldenström's macroglobulinemia. I convinced Brian that we needed a third editor. He had worked at the Charing Cross Hospital in London for a couple of years and had worked with Diana Samson, who was a good friend of mine from my EBMT days. She agreed to join us, and I knew that she was a good writer, a good scientist and a very reliable person that I could trust. We had worked together on several projects in the EBMT, and we had the best editor team in place. Brian contacted the Americans and Diana Samson and I contacted the Europeans. Each of us would also write at least one chapter. After some delays we eventually published the book in 2004[129].

Editing a textbook is not without its difficulties. I cannot deny that sometimes there was minor friction between Brian and myself. Brian was indispensable when it came to recruiting the American authors, but he had a tendency not to produce his own chapters. I had to convince his wife Susie, my continuous supporter, to push Brian to write one of his promised chapters. Brian was an excellent writer, but either had too much to do or had other priorities.

Instead, our co-editor Diana Samson wrote two chapters, the very heavy ones about treatment. She did a fabulous work of the editing and proofreading. The book published in 2004 provided the most comprehensive text about myelomas for some years and it stayed current for much longer than the one published in 1996. The review in *New England Journal of Medicine* on 9 June 2005, ended *"A copy of the book should be available in every hematology department and on the shelf of every specialist in this field"*.

My interest in treating multiple myeloma persisted. Allogenic transplants were my topic, and my base was the Myeloma Subcommittee of the EBMT. We carried out many retrospective studies using the EBMT Registry, which was based in Leiden in the Netherlands. Simona Iacobelli was the statistician and a key contributor to most of these studies and is a wonderful person with a competence that cannot be overestimated. She also dealt patiently with my continuous efforts to find ways to analyze the material in a different way if I did not find the statistically significant difference I had predicted and hoped for. Before Simona took over as a statistician for the myeloma studies, I had employed a young newly-examined statistician at the Huddinge Hospital, Hanna Svensson. She was super intelligent and performed the statistics in the earlier registry studies, which showed excellent results in twin transplants and improved results over time. We were also able to show that transplants using peripheral blood stem cells provided the same good results as bone marrow transplants. This was very important for the donor, as well as for the transplant team, because the peripheral blood technique did not need an operating theater and there was no need to anesthetize the donor.

In the 30 years that followed the workshop at Blenheim Palace, I travelled about 20 times a year to workshops, meetings and congresses all over the world. It was always about transplants for multiple myeloma. We planned a prospective study that compared combined autologous/allogeneic transplantations to single or tandem autologous transplants in the late 1990s, but did not manage to start it until the year 2000 under the name A Phase-II Study Comparing Non-Myeloablative Allogeneic Hematopoietic Stem Cell Transplantation Following Autologous Transplantation to Autologous Transplantation Alone in Multiple Myeloma (NMAM 2000). This comprised 23 EBMT centers and 357 patients. The findings were reported at intervals at congresses throughout the world and published twice, first in *Journal of Clinical Oncology* (Chapter 34) and a few years later with a longer follow-up in *Blood*. It showed that Auto/Allo was superior. Two other studies supported our results. However, the number of allogeneic transplants performed for myelomas decreased to a few hundred a year worldwide. This was because one large American study, and another study by a group from Europe and the Netherlands, did not find a difference in outcome between the two treatments.

One problem with all cancer studies is that long-term follow-up studies are needed to know if one treatment is better than another. Early responses do not provide firm confirmation about whether they are sustainable. Diseases can recur late in both compared groups or earlier in one of them. The early recurrences may occur in patients with low transplant-related mortality, which means that without a long follow-up period it may be difficult to assess the results correctly.

There are many other difficulties in performing long-term studies. New treatments that seem promising may prevent the ongoing studies to continue long term, since the patients are entered in studies with the new treatments before the long-term result with the initial study has been obtained. New myeloma drugs appear very frequently. Some that build on principally new ideas are very effective initially. Others build on old ideas, but with additional ones added. The newest one at the moment builds on the idea that the body has T-cells that can attack cancer cells. However, when the cancer is established the patient's own (autologous) T-cells are not strong enough to kill the cancer, or there are not enough of them. Allogeneic transplantation is one way to give the patient fresh, strong T-cells to fight the cancer. However, the problem is that these cells also attack the other cells in the body and cause graft versus host disease, which can be deadly. The new idea is to genetically manipulate the T-cells so that they only kill cancer cells. These cells are called chimeric antigen receptor-T (CAR-T) cells.

CAR-T cells can kill certain cancer cells extremely effectively, including myeloma cells. Hundreds of studies are going on to see if the dramatic responses are sustainable. The first two CAR-T cell products for treating myeloma have been registered in many countries and there are more to come. The research on this type of cell therapy is exploding. In addition, natural killer (NK) cells can be manipulated in the same way as T-cells. Evren Alici's research group at the Karolinska University Hospital, Huddinge, is focusing on this cell and in 2022 we published a study on treating patients with NK cells, together with Hareth Nahi's clinical group. The results look promising[130]. It is too early to judge whether these approaches will produce sustained remission and cure of the disease. With current CAR-T cell therapy of multiple myeloma all patients seem to relapse, in contrast to results in lymphomas and acute lymphoblastic leukemia where many patients seem to be cured. However, combining these approaches with current drug treatments are likely to improve results and maybe eventually cure patients with multiple myeloma. Autologous T-cells are currently being manipulated to CAR-T cells which are expanded and returned to the patient, but allogeneic T-cells seem to me to be the favored approach. The future for cell therapy, which can be seen as a further development of allogeneic and autologous stem cell transplantation, looks bright.

After the first IMW meeting at Blenheim Palace, I participated in most of the subsequent meetings and presented the results of allogeneic stem cell transplants, mostly from our joint EBMT studies. We met at exiting places outside Europe like Banff in Canada, Sydney in Australia, Kyoto in Japan, New Delhi in India and Boston in USA. But we also met in Europe, in Torino and Rome in Italy, La Baule in France and Salamanca in Spain.

My latest presentation was in September 2021 during the Controversies in Stem Cell Transplantation and Cellular Therapies meeting. It is usually held in Berlin, but this time it was a digital meeting due to the COVID-19 pandemic. The meetings only include pros and cons debates. My opponent this time was Philippe Moreau, Professor of Clinical Hematology at the University of Nantes and Head of Hematology at the University Hospital. He is also a leading international myeloma clinician, and I must admit that, despite our opposite views on transplants, I appreciate him very much. However, he has gone from being one of my strongest opponents to allogeneic stem cell transplantation to an equal fan of CAR-T cell therapy, maybe both allogeneic and autologous ones.

Highly valued prizes have been awarded to many specialists in the myeloma field. Prizes have also been designed for this specific field. Brian Durie has a long list. So have Robert Kyle, Kenneth Anderson, Jesus San Miguel, Bart Barlogie and my latest friend in this field Nikhil Munshi, now president of IMS, professor at Harvard Medical School, and the leading scientist in myeloma research at the Dana-Farber Cancer Institute, my workplace in the 1960s, and many others. Robert Kyle has also given his name to a very prestigious prize. Everybody is proud of their prizes and honors. When I got His Majesty the King of Sweden's Medal 12th size, blue ribbon, for contributions in medical research I was very proud. Even more so when I received the Robert A Kyle Lifetime Achievement Award.

But which one of the myeloma researchers would be worthy of the Nobel Prize? Frankly speaking, I do not know if any of them would be. To be the co-author of 10 publications about industry-sponsored clinical trials of new drugs or drug combinations in the *New England Journal of Medicine* is not uncommon among leading myeloma clinicians. But they do not count very much in Nobel Prize terms. You need to make a paradigm shifting new discovery. The survival of myeloma patients has increased dramatically from a few years to a median of close to ten years during the last thirty years. Many myeloma patients live with treatment for more than 20 years. But who is the main contributor to this development and has made the paradigm shifting discovery? I think the most rewarded one is probably Ken Anderson at the Dana-Farber Institute. He and his team have been very successful in developing the myeloma drugs lenalidomide, an immunomodulator, and bortezomib, a proteosome inhibitor, to approval by the FDA (Food and Drug Administration, responsible for approval of drugs in USA) and have established a big laboratory for translational research about myeloma focusing on the microenvironment. However, many other important scientists have been participating and added to the knowledge and success in myeloma treatment. One paradigm shifting discovery that later was applied to myeloma treatment was that T-cells could be genetically manipulated to target antigens on cancer cells. But this discovery was made experimentally by Zelig Eshhar at the Weismann Institute in Israel, who does not belong to the myeloma "lobby"; and the first to use it against an antigen, BCMA (B-cell maturation antigen), on myeloma cells was James N Kochenderfer and his group at NCI (National Cancer Institute in USA), also rarely seen at myeloma meetings. Their contributions have shifted our view on how to treat not only myeloma but also other tumors in the future, i.e., by using genetically manipulated T-cells (CAR-T-cells) to specifically target antigens on the tumor. Many groups are advancing their myeloma research in this field. One of the leading ones is headed by Professor Hermann Einsele at the University Hospital of Würzburg in Germany.

It is important that people who nominate others for the Nobel Prize read Nobel's will. Then they can propose someone accordingly, if they are invited to. The most important universities worldwide are invited to nominate people for Nobel Prizes. That is why many of my friends in the myeloma field may already be, or become, nominators. The next step is to look for those with new paradigm shifting ideas and who have shown them to be right.

45 Kuwait, Pakistan, Egypt, Saudi Arabia and Turkey

Muslim or primarily Muslim countries, namely Kuwait, Pakistan, Egypt, Saudi Arabia and Turkey, may not have suitable candidates that would qualify for the Nobel Prize in Physiology or Medicine at the moment. However, scientists from those countries who have moved to the USA or Europe may well have been worthy of the Prize. Uğur Şahin and his wife Özlem Türeci are second-generation immigrants from Turkey to Germany who developed the messenger RNA COVID-19 vaccine Comirnaty[131]. Their pharmaceutical company, BioNTech, teamed up with Pfizer to produce and distribute the vaccine, which is now the dominant COVID-19 vaccine on the market. However, the vaccine was based on the earlier discovery of mRNA as the key substance for its production[132], which was awarded with the Nobel Prize to Katalin Karikó and Drew Weissman in 2023 *"for their discoveries concerning nucleoside base modifications that enabled the development of effective mRNA vaccines against COVID-19"*. The importance of Şahin and Türeci, who were instrumental in the development of the vaccine, was mentioned and shown in the last slide at the Nobel lecture presented by Karikó on the 7th December 2023 in Stockholm. Thus, researchers from these primarily Muslim countries have ambitions to perform important science and I write briefly about my experiences of my many visits to them for lectures and meetings.

The Union International Contre le Cancer (International Union against Cancer) has an ambitious international educational program and is represented in 172 countries. I became involved in their program in the 1970s when about 90 countries were members. One day, the Head of the Department of Oncology at the Karolinska Hospital, Professor Jerzy Einhorn, asked me if I had the time to go to Kuwait to participate in an educational program for cancer physicians organized by the Union. The plan was for researchers, primarily from Europe, to give lectures on malignant blood disorders, mainly leukemia and lymphoma. Our project at that time dealt with immunotherapy for acute leukemia and it was perfect for a core presentation that could be used to discuss other treatment options.

Although I understood that I was a stand-in for someone who had pulled out, and it was short notice, I accepted and managed to get a leave of absence from my residency at the Department of Medicine at the Karolinska Hospital. I joined the Union's teacher group in Kuwait and spent a few days in this interesting country. I gave my lectures and was impressed by the informed questions that were asked and the enormous interest in what we had to say. Kuwait had recruited many foreign specialists to their hospitals and their cancer care was undergoing rapid development. The country had not yet been invaded by Iraq and the atmosphere was good. Many physicians had come from Palestine and wanted to settle down in Kuwait, but they were never granted permanent residence. The Israel-Palestine conflict had put a real damper on their views on the Middle East situation. Kuwait was still a rich country, in contrast to Palestine, and the future was considered bright. A faculty of medicine was established in 1973, but so far international top-class research has been limited or lacking.

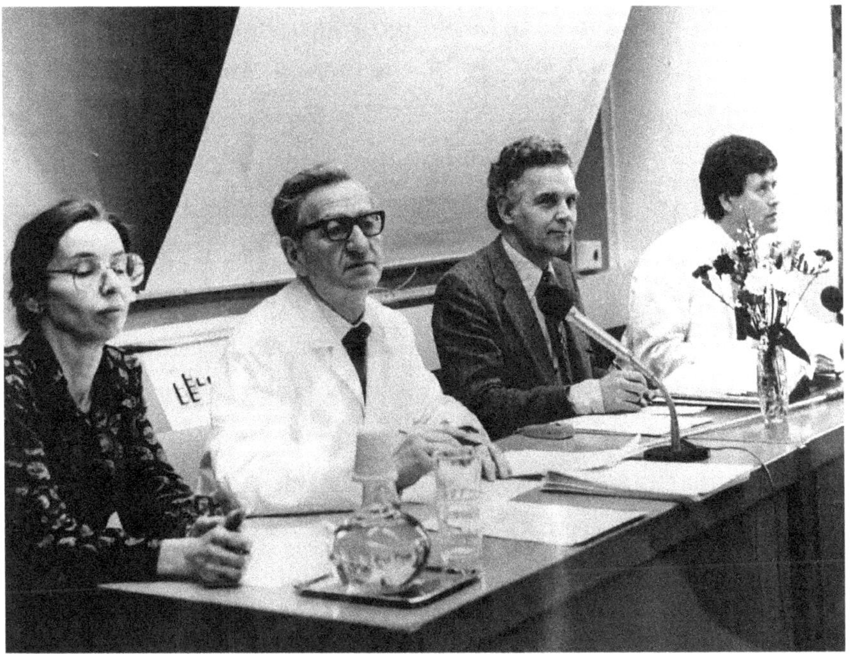

Jerzy Einhorn (second from left), Professor of Oncology at the Karolinska Institutet, member of the Nobel Assembly and Head of Radiumhemmet, the Department of Oncology at the Karolinska Hospital, was my friend and supporter. He invited me to participate in an oncology course in his department, which led to my involvement in the International Union against Cancer and my first engagement as a teacher in Kuwait. We are pictured here, together with his administrator Evy Kadaka (left) and Ulrik Ringborg (right), later his successor as Head of Radiumhemmet.

I soon became a regular member of the Union group that gave lectures about malignant blood disorders. In 1982, it arranged a course in Cairo, Egypt. Our host was Mahmoud Mahfouz, who was the ambitious Professor of Radiation Therapy and Director of the Nuclear Medicine and Radiation Oncology Cancer Center at Cairo University Hospital. He had decided to start a bone marrow transplant program and wanted to be updated on all that had happened in bone marrow transplants. It turned out that a few transplants had already been performed at the competing National

Cancer Institute, but with very high transplant-related mortality. I learned that the educated elite in this otherwise poor country wanted to engage in the newest technology, even if it could not afford to provide the most elementary health care to most of the population. At one of our conferences, one of the leading cancer surgeons in Cairo, Professor Ismail El Sebaie, Dean of the National Cancer Institute, brought the issue to the table. He asked whether it was better to spend the limited resources the country had on cheap drugs for the majority of the population rather than spend enormous amounts of money on high-cost specialty treatments, like bone marrow transplants, for a few rich ones. He stated that the National Cancer Institute lacked the resources it needed to efficiently support highly specialized treatments, and this resulted in poor outcomes for the patients. None of his Egyptian colleagues agreed, even if they knew that he was right. Instead, they wanted to discuss new clinical research projects with us, and I must admit that we were probably of little help. Many of the Egyptian physicians were well educated, but they lacked the resources to perform high-quality research at that time. Egypt was a long way off when it came to producing discoveries worthy of a Nobel Prize.

However, I visited Egypt and Cairo several times after that to attend international congresses. In 1989, I was invited to the first National Cancer Congress in Egypt and was greeted by no less than the Egyptian Prime Minister Atef Mohamed Naguib Sedky, who was serving under President Hosni Mubarak.

I had the impression that much had improved since my visit in 1982. More patients could receive adequate treatment and the physicians' knowledge had increased.

In 1990, we went to Lahore in Pakistan and were well received. The hospital was much better equipped than I had dreamed. The audience was interested and knew a lot about cancer treatment,

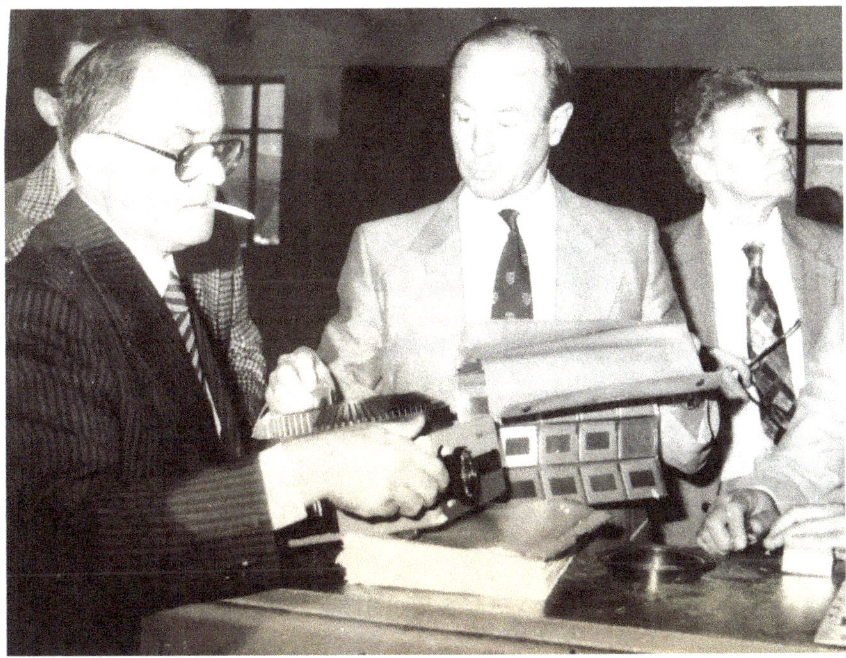

Mahmoud Mahfouz (left), Professor of Radiation Therapy and Director at the Nuclear Medicine and Radiation Oncology Cancer Center at Cairo University Hospital, was our host in Cairo. Sidney Whitehouse (middle) from Southampton, UK, and the author (right) were teachers on the International Union Against Cancer course in 1982.

but their experience of using new treatment methods was limited due to lack of resources and drugs. Research in medicine seemed absent.

Pakistan was a troubled country and Lahore was close to Peshawar, which was on the other side of the border to Afghanistan. Some of my faculty colleagues wanted to go there to look at the place, which was considered both dangerous and a location for smugglers of goods and people. I was not one of them and thought that it was a bad idea. They would not be able to see much of what really took place at the checkpoint in the afternoon and our friends at the hospital warned us that it was not safe to go there. Foreigners being kidnapped was a real threat. In the end we all

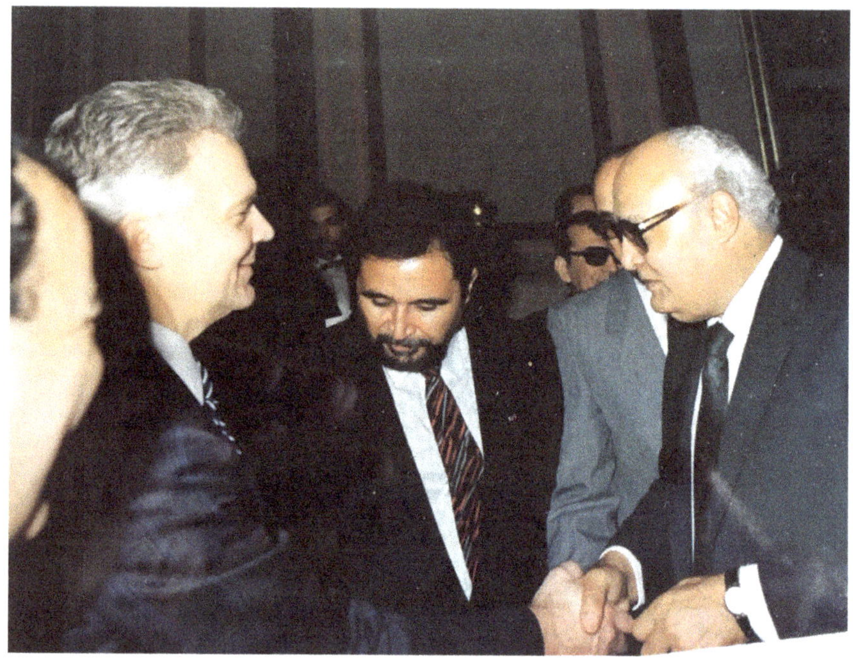

The author (left) is welcomed by the Egyptian Prime Minister Atef Mohamed Naguib Sedky (right) and the General Secretary at the first National Cancer Congress in Cairo in 1989.

stayed in Lahore and returned home through Karachi a few days later.

Saudi Arabia was very different to Pakistan and Egypt. Some of my friends in the EBMT had been recruited to well-paid positions in hospitals in Riyadh. One of them, Peter Ernst, who was still the Treasurer of the EBMT, invited me to an international conference arranged by the King Faisal Specialist Hospital and Research Centre. I was asked to speak about our bone marrow transplant program. It was an interesting experience, in terms of the country's medical research and the life that people led in a strict Muslim country governed by a family.

The adventure started when we arrived at the customs check at Saudi Arabia airport. I was planning to spend my visit at the home of the Head of the Hematology Unit, who was a physician from Canada. I had brought a large, nicely wrapped box of chocolates from Arlanda airport before I left Sweden and had put it in my hand baggage. The custom officer asked me to open my bag and asked me to open the chocolate box and show him what was in it. I tried to tell him that I did not want to destroy it because it was a present for my host. He pretended not to understand, took the package, tore the wrapping paper apart and opened the box. He immediately seemed to find what he had expected, namely punch praline. Then he removed three or four, smelt them, threw them away and then gave me the box back, with the rest of the chocolates. He seemed satisfied. The Saudi Arabian princes toasted people with whiskey, but the people were not allowed to eat punch pralines.

The program included a trip to the desert. We travelled in Jeeps and drove several miles in the sand, past herds of camel and ended our journey when we reached a tree that provided shade. Our hosts spread out blankets on the sand and served us an outstanding meal. Then I noticed that the children in the group were picking at the sand with small sticks. I looked in the sand and saw some insects and asked them what they had found. It was nothing special they said, only scorpions, but you have to be careful and not touch them with your hands.

Most of the specialists in hematology and transplants were foreigners. The goal was to educate the domestic physicians, but that was rather difficult. My impression was that all of them were very wealthy and did not need to work. Many of them came and went as they pleased, while the foreign doctors were working hard and had access to whatever equipment they needed to successfully perform the most difficult operations. Saudi Arabia was the opposite of Egypt, and it could not have been more obvious. They could dedicate enormous resources to infrastructure, material, drugs and not least on knowledgeable foreign doctors and nurses. In contrast, Egypt had shortages of practically everything they needed.

The women had not yet started their struggle for independence. The foreign families lived in fenced villa areas, where the women enjoyed their own lives as Europeans or Americans with swimming pools and amenities. However, if they drove outside their living quarters, they had to have a man by their side. I had the pleasure of keeping my hostess company for a few days, when we visited Riyadh's bazaars and other exotic attractions.

46 Gene Therapy

No Nobel Prizes have so far been awarded for clinical gene therapy. I am sure that it will happen, because the field is developing very rapidly.

Soon after I had become Professor of Medicine at the Karolinska Institutet in 1985, I went to a lecture on gene therapy. The College of Professors had invited a Swiss researcher to talk on the subject. He presented a lecture about using a virus carrier to transfer genes to experimental animals. His key point was that it would be possible to cure a disease by transferring a normal gene to an individual with a sick gene. There are many blood and bone marrow disorders that are caused by either an inherited or acquired abnormal gene. I was fascinated by the lecture and asked him for his opinion on the practical application of the experimental results in humans. He gave a very pessimistic answer. *"Only idiots are spending their time on gene transfers. Nobody believes that it will ever be possible to cure human diseases with gene therapy"*. He was wrong.

Gene therapy had not been successful in humans by the mid-1980s. However, at the beginning of the molecular revolution, many had great hopes that it would be possible to cure diseases with gene therapy. I was one of them.

In 1987, my enthusiasm for the possibilities offered by gene therapy encouraged me to gather some of the most competent scientists at the Karolinska Institutet together, to start a pressure group to get funding for this futuristic area of medical science. They were all members of the Nobel Assembly, and I knew them well or very well. The first one was my old friend, Professor Nils Ringertz, who had succeeded my previous boss Torbjörn Caspersson as Head of the Department of Medical Cell Research and Genetics (Chapter 19), and also succeeded Professor Jan Lindsten as Secretary of the Nobel Assembly and Committee. The second was Jan Lindsten, Professor of Clinical Genetics and previous Secretary of the Nobel Assembly and Committee. The third was Jan-Åke Gustafsson, Professor of Nutrition, a well-known researcher in the molecular field and initiator and head of the new research institutions at the Huddinge Hospital. The fourth one was Håkan Eriksson, Professor in Reproduction Endocrinology, who collaborated with Jan-Åke Gustafsson and was the Assistant Secretary of the important Swedish Medical Research Council (Chapter 35).

At the first meeting on 22 December 1987, a formal Karolinska Institutet Planning Group for Gene Therapy was established and I was elected Chairman. The goal was to convince the Karolinska Institutet and then the Swedish Medical Research Council to start a special gene therapy program. The most important members of the group were, in my opinion, Gustafsson and Lindsten and I was very disappointed when they showed little interest. They claimed that gene therapy was part of molecular biology and if a special program was created it would include all kinds of molecular biology. Håkan, who was representing the Council, was more positive. Despite these hurdles, I managed to ensure that we reached a consensus. I had to give in on many points, but eventually we suggested that research professorships that focused on genetic engineering and molecular biology would be established at clinical institutions. However, the post holders would not have clinical responsibilities. This was a typical ploy by Gustafsson to make it possible for theoretical medical researchers to apply for the positions. I agreed to some extent. The field was very new, and the gene technology methods were not yet applicable for clinical use. We also suggested positions for associate professor and research assistants. Eventually I managed to include proposals for clinical researchers and a couple of stipends for guest researchers attached to clinical departments. I wrote the final proposal and sent it to the Dean of Karolinska Institutet, Sten Orrenius. The planning group was then formally terminated. However, at the last minute I managed to include a sentence asking the group to continue to meet up to follow the developments in the field.

Years passed without a decision, but 10 years later the document was once again put before the administration of the Karolinska Institutet, thanks to my friend Professor Ralph Pettersson, who died many years ago. He finalized the proposal and secured 20 million Swedish Crowns, which was 2.5 million US dollars. It was not a large sum of money in research terms, but at that time it was not too bad. Most importantly, it was a sign that this was a developing field.

However, back in 1987, when the proposal was finalized, I was impatient and not prepared to wait for a decision. Instead, I teamed up with Edvard (Ted) Smith who was docent in clinical immunology at the time and later became one of the leading professors at the Karolinska Institutet and Huddinge Hospital. We agreed to focus on two projects. One was a clinical gene marking project to find out more about the cells that appeared at relapse following an autologous stem cell transplant for multiple myeloma. We wanted to know if they were derived from cells that were returned to the patient with the transplant or whether they came from cells that persisted in the patients despite the high-dose cytotoxic drug treatment. The current method used for multiple myeloma was to treat the patients with a lethal dose of melphalan and then save the patients with bone marrow or peripheral blood stem cells that had been collected, frozen and stored before the drug treatment. After the high-dose treatment, the rescue treatment involved giving the thawed autologous stem cells back to the patients, in order to produce new, normal bone marrow and blood cells. The question we wanted to answer was whether these transplanted stem cells also harbored malignant myeloma cells that could proliferate later and be the reason why the disease recurred, often many years after the transplant. Alternatively, it could be that the cells had survived the high-dose treatment that caused the relapse. We felt that it was possible to determine this by marking the cells that were infused after the high-dose treatment with a gene that could be identified in the myeloma cells that appeared at relapse. If they contained the marker gene, then it would be clear that the transplanted product had caused the relapse and measures could be taken to get rid of the affected cells. If not, the induction treatment carried out before the transplant could be modified or intensified.

Bo Björkstrand, who had now passed his dissertation, became principal investigator for the project (Chapter 34). It was a long-term study, but we thought it was worthwhile because it could help us to modify and improve the treatment of patients with multiple myeloma. After several years, we concluded that the gene marked cells could not be identified among the cells that appeared at relapse. These were more likely to have come from cells that had not been killed by the high-dose treatment before the transplant.

We concluded that we needed to focus on modifying the induction and conditioning treatments before the transplant to improve the outcomes for patients[133].

For technical reasons, including the efficacy of the gene transfer, the study was only partly conclusive. However, one important message was that gene marking did not have any side effects and an autologous transplant with gene marked cells was as effective as transplanting non gene marked cells for myeloma patients.

It took a long time until the study was published. After Bo Björkstrand went to work in industry, the study was eventually finalized in 2007 by my new collaborators Evren Alici and his tutor Sıraç Dilber[134]. They were both talented immigrants from Turkey.

The second project that I planned with Smith was to build a gene therapy center at Huddinge Hospital. Its primary purpose was to produce the viruses that were key to transferring genes to the cells that would be used for treatment. It had to have a high security laboratory that was certified according to the so-called good manufacturing practice (GMP) regulations, but building it would not be cheap. I negotiated with the Hospital Director that we could use a share of the money that the Government provided to the hospital to educate medical students and research. The Hospital Director oversaw this money. The education funding was distributed to the clinical departments, based on the number of medical students and the time they spent in departments. However, the system for spending the research funding was less clear at the time and the Hospital Director had some freedom to choose how it was allocated.

It took some years before we started to plan for the second part of our goal. This happened in 1993 and Birgitta Böhlin was the Hospital Director at the time (Chapter 33). I had agreed with her that I would present a plan for the project, which I did in 1994. This claimed that we were at the forefront of gene therapy research and pointed to several areas where it could be of value. In addition, the center could also produce virus vectors that could be sold to other researchers and generate income for the hospital. It could even be self-supporting in the future. She probably understood that the plan would circumvent the Karolinska Institutet, but that was not discussed. No decisions were made at the meeting. After the meeting with Böhlin and Smith we had the vision that the hospital would allocate five million Swedish Crowns to build the center and then five million a year for the next couple of years, to cover the running costs.

When we were close to finalizing our agreement in late 1994, I heard that Böhlin was going to resign as she had been appointed Head of the Swedish Defense Materials Agency. Time was running out. I created a summary of the project for her and why I felt it should be allocated five million for building the facility and five million a year for the ongoing costs. I rushed to her office with the paper the day before she was due to leave. She signed it and the final decision to build a gene therapy center with a high security laboratory that met the good manufacturing practice regulations was taken in 1995. It was inaugurated and functioning by 1996, with the support of the new Hospital Director, Sören Olofsson. It is still there and very active.

47 Gene Therapy Supported by the European Commission — Odile Cohen-Haguenauer and Zelig Eshhar

I recall attending a lunch where a few hematology researchers were discussing gene therapy. That was the first time I met Odile Cohen-Haguenauer from the St Louis Hospital in Paris. After the lunch she asked me to become a partner in an application for EU funding to form a network of centers interested in gene therapy. The first network, Euregenethy, was followed by Euregenethy 2 and Clinigene. Most of the important gene therapy research groups in Europe were included. Odile, who was one of the founders of the European Society for Gene Therapy, later the European Society for Gene and Cell Therapy, was the principal investigator and eventually raised 12 million Euros for the three network programs. The initial goal of the first Euregenethy project was to harmonize national regulations on gene therapy in Europe.

I had previously received grants from the European Commission and knew that a good application could result in very large funding. However, I was also aware that the bureaucracy was enormous (Chapter 41) and that this was even worse for Swedes. Despite being part of the EU, the Government had been stupid enough to keep the Swedish Krona instead of adopting the Euro.

I promptly accepted the invitation, and I gathered a few centers at Huddinge Hospital interested in gene therapy. They had to describe the projects that they planned or had started. The grant was not supposed to finance their projects, but to support joint meetings with European groups, create joint projects and harmonize European regulations that could facilitate the projects.

Eventually, we attracted 15 partners from most European countries. We called our network *Euregenethy/Regulation of Gene Therapy in Europe — a scientific network of users.*

Odile's energy was enormous, but she also required hard work from the partners and for them to be on the same page. The meetings were frequently charged with emotion and unfortunately some partners left. One of them was from the Weizmann Institute in Israel, represented by Zelig Eshar. Israeli groups were often allowed to be part of European activities. Looking back, I must admit that I had not predicted that his discoveries of chimeric antigen receptor T-cells (CAR-T) would provide a breakthrough in cancer treatment (Chapter 44).

This first application eventually lead to a grant of 280,000 Euros[135], which was not a huge sum once it had been split between the 15 partners. However, after many meetings in Paris and Annecy in France, between us and representatives from the European Commission, we filed a report that became the basis for a new application. We called this *Euregenethy 2, Establishment of a European scientific Expert System to facilitate clinical implementation of gene transfer technology (gene therapy)*[136]. This application was written in 1999 and the decision was taken by the European Commission at the beginning of 2001. Now there were 20 partners, and the grant was 760,000 Euros for three years. I received 47,000 Euros for our group at the Karolinska Institutet and Huddinge Hospital. The most important outcome of this grant was probably creating European collaboration on gene therapy, rather than promoting individual projects.

By 2002, Odile had persuaded us to support her with material for a new application. Our present grant would only last until 2004 and it would take time to plan for a larger grant. Special companies had been created in Europe to write the final application to the European Commission, because the language that the EU used was very special. If you had not learned how to use it, it was better to employ these companies to phrase everything correctly and not forget any formalities that were required. The EU now had a new program called Life Science, Genomics and Biotechnology for Health. We applied to this using the title the *European Network for Advancement of Clinical Gene Transfer and Therapy*, which was abbreviated to Clinigene. The EU had a requirement that industry, primarily small innovative companies, would be partners in the network and Odile managed to involve many of those interested in the field. One proviso was that they would not share the funding, as this was for the academic institutions. Many of the important groups and small companies in the field in Europe became partners. This meant that there were 25 academic partners and 10 from industry.

The new ambitious application aimed to collect information about all ongoing gene therapy experimental and clinical projects in Europe. Results from these projects to date would form the basis for regulations about vectors for gene transfer and all other technical, clinical and ethical aspects on gene therapy. We also included cell therapy, even though it did not necessarily involve gene transfers.

The Department of Hematology was not the only department at the Huddinge Hospital to use gene transfer technology

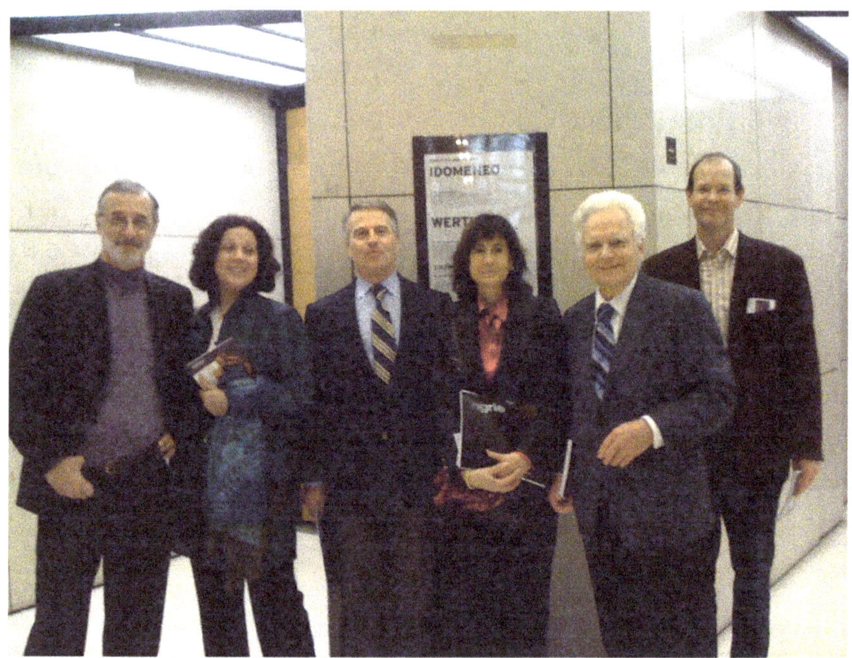

Odile Cohen-Haguenauer, clinician at Saint Louis Hospital and leader of three EU networks for gene therapy, together with a few of her 35 partners in the Clinigene Network. Pictured after a visit to Opera Bastille in Paris on 23 January 2010, to see Werther by Jules Massenet, with the world-famous tenor Jonas Kaufmann in the lead role.

From left: Bernd Gänsbacher (Professor at the Technical University of Munich, Germany, and Director of the Institute for Experimental Oncology and Therapy Research), Odile, Manuel Carrondo (Senior Professor at the University of Lisbon and former Director of the Instituto de Biologia Experimental e Tecnológica, Oeiras, Portugal), Fatima Bosch (Professor and Director of the Center of Animal Biotechnology and Gene Therapy, University of Barcelona, Spain), the author, Stefan Kochanek (Professor and Director of the Department of Gene Therapy, University of Ulm, Germany).

for clinical use. The Department of Geriatrics had a collaboration with the Department of Neurosurgery at the Karolinska Hospital, led by Maria Eriksdotter-Jönhagen. It involved transferring cells that produced nerve cell growth factor into the brains[137] of patients with Alzheimer's disease. The cells had received a gene that resulted in the production of nerve growth factor that was lacking or underproduced in the brain of these patients. This deficit had previously been shown by the 2000 Swedish Nobel Prize Laureate, Arvid Carlsson (Chapter 35). The gene transduced cells were introduced with a tether into the forebrain of six Alzheimer's patients. It was an advanced intervention carried out in an operating theater by a neurosurgeon. After about a year the incapsulated cells were retrieved and the nerve growth factor production was measured. Several tests were made on the six patients and some improvements in the disease could be seen in three of them. The cells appeared to have produced nerve growth factor, as predicted.

Sıraç Dilber from Turkey joined my hematology group in 1992 (Chapter 34). After he had passed his thesis on *Experimental gene therapy, with special reference to plasma cell tumors* in 1996[138], he, in turn, recruited several students to work in the gene therapy field. They included Evren Alici, whose dissertation project concerned the natural killer cell, which is a special cell in the human body that participates in killing cancer. Alici's thesis concerned how to expand and make more natural killer cells for cancer treatment, so that they could specifically be used to treat multiple myeloma. This was my main interest, as we had performed one of the first successful bone marrow transplants in a patient with this disease (Chapter 28). After Dilber left the Institution, Alici formed his own group and focused on making the natural killer cells more effective by using the most advanced gene manipulation methods[139].

The initial natural killer cell projects became part of the Clinigene application that eventually resulted in a six-year budget of 12 million Euros that had to be split by the 25 academic partners, after expenses. These expenses covered the administrative team of Cohen-Haguenauer and four employees and the fee charged by the company that had written the final application and the 140-page Consortium Agreement.

Looking back on the enormous efforts involved in promoting these joint European actions in the gene therapy field, I wonder if this overwhelming bureaucracy was necessary. Maybe it was. Maybe four administrators had to be involved to avoid financial fraud, and maybe the requirements of a particular number of participating countries were necessary to obtain the goal of successful European collaboration in the field. On the other hand, the projects that were included to the final report, the CliniBook, mainly seemed to have started, and were ongoing, without too much reliance on the grant. Each group had its own grants for specific projects. Despite this, I have a positive view on the initiative and learned a lot and made many friends at the many constructive scientific meetings arranged by Odile.

In 2011, a few of us had to say a final goodbye to each other and to the EU grant that had been spent. My group at the Huddinge Hospital had received 400,000 Euros and it was used to support a number of the centers at the hospital, including my own. However, perhaps the most important impact was that it had helped to put us on the map of qualified centers for gene therapy in Europe and it gave us new ideas that we included in our own projects. In addition, we had participated in establishing a regulatory framework for gene therapy in Europe. We had also showed that we were ahead in Sweden, by creating a good manufacturing practice facility for producing gene manipulated therapeutics (Chapter 46).

The number of partners in the Euregenethy and Clinigene projects successively increased, but only three of the founding partners stayed on to the *"bitter end"*: me, Odile and Klaus Cichutek from the Paul Ehrlich Institute in Langen, Germany. New partners were successively added to the projects and were, of course, not aware why the early participants had left. Klaus Cichutek was a very able and diplomatic person who later became Head of the Paul Ehrlich Institute, founded by the Nobel Prize winner Paul Ehrlich in 1896, which had the same standing in Germany as the Food and Drug Administration in the USA. We both remained calm during Odile's emotional outbursts, because we both appreciated her enormous efforts and knew that she meant well, even when it did not seem like that. We frequently managed to calm situations when other partners could not accept the way they were treated.

At our last meeting in April 2011, I had brought a couple of Nobel Prize champagne glasses, designed by Gunnar Cyren and produced by the Orrefors Glass Factory. Odile seemed to be happy. She was probably even happier because she had managed to get us all to summarize all of our projects in a 545-page book: *The CliniBook — Clinical Gene Transfer — State of the Art*. I had been responsible for the chapter called *Highlights on gene-modified cell therapy*, which summarized six cell therapy projects by 26 authors[140].

Zelig Eshhar from the Weizmann Institute in Rehovot, Israel, left after the end of Euregenethy 2. I do not think that we fully appreciated, or predicted, the value of his discoveries, which have led to breathtaking successes in cancer treatment, namely CAR-T cell therapy. Although we all used gene transfer in the hope of creating effective therapy, Eshhar was definitely the first to transfer genes to the lymphocytes that are called T-cells, with the aim of making them specific for certain cancer cells. By identifying specific structures, called antigens, on the cancer cells, he could use gene transfers to create receptors on the T-cells that were directed against these cancer cells and kill them. Eshhar had shown it in experimental systems as far back as 1989[141–143].

The clinical effects of Eshhar's CAR-T therapy were shown many years later by others. Malignant diseases dramatically and astonishingly disappeared when CAR-T cell therapy was used in patients with lymphoma, leukemia, myeloma and other tumors. By 2022, a few CAR-T cell products had been approved for clinical use by the European Medicines Agency, the American Food and Drug Administration and in many other countries. Numerous clinical studies of CAR-T cell therapy for other tumors are ongoing all over the world.

There is no doubt that Zelig Eshhar was the original inventor, and this is something for the Nobel Committee to consider. He is now 83 years old (born 1941), so they should not take too long to make a decision.

48 Gambro

Gambro was a Swedish company that was founded in 1964 by the businessman Holger Crafoord and was based on Nils Alwall's discovery of the artificial kidney[144] (Chapter 12). Crafoord had been the Chief Executive Officer (CEO) of Åkerlund & Rausing and had also co-founded Tetra Pak with Ruben Rausing in 1951. Tetra Pak became a world-leading packaging company and Crafoord became a wealthy man when he sold his shares in the company.

Alwall had become Professor of Medicine, with a particular focus on renal disorders, at the University of Lund in 1957. He had invented a dialysis machine in 1946 when his first experiments with rabbits was followed by his success with human dialysis. Crafoord had heard about the invention and became interested in commercializing dialysis and the artificial kidney. He met with Alwall and they teamed up to develop dialysis. The new company was named Gambro after the street in Lund where Crafoord's technical medical products store *Gamla Brogatans* Sjukvårdsaffär Aktiebolag, which translated as The Old Bridge Street Medical Supplies Company, was based. The first commercial artificial kidney machine was produced by Gambro in 1967. It was based on a relatively primitive machine that was built and used by Alwall at his department for renal disorders at his university hospital.

The Gambro company did very well, expanded, and produced artificial kidney machines that were sold all over the world. They also started special private clinics for dialysis in many countries and soon had more than 400 clinics in the USA.

It is no secret that Alwall was nominated for the Nobel Prize several times for the development of the artificial kidney. However, he had a competitor. The Dutch physician Willem Johan Kolff had presented a different artificial kidney machine in 1943. He treated 15 patients during the following two years, but all died. However, in 1945, one year before Alwall presented his device for the first time, Kolff successfully treated a 67-year-old woman with renal failure[145]. Kolff's artificial kidney machine was principally different from the one presented by Alwall in 1946 and from the one developed and produced by Gambro in collaboration with Alwall. Whatever the reason, neither Alwall or Kolff were awarded the Nobel Prize. Alwall died in 1982 and Kolff in 2009, which means that the discovery of the artificial kidney machine will never be rewarded with a Nobel Prize.

In 1994, I got a telephone call from the CEO of Gambro, Berthold Lindquist. He asked me if I would consider joining the board. There would be an election at the annual shareholders' meeting, and he would arrange for me to be proposed. I had the support of the board and the Chair of the Board, Lennart Nilsson, who was one of the big shareholders. He was married to the daughter of the then-deceased founder, Crafoord.

I did not know too much about Gambro, but I knew a lot about Alwall. During my internship at the Department of Medicine in Lund during 1959–1961 there was a joint emergency service between Alwall's Department for Renal Disorders and the large Department of Medicine where I served under Professor Haqvin Malmros (Chapter 15). Although Alwall was never on call to back up the emergency doctors at night, you could always talk to him later about any patient you had admitted at night for dialysis. During the night you had to call his frontline doctor, Per Erlandsson, who told you how to handle the patient for dialysis or did the job himself.

By 1994, Gambro was a big international company with its headquarters in Lund. Alwall had died, but the main company's assets were still based on producing artificial kidney machines and selling them to their own dialysis clinics. Running the private clinics was also part of the business.

I asked Lindquist how he thought that I could contribute. I had no specific knowledge in the renal field, because I was a hematologist. It turned out that they needed a hematologist. In 1990, Gambro had bought COBE, a company that developed machines that could collect peripheral blood stem cells for transplants. In the same year, Donnall Thomas received the Nobel Prize for *"his discoveries concerning cell transplantation in the treatment of human disease"*. Until then, bone marrow had usually been used for allogeneic transplants to treat many blood disorders like leukemia, but stem cells in the peripheral blood had recently been shown to work as well. Buying COBE meant that Gambro had a third area of expertise, and the question was if this one could be developed further and what the prospects for peripheral blood stem cell transplants were. One of my roles on the board was to advise on this area. Lindquist knew very well that I had given the celebration speech to the two Nobel Prize winners, Joseph Murray and Donnall Thomas, in the Concert Hall in Stockholm in 1990.

I agreed and was elected to the board at the annual meeting in 1994, as planned by Lindquist. Bengt Samuelsson, the President of the Karolinska Institutet and Nobel Prize winner, provided his permission and so did Birgitta Böhlin, the Director of the Huddinge Hospital. I was congratulated by both, who thought that collaborating with this important medical company at the forefront of science could benefit academia.

I entered a new world, which was different to the one I was used to. Gambro was listed on the stock exchange, but the big shareholders were the two daughters of the founder, Crafoord. The Chairman of the Board was Lennart Nilsson and his wife, Crafoord's daughter Margareta, was also a board member.

I enjoyed entering this new world of thinking and rapid decisions. New dialysis clinics were set up around the world with amazing speed. I was not familiar with private dialysis clinics, but all the figures in the annual report showed that they were important and good business for the company. Like the other board members, I supported this part of the company's activity.

However, I was not expected to have specific knowledge in kidney disease or dialysis, as there were other members of the board who were recruited for this purpose. My role was to judge the future for cell therapy and the cell separators produced by the recently acquired COBE company. But what was the future for this therapy? The switch from bone marrow transplants to peripheral blood stem cell transplants for treating many blood cancers had just started. I was convinced that it would expand. This was one of the first questions asked by Lindquist at our first encounter and I repeated my answer at the first board meeting. History has shown that I was right. Some 30 years after I joined the board, autologous transplants using peripheral stem cells collected from the patient are still the key treatment for multiple myeloma, despite all the new drugs. Allogeneic transplants with donor peripheral blood stem cells are still important and often the only treatment that can cure patients with acute leukemia (Chapters 28 and 29). COBE's cell separator was needed to collect both types of cells.

Gambro expanded and soon became attractive for potential big buyers. A few years after I joined the board there was a bid from a Swedish company, Incentive, that was dominated by the Wallenberg family (Chapter 49). The bid was too good for the Crafoord family to refuse, and Gambro was delisted on the stock exchange and incorporated into Incentive, which was a very diverse company, composed of a conglomerate of minor companies. Gambro became one of the biggest companies in the Incentive group, after it had sold off their smaller companies, and Incentive changed its name to Gambro, which was once again listed on the stock exchange.

It was quite clear to me that the old Gambro board would dissolve after the acquisition and my time in the industry would come to an end. We were thanked at the last board meeting and received a nice goodbye present. However, I was wrong about my involvement. Incentive, or rather the new Gambro, appointed a new board and the CEO Mikael Lilius called me, invited me to join it and I had no problem accepting. Lilius was already in that role at the time of the takeover, and we had served on the old Gambro board together. My main role would be the same as before, but there would be new faces around the board table. Claes Dahlbäck became Chair of the Board. He was a well-known industry figure in Sweden, with a long career in the USA, where he worked for the Swedish company Investor and was later its CEO. This company is dominated by the Wallenberg family and its Foundations (Chapter 49) and is probably the most important one in Sweden.

The new Gambro would have the same focus as the old one and focus on medical technology, dialysis and cell separation, with an eye on new developments in transfusion technology and cell therapy. It would continue to operate and develop private dialysis clinics. I felt that Gambro was a brilliant company of the future, particularly in the cell therapy field. Gambro bought a small new company dealing with regenerative medicine, namely with cells that could be substituted for a damaged kidney. Another company tried to make hemoglobin out of red blood cells. The idea was that this would make it possible to store the substance that was so important for transporting oxygen, which could be an alternative to blood transfusions. Maybe this idea was too optimistic, as blood transfusions are still necessary when large amounts of blood have been lost. Another idea was to make it possible to prolong the storage of platelets, without losing too much of their ability to prevent bleeding.

I got to know Lilius relatively well. He came from the Swedish speaking part of Finland and his parents had experienced World War Two. He was a very effective leader but could be very tough when people in the organization did not deliver things the way he wanted or tried to do things their own way. He fired the CEO of COBE and appointed David Perez, who was very able and already working for the company. At the same time, Lilius could show warmth and appreciation for previous retired or fired employees. During a meeting in Denver, Colorado, where Gambro had a production plant, we were invited to visit a previous member of the "*Gambro family*". During the taxi ride, Lilius stopped to buy a large bouquet of flowers for the wife who was the hostess for the event.

All the board members were very disappointed a few years later when Lilius announced that he had decided to resign because he had been offered the role of CEO of the Finnish energy production company Fortum. It meant he could return to his home country and that was probably a major reason for his decision.

Lilius recommended his previous Chief Financial Officer at Incentive, Sören Mellstig, as his successor. I knew him from before. He was a good friend, very able and someone you could trust. Claes Dahlbäck and the board thought the same and he was appointed.

Mellstig had to spend quite a bit of time addressing an issue that he probably did not want to. A whistleblower had claimed that there was a fraud issue relating to debits and record keeping at Gambro's dialysis clinics in the USA. A subpoena was issued by the United States Justice Department. This was extremely serious and threatened Gambro's existence. Mellstig had to present numerous documents and it took about two years of negotiation until they reached arbitration. Gambro had to pay $200 million, which was an enormous amount of money, even for a successful company.

I retired from the Gambro board when I had passed 70 years of age, but I stayed on for a few years as an advisor at Mellstig's request. Gambro's successes continued and it became attractive to larger companies. It was acquired by Baxter International Inc. in 2013, long after I left.

The Gambro-Alwall concept of dialysis persists, and artificial kidney machines are still produced for patients with damaged kidneys. The need for separated cells for therapy is rapidly expanding, after it was shown that leukemia and other malignant blood disorders could be cured by CAR-T cell therapy (Chapter 47). When I look back at the time I spent with Gambro, I am thankful for all I learned, and I hope that some of my advice helped it to carve its successful path in the cell separation and cell therapy business.

Alwall's discoveries about dialysis, and his invention of the artificial kidney machine, developed in collaboration with Gambro, was never awarded the Nobel Prize. Donnall Thomas received it in 1990 for cell therapy, but this was not due to Gambro. However, Gambro did help to develop the field by producing and developing the machines necessary for the therapeutic application of cell therapy.

49 The Wallenberg Foundations

"It is people that act like you that support a disaster". I was at a dinner celebrating the Nobel Prize winners when the incoming Chairman of the Nobel Foundation approached me with this claim because I had joined the board of the Marianne and Marcus Wallenberg Foundation. He was a good friend of mine and we had worked on another foundation board, and he had also been instrumental in forming an organization for building a register of voluntary cell donors for allogeneic transplants.

His claim was totally wrong, and I understood that his anger was directed against Jacob Wallenberg, who he had met when he was a board member for the Nobel Foundation. I could only guess that they had clashed for some reason. Jacob Wallenberg was one of the most successful industrial leaders in Sweden at the time. His father Peter Wallenberg senior, mostly called Pirre, was the Chairman of the Board of the foundation that I had just entered.

The Wallenberg family had created a fortune over many generations by developing Swedish industry and banking. The main part of the fortune had been established by earlier generations, in particular Knut Wallenberg, who had no children. He and his wife founded the Knut and Alice Wallenberg Foundation in 1917 to support research into natural sciences, technology and medicine. Later generations created new foundations and one of them was the one I had just joined. The Marianne and Marcus Wallenberg

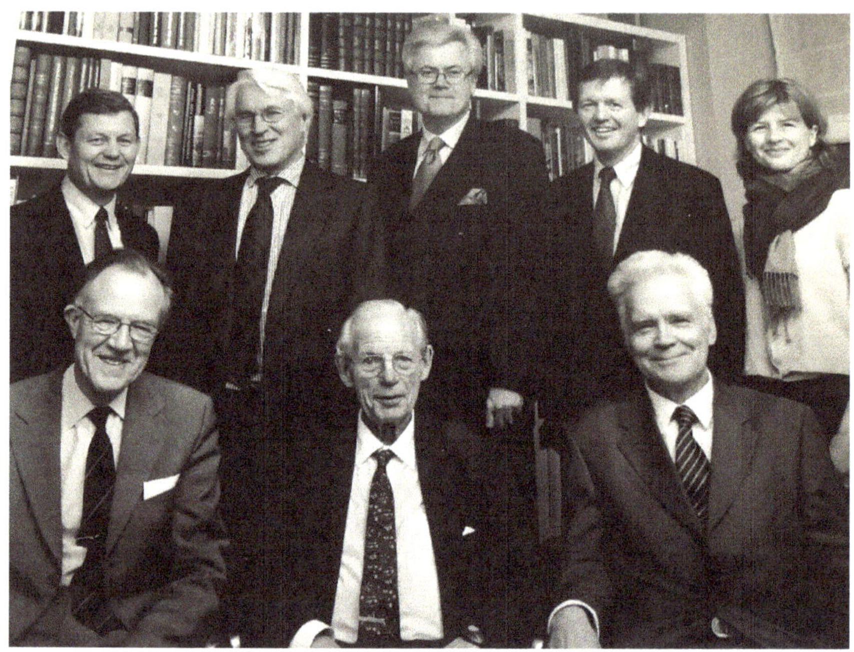

The Board of the Marianne and Marcus Wallenberg Foundation in 2002.

Sitting from left: Inge Jonsson (Professor of Literature and former Rector of Stockholm University), Peter (Pirre) Wallenberg Sr (Chairman of the Foundation) and the author Gösta Gahrton.

Standing from left: Jacob Wallenberg Jr (Chairman of the Investor company board), Johan Stålhand (Secretary of the Wallenberg Foundations), Håkan Mogren (former CEO of the ASTRA company), Marcus (Husky) Wallenberg (Chairman of the SEB Bank board), Mariana Risberg (MSc in Economics).

Foundation was created in 1963 to celebrate the 70th birthday of Marcus's wife Marianne.

During the 20 years I was on the board, the 16 Wallenberg Foundations granted billions of dollars to Swedish research. In the last two years of my membership, the three largest ones, including the Marianne and Marcus Wallenberg Foundation, granted about $400 million.

For many years, the Marianne and Marcus Wallenberg Foundation allocated the majority of their grants to research in natural sciences and basic medicine. However, during my time we started a program called Wallenberg Clinical Fellows, which supported talented young doctors working in clinics. For three years they could spend half of their time in the clinic and half in clinical research. Each year they were supported by a research grant, in addition to their half time salary, of about $90,000.

I joined the Marianne and Marcus Wallenberg Foundation in 1998, the year after I had formally retired from the Huddinge Hospital and the Karolinska Institutet. I was still a board member of Gambro, which at that time was a Wallenberg dominated company. Both the Chairman of the Board and the CEO, Claes Dahlbäck and Mikael Lilius, were closely connected to the Wallenberg companies and the Wallenberg family (Chapter 48). Although they had obviously told Pirre Wallenberg about me, I was asked to come to an interview with the father and son and a few others from the board. If it went well, I would substitute for a board member I knew, Bengt Pernow, who had been Rector and President of the Karolinska Institutet. He was now 70 years old, which was the normal retirement age for industry board members and many Swedish foundations.

At the interview I was asked about my previous career and my view about medical research in general and in my specialist fields. Jacob made some references to his grandfather's brother Jacob Wallenberg, who he simply called JW. He was regarded as one of the most important earlier members of the family. I thought they were talking about JP, Jacob Palmstierna, who had been CEO of the Scandinavian bank SEB for a long time, which was mainly controlled by the family. I answered *"Yes of course I know Jacob Palmstierna, we collaborated in the Royal Gustav V Jubilee Foundation"*, which was attached to the Radiumhemmet, the Department of Oncology at the Karolinska Hospital. It suddenly became very quiet. Jacob Palmstierna had recently had problems with the tax authority concerning the rental of his home and it had led to negative publicity in the press and Swedish Public Service. This, in turn, had led to a schism between him and the family and he had been fired from his business with the family and from his position as CEO of SEB. Sometime later he was recruited as CEO of the competing Nordea Bank. He then fought back by writing a book: *The ladder of Jacob: triumphs and defeats in a banker's life*[146]. The book criticized Pirre for not supporting him when he was in trouble.

My misunderstanding during the interview was resolved by Pirre, who simply corrected me, saying *"We meant Jacob Wallenberg senior"*. The interview then continued without any further problems.

I was warmly welcomed by Pirre at the first meeting with the board. My mistake during the interview seemed to be totally forgotten, not by me, but seemingly by the interviewers. After the meeting, Bengt Pernow, who was participating for the last time, told me what I could expect in the future *"When Pirre invites you to a private lunch, then you know that it is time for you to resign"*. Since my 70th was in four years, I knew I could expect to be invited to lunch, like Bengt had been recently.

Bengt was totally wrong about my future in the Foundation. When I was approaching 85, after 20 years on the board, the new chair Peter (Poker) Wallenberg Junior wished to change direction of the Foundation and support mainly social science research. I thought that this was the right time for my resignation. Poker thought there was no hurry and I stayed on for another six months and then resigned. I was happy that I had made the decision myself and had done so without a lunch with Pirre Wallenberg or Poker. Instead, the new Chair invited me for a private lunch sometime after my resignation. I had experienced 20 interesting years with the board and had hopefully had some impact on medical research in Sweden.

The warmth and the positive spirit I felt throughout the years on the board was to the greatest extent due to Pirre Wallenberg. In contrast to the picture painted by journalists, Pirre was a warm and welcoming person toward the three experts on the board, including me. The other four were all family members. He was about six years older than me, but he was crystal clear and decisive, despite his age. He often cheered us up with stories, sometimes about some controversy with the Government. He was proud that he had a basic technical industrial background, in contrast to many other industrial leaders in the country. It was easy to forgive him for smoking his pipe for most of the meeting, despite having undergone more than one heart bypass operation.

I cannot remember that he ever questioned my assessment of an application in medical research, even though I criticized other expert opinions. Pirre got straight to the point when he wanted more information, but still respected those who had more knowledge on a subject than himself. I was privileged in this respect when I was judging medical research projects.

Pirre could sometimes make drastic statements and annoy journalists. It did not mean that he discriminated against certain people, but he was sometimes misunderstood in this respect.

His contribution to Swedish research was enormous. At his funeral in the Katarina Church in southern Stockholm, his son Jacob presented a brilliant personal eulogy to his father to the Swedish establishment, including the King and the Queen. *"Everybody is here"* said the previous President and Rector of the Karolinska Institutet.

His sense of tradition, objectivity and positive spirit continued in the Foundation under the leadership of his youngest son Poker. Poker's older brother Jacob is still Chairman of the Board of the most important company in Sweden, Investor, and his cousin Marcus is Chairman of the Board of the SEB bank. Both are still board members of the Marianne and Marcus Wallenberg Foundation.

It is no secret that the Wallenberg Foundations have supported many of the Nobel Prize worthy Swedes that have not been awarded the prize. They have also supported those that have received it, like Arvid Carlsson, Bengt Samuelsson, Sune Bergström and Ragnar Granit. Although the Wallenberg Foundations have displayed their national character, by mainly supporting Swedes, they have also promoted international science by giving Swedes the possibility to lead international scientific collaborations. It was a privilege to be part of the evaluating body that supported this research.

Chapter 50

Japan and the Fujimoto Pharmaceutical Corporation

I visited Japan for the first time in 1966, for the 9th International Congress of Cancer in Tokyo from 23–29 October. I had submitted an abstract entitled: *DNA, RNA and proteins in lymphoid cells from normal, preleukemic and leukemic mice*. It had been accepted as an oral presentation in a section called: *Biochemistry of Cancer cells — Nucleic acids*[147]. It was a piece of work that reflected the spirit of Caspersson, but during the period of his life when he had got stuck trying to use microspectrophotometric methods in the clinic. The idea was to identify a greater variation in the content of nucleic acids between individual cells in malignancy and premalignancy than in normal cell populations from which the cancer had developed.

I had adopted the idea using an experimental mouse model to prove the case. It was known that a high percentage of AKR mice (inbred mouse strain, originally developed at Rockefeller Institute with a leukemia incidence of 60–90% , frequently used in cancer research) developed leukemia. I was able to show how the intercellular variations in the amounts of the nucleic acids, DNA, RNA and proteins in the peripheral blood lymphocytes increased when the mice first developed a stage of preleukemia and then leukemia. The conclusion was that the increasing intercellular variation was a sign of malignant development. Perhaps it could be used as a marker of malignancy in the clinic. However, the increasing variability occurred relatively slowly in comparison to other cellular changes, like the antigens on the cell surface that had been measured by my collaborator Britta Wahren. The practical use of the measurements of the nucleic acids were questionable and were never transferred to clinical practice. The hard work of measuring the cells was performed by a German guest researcher in my laboratory, Wolfgang Habicht (Chapter 34), who spent about a year with me. Unfortunately, I lost contact with him after he went back to Germany.

The Swedish Cancer Fund had announced 15 travel grants for participation in the Congress. The announcement made it sound very attractive, but the regulations for Swedish travel were very strange. The Fund said it was cheaper to join an organized tour for two weeks, arranged by the Fund, including the time at the Congress, than just to travel back and forth to the Congress by regular flights. Those who were awarded a grant from the Fund were encouraged to join the tour and the cost was completely covered by the Fund for the two weeks. All the people who received a grant agreed and were able to visit Osaka, Hong Kong, Thailand and India after the Congress. I joined them.

The first stop after the Congress was a large bath facility up in the mountains south of Tokyo. They were similar to Polynesian baths, supported by hot springs. Families walked around naked and so did some of us, while others hesitated or abstained.

From there we took the rapid Shinkansen train, which travelled at nearly 200 kilometers per hour to Osaka. The journey then continued with a flight to Hong Kong. Mao was ending the cultural revolution and we manage to go on a sightseeing trip to the fence at the border with China. We saw a nice forest landscape, but without a single human being in sight on the other side of the fence. Hong Kong still belonged to the UK and the inhabitants were worried about what would happen in the future. They had every reason to be worried. In 1997, Hong Kong became part of China and anyone following the media coverage can see how much trouble there has been since then.

In 1966, everything was cheap in Hong Kong. We bought custom-made clothes that were sewn overnight. After some more sightseeing we left for Bangkok, where we went on a nice river boat trip, looked at palaces, visited temples and looked at snake artists.

The next stop was New Delhi, where we were invited for an Indian dinner at the Swedish Embassy. We also took the train to visit the famous Taj Mahal, one of the wonders of the world. On the train I happened to sit opposite another Congress participant on the trip, the controversial Swedish Professor of Medicine, Erik Ask-Upmark, who was often called Ask-U. He was born in 1901 and educated in Lund, where he had defended a thesis in anatomy, but he later turned to internal medicine.

He had applied for a professorship in Lund but lost the battle after a tough fight with his competitors. However, he managed to secure the same position in Uppsala in 1946, despite tough competition from Jan Waldenström. Instead, Waldenström became the second Professor in Medicine at the University of Lund, in parallel with Haqvin Malmros, but his Department of Medicine was located in Malmö General Hospital, 20 km south of Lund (Chapter 18).

Although I had heard about Ask-Upmark and seen him present at a congress arranged by the Swedish Society of Medicine, I did not know him.

There were many stories about Ask-Upmark. He was extremely conservative, there was a rumor he did not like women, and he required his students to go to extremes. For example, he expected all of them to be at the hospital on Christmas Eve. He was against abortion and claimed that contraceptives were dangerous. At a symposium he stated that contraceptives increased the risk for stroke and thrombosis, but when a psychiatrist claimed that he was wrong his reaction was to leave the floor.

Despite these extremes, no one denied that he was extremely knowledgeable in internal medicine, and he was considered to be one of the last ones that mastered the whole subject. He wrote excellent educational textbooks, particularly one on emergency medicine, which I have used many times.

I talked with Ask-Upmark for the first time on the train to Taj Mahal. I presented myself and when he heard my name he said: *"Well, are you the son of the tall and handsome doctor Gahrton?"*. I was totally surprised, because I had never heard my father talk about Ask-Upmark and did not think that he knew him. My father was eight years older than Ask-Upmark and had finished his short academic career in the late 1920s when he had just started his. Ask-Upmark started his postgraduate education at the Department of Medicine in Lund shortly after my father had left for Kristianstad.

Ask-Upmark knew a lot about my father's career at Lund, under the late Professor Karl Petrén in the 1920s, and he told me about the old times and his colleagues in Lund. However, he did not mention his competitor Haqvin Malmros, a friend of my father and my previous boss, who to his annoyance got the professor position in Lund that he had longed for.

I was astonished that this man was so nice and nonconventional during our chat, because practically all my colleagues only told bad stories about him. During the sightseeing visit to the Taj Mahal, he walked around with an American shirt hanging outside his trousers. He was very overweight and had some difficulties walking. Sometimes he had to be helped by either his charming young wife or our unofficial leader, Karl-Ludwig Wiechel, Head of Surgery and a specialist in hepatic disorders at the South Hospital in Stockholm. Maybe he had calmed down over the years, as he only had two years to retirement.

However, Ask-Upmark was far from burned out. After we had visited the Taj-Mahal and New Delhi, he and his wife left the company. Ask-U had a patient in Afghanistan that he needed to visit. I later heard that the patient was King Mohammed Zahir Shah. I am not sure if it was true or not, but his reputation outside Sweden was obviously better than it was at home.

After New Delhi, we went to Bombay, now Mumbai, where we visited an area around the mountain where the Parsis left their dead relatives to be eaten by the vultures. On the evening before we left for Sweden, we had a splendid dinner, which gave me terrible diarrhea the next day. That gave Karl-Ludwig unexpected work. He arranged for me to lie comfortably over a couple of seats in the plane home. It took me about two weeks to fully recover. My first encounter with Japan and Asia, and its consequences, was over.

I did not return to Japan until many years later. My involvement in the World Marrow Donor Association (Chapters 42–43) resulted in a number of new friends. One of them was Shinichiro (Shin) Okamoto, who was head of the bone marrow transplant team at Keio University Hospital in Tokyo. Shin and I became very good friends. One day he invited me to give a lecture on allogeneic transplants in multiple myeloma at the annual meeting of the Japanese Society for Hematology in Yokohama in September 2002. It was a surprising experience. I had expected an auditorium of a couple of hundred people, but there were more than 1,000. Shin thought that I could also listen to the lectures by the

Japanese doctors, which he would translate into English. I and a few other non-Japanese scientists from the USA and Europe gave our lectures in English, while all the inborn Japanese speakers presented theirs in Japanese. I was foolish to think that I would understand the pictures shown on the screen, but the Japanese text made it impossible. There was only a short discussion following the lectures. Most of the Japanese academics understood English well, but very few spoke English well enough to participate in a discussion. Shin was an exception, but he had spent four years in the USA.

The next day I gave a second lecture on the same topic, but this time it was for a small group in Shin's department at Keio and there was more discussion under his leadership. I also went on a clinical round on his ward and concluded that his transplant department was of the best international class and not that different from our own.

From then on, I met Shin about once a year during the annual EBMT meetings (Chapter 41). It was during one of these that I told him about my grandmother's uncle, Edvard Hernsheim, who had been rescued by the natives on the island of Miyako-jima (Chapter 6). Shin was extremely interested and revealed that he had spent his honeymoon on the island and had, for a long time, planned to go back to the island with his wife to experience old memories. This was how we ended up planning a joint visit to Miyako-jima in the spring of 2007. He prepared everything and became aware that lots of Japanese journalists, and especially the native islanders, knew the story about the German ship Robertson. It had run aground and been destroyed by a typhoon on the coral reefs outside the island. The crew had been rescued in canoes by the inhabitants of the island.

My wife Astrid and I went to Tokyo and then continued, together with Shin and his wife Keiko, to Miyako-jima. They revisited the places that they had seen and loved when they were first married, and we all got together for a reception in the German Village, hosted by the fifth-generation heirs of the lifeguards who saved Edvard Hernsheim and his crew.

Astrid and I were totally dependent on Shin and his friend Ito, who drove us around the island and guided us to the right places. All the road signs and road names were written in Japanese, with one exception. The last stretch of road to Ueno had been given a non-Japanese name, Gerhard Schröder Road, the name of the German Chancellor. He had visited the village on his way to the 28th Group 8 meeting, which brought together the leaders of the eight most industrialized countries in the world. They were meeting in Nago on the island Okinawa in July 2000. This gave him the opportunity to visit both the village to see the monument that had been donated by the German Emperor Wilhelm I in 1876 and the museum that paid tribute to Edvard Hernsheim (Chapter 6).

At the party in our honor, Astrid and I were first greeted by welcome banners with our names and then a speech by the Chairman of the Japanese–German Society. After the dinner a half-hour movie was shown. Japanese and German movie stars described the shipwreck, the crew's rescue and Edvard Hernsheim's time on the island until he eventually managed to borrow a ship to take him back to the island of Formosa, which is now Taiwan. Shin once again had to be the translator. Only Japanese was spoken at the table and in the movie, with one exception, and that was a young German woman who was affiliated with the Japanese–German Society. She had translated the movie text into English and tried to translate when needed during the dinner and while the movie was shown.

Shin was not the only doctor in Japan that knew about our transplant projects with multiple myeloma. In 1998, I was contacted by Dr Kazuyuki (Kaz) Shimizu who was Head of Medicine in a hospital in Nagoya and had a special interest in multiple myeloma. My daughter was an exchange student with Nagoya during that summer and Astrid and I had traveled to see her. We also planned to see Kaz at his hospital. He was in contact with many academic colleagues in the myeloma field and with the pharmaceutical industry in Japan. He had particularly good contacts with the family-run Fujimoto Pharmaceutical Corporation. They had the monopoly in Japan when it came to the production and distribution of the drug thalidomide, which has immunomodulatory effects and has proved effective in treating multiple myeloma. The drug was originally introduced in Germany in the 1950s as a tranquilizer and could be bought over the counter. It was later shown to have serious side effects, including birth defects, when it was used by pregnant women. However, a pivotal trial by my friend Bart Barlogie and his team in Little Rock, USA, found that it had an amazing therapeutic effect on multiple myeloma. Having been prohibited, it can now be used to treat myeloma, under strict regulations and in combination with other drugs (Chapter 44).

Kaz arranged for me to talk to the main owner of the company, Mr Kuniyoshi Fujimoto, which resulted in an invitation to serve as an advisor to the company. I made it very clear that I accepted the invitation on the condition that I would not participate in marketing to promote thalidomide and that I would just be an advisor on the treatment options and scientific background for the present state-of-the-art. I joined the company as an advisor in 2011 and my involvement was ongoing until the end of 2023.

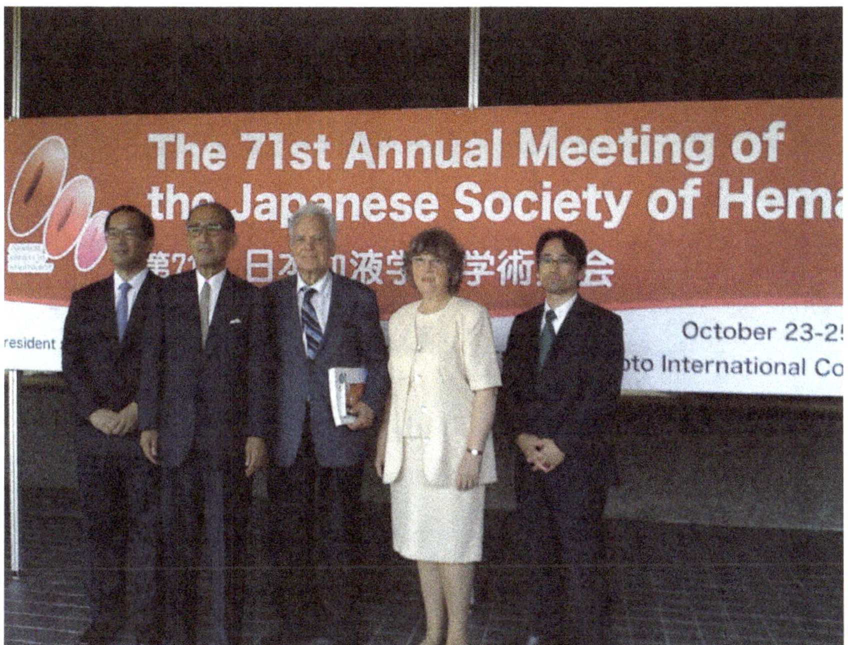

The Chairman and owner of the Fujimoto Pharmaceutical Corporation, Mr Kuniyoshi Fujimoto (second left), together with his two sons (left and right), the author and wife Astrid during the 71st annual meeting of the Japanese Society of Hematology in October 2009.

I also met Fujimoto's wife and his two sons, who both worked for the company. One was the CEO and still is. The other was a physician who was very involved in looking at scientific developments in the field, travelling to congresses and meetings all over the world and being a very nice host to visitors like me. We became very good friends during my many visits to the country and to the family. Kaz Shimizu eventually became President of the Japan Myeloma Society and, thanks to this position, he also became the President of the International Myeloma Workshop meeting in Japan many years later.

The Fujimoto family were charming and generous during my many visits to Japan. I also got to know some of the top scientists in

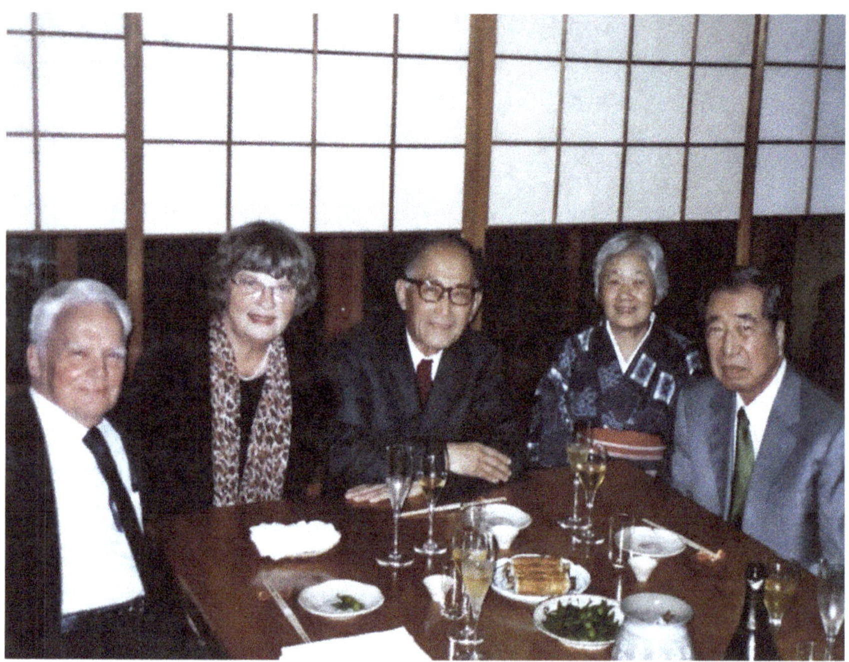

Professor Tadamitsu Kishimoto (right), considered by many a Nobel Prize worthy scientist, during a dinner at the home of Mr Fujimoto and wife (middle) in Nara, Japan. The picture was taken after my lecture, chaired by Professor Kishimoto, during the 36th annual meeting of the Japanese Society of Myeloma in November 2011. The author and his wife Astrid are to the left of the picture.

Japan through the family. I was invited to give a lecture at the 36th annual meeting of the Japanese Society of Myeloma, in November 2011, about treatment progress in multiple myeloma. The lecture was chaired by one of the most famous scientists in Japan, Professor Tadamitsu Kishimoto from Osaka University. In the 1980s, he led a group that discovered a factor of great importance for myeloma development, namely cytokine IL-6[148]. He very soon managed to synthesize an antibody to this cytokine, in the hope that it would provide a drug for treatment of the disease. This mono-clonal anti-IL-6 antibody did not turn out to be very effective in treating multiple myeloma. However, it was shown to be the most important one to treat the so-called cytokine release syndrome that occurs, and is sometimes life threatening, after CAR-T cell treatment of malignancies, including myeloma (Chapter 44). The monoclonal anti IL-6 antibody is now called tocilizumab and is marketed as RoActemra by Chugai and Roche. It is also registered for treating other disorders with an immunological etiology, like rheumatoid arthritis, and seems to be well placed for treating severe COVID-19 disease.

Kishimoto's discoveries have opened the door to develop other monoclonal antibodies, and many have already been shown to be extremely effective in many types of cancer. For example, daratumumab, marketed as Darzalex, was the first monoclonal antibody registered to treat multiple myeloma. It is directed against the protein CD38 on the surface of the myeloma cells.

Many scientists consider Kishimoto's discoveries worthy of the Nobel Prize. In 2020, he received the Tang Prize in Biopharmaceutical Science, which is worth considerably more than the Nobel Prize. Three awardees share 50 million Taiwan dollars, which equates to about 1.63 million US dollars. Kishimoto was born in 1939 and is now over 80 years old, which is something for the Nobel Committee to consider.

My lecture about multiple myeloma treatment went well, Kishimoto asked a number of relevant questions and an interesting discussion followed in the auditorium. In the evening Astrid and I, and Professor Kishimoto, were invited to Mr Fujimoto's home in Nara, Japan's capital in the 8th century, for a nice, informal dinner with his wife and sons. During the dinner he was amused at our reactions when we ate the potentially deadly Fugu fish, hoping that the poison had been removed. Only special distributors had the right to sell the fish after they had removed the toxic organs, especially the gall bladder. We survived and stayed overnight as honored guests in Fujimoto's house.

51 China

I saw China for the first time from the border with Hong Kong in 1966 (Chapter 50). The cultural revolution in China was ongoing, but the British Crown colony of Hong Kong did not seem to be affected.

The next time I saw China again was in 1992 and this time it was from the inside. I had been invited by the only known physician performing bone marrow transplants in China, Cao Lu-Xian in Beijing. He had invited a small international group to give lectures on bone marrow transplants at a symposium organized by the China International Exchange Center at the Bei Tai Ping Lu Hospital. Most of the other invited speakers were friends of mine. They included the American Robert Peter (Bob) Gale (Chapter 40), the head physician and bone marrow transplanter at Hammersmith Hospital in London and the previous President of the EBMT, Ted Gordon Smith, and the Australian physician Kerry Atkinson. He later edited the most comprehensive textbook about the subject, and I was one of the co-authors. We were also joined by the Danish-American physician Finn Bo Petersen, later head of this activity in Salt Lake City, which was the home of the legendary hematologist Maxwell Wintrobe, and finally my later friend the Japanese physician Shinichiro (Shin) Okamoto (Chapter 50). We gave a series of lectures for some 100 Chinese doctors. Our

English had to be translated to Chinese by Xiang and this meant that the lectures progressed slowly. The slide projections were primitive, but worked, Xiang led the discussion and questions and translated them for the audience.

We were always monitored by a politician from the Communist Party. It took a while for us to understand who he was. It wasn't until Finn started a campaign for us to be allowed to see the hospital from inside and participate in a round to see patients on the wards that we realized. Finn tried to persuade Xiang to give us permission, but soon realized that he was not the person who made decisions. After a while he directed us to the politician, who turned out to be the man who could decide. He said no for three days, then suddenly said yes.

We followed Xiang on a round, where he reviewed patients who had received transplants and patients with leukemia. The patients' rooms were very primitive. They had cement floors and an open well in the middle. The patients lay in primitive steel beds and there appeared to be no special arrangements for air conditioning or filtering. We were amazed that severe infections or other complications did not seem to be a greater problem here than at home. The results of the bone marrow transplants were, according to Xiang, about the same as in Stockholm or in the USA. About 50% of the patients with the deadly disease CML survived and were apparently cured. Not much different from Europe or the USA.

I cannot deny that we were skeptical about the results, although we did not argue, for obvious reasons. On the other hand, I must admit that later studies showed that filtered air and many other measures that had previously been used to prevent severe infections had failed and the most important measure seemed to be to wash your hands with disinfectant between every patient contact.

It appeared that we had unlimited freedom to do what we wanted in between our lectures. I could observe the traffic from the window of our hotel. It was dominated by a stream of hundreds, maybe thousands, of cyclists. I borrowed a bicycle and joined the stream. Some years ago, the Chinese had stopped the requirement for revolutionary uniforms and residents could now wear all kind of clothes. There was a pinup girl in high-heeled shoes cycling to a party and a brick conveyor with a brick-laden bicycle trailer.

There was a traffic light on the street outside the hotel and below my window. The cyclists crowded together in a large lump at the red light, while the green light stretched out like a long snake. At Tiananmen Square the stream dissolved and spread out in different directions. It was there that I met a couple of girls who were cycling. They waved to me and seemed to look upon me as some kind of exotic individual. When I was in the crowded stream I did not stand out, but when it spread out, I was clearly visible and strange and different from them. I parked my rented bicycle in a guarded parking lot for bicycles that cost less than a nickel. I did not want to risk losing it among the thousands of bicycles parked around the business street while I was buying a silk robe for my wife.

After the meeting, I visited the Great Wall of China, The Forbidden City with the Imperial Palace and the sleepy pandas at Beijing Zoo. I also attended an exclusive dinner with the faculty, including Bob Gale, who appeared tie-less and jacket-less with shorts and wooden slippers. Meanwhile the hosts wore proper dark suits and ties. I left the company to visit the old city of Xi'an and the Terracotta Army. My final impression about Beijing was mainly positive and it seemed that China under Deng Xiaoping had finally emerged from the Cultural Revolution. But what about the Tiananmen Square incident in 1989?

At the airport in Xi'an, I was picked up by a prebooked taxi with an English-speaking guide. The guide was a young student who spoke excellent English. He seemed to know that the chauffeur did not understand English, because before I had asked him about the present situation in China, he started to talk about what had happened in Tiananmen Square three years earlier. Students in Xi'an had continuous telephone contact with those on the Square, who they had supported and encouraged to maintain the rebellion. He suggested that there would be new riots against the Communist Party and demands from Chinese youths for freedom and democracy.

I was amazed by his openness and that he dared to talk about riots against the regime with the chauffeur listening, even if he was sure that he did not understand English. Single words to a foreigner could be picked up and create suspicion.

I returned to Sweden with the impression that China was developing rapidly, but the youths were dissatisfied and wanted freedom and democracy. However, my guide was not right about the riots by 2023, except for those in Hong Kong.

I did not visit China again until February 2003. The Karolinska Institutet had taken the initiative to lead a couple of research symposia. One was at the Cancer Center at the Sun Yat-sen University in Guangzhou, previously Kanton, and the other one was at the Faculty of Medicine at Hong Kong University, which had been part of China since 1997. The Karolinska Institutet had gathered a large group of professors in theoretical and clinical medicine, mainly cancer medicine, and the aim was to establish collaborations or extend existing ones. In addition to me, the group included Professors Ingemar Ernberg and Hans-Gustaf Ljunggren from the Department of Tumor Biology, which was previously chaired by the well-known cancer researcher Professor George Klein. It also included Hans-Olov Adami, a specialist in epidemiological cancer research, Juleen Zierath, who was later Chairman of the Nobel Committee for many years, and Urban Lendahl, later Secretary of the Nobel Committee. Completing the line-up were Christer Betsholtz, Per Artursson and Lars Engstrand, who were all well-known scientists, and Annika Tibell, who was Head of the Department of Transplantation Surgery. In addition, the administration was represented by the Dean of Research, Jan Carlstedt-Duke, and the future President (Rector) of the Karolinska Institutet, Harriet Wallberg-Henriksson.

I had been asked to give a presentation on gene therapy in both Guangzhou and Hong Kong, based on our experimental and clinical work. The title of the symposium in Guangzhou was the *Chinese and Swedish Bioscience Forum* and in Hong Kong it was the *Biotechnology Forum — from Scientific Innovations to New Medicines*. I was also asked to talk about *How to be awarded the Nobel Prize in Physiology or Medicine* in Hong Kong.

I chose to adopt a broad perspective on gene therapy. This included talking about our own studies on gene marking of peripheral blood cells from myeloma patients used for autologous transplants (Chapter 46). I also talked about gene therapy studies performed within the Euregenethy and Clinigene networks. Unfortunately, the technical arrangements for simultaneous interpretation did not work at Sun Yat-sen and the interpretation had to revert to the old-fashioned way it had been handled 10 years earlier in Beijing. However, we worked with our Chinese colleagues, managed to handle it and everybody seemed to be happy.

I had been told that the University Hospital attached to Sun Yat-sen performed bone marrow transplants and wanted to see the wards and patients and talk with the doctors working with the patients. This was arranged and I could see that the transplant unit was modern, and the activity was similar to any European or US transplant department. The difference between what I saw now, and what I had seen more than 10 years earlier in Beijing, was enormous.

However, what I did not know during my visit was that on the floor above the bone marrow transplant unit was a ward for many patients with a deadly disease that was not well known at the time. It was the severe acute respiratory syndrome (SARS).

A few days before our departure from Sweden on February 27, the administration of the Karolinska Institutet sent a letter to all the participants saying that they had received informal information that cases of an unknown severe lung disorder had been discovered in China. They did not know where the patients were being cared for or the degree of severity. We were informed that they could not verify the accuracy of the information and the Institutet had decided that the visit should take place as planned. However, they said that if any of the participants wanted to forgo the visit it was perfectly OK. None of us took the information seriously and not one of us abandoned our plans.

It later emerged that the Chinese authorities had failed to provide information about SARS, that was first discovered in the province of Guangdong in November 2002. It wasn't until we had returned to Sweden that Dr Carlo Urbani, a World Health Organization physician working in Vietnam, alerted the world about the serious illness. The virus that caused the disease was the SARS coronavirus (SARS-CoV). Urbani became the first victim of the disease outside China. Thousands of cases were soon diagnosed in China. The mortality rate in patients above 65 years of age was more than 50% and many younger patients also died. There was no treatment available for the disease at the time. However, the spread was limited due to patients being placed in strict isolation.

About a year after our return to Stockholm, we were all invited to the Chinese embassy. The Ambassador gave a speech in which he apologized for the lack of information from the Chinese Government about the disease at the beginning of 2003. There had been many cases diagnosed in China before our arrival, but because the cause of the disease was unknown, and there was uncertainty about the effect on tourism and trade, the Government had decided to keep all the knowledge secret. He admitted that this had been wrong. It was to his credit that we had now received an apology and clear information.

We had a few delicious dinners and admired the tens of thousands or more lights that lit up the bridge over the Pearl River, or Zhūjiāng in Chinese, and its surroundings at night. Then we left in buses on the 2 March for Hong Kong. The trip was on a two-lane highway that could compete with any such motorway in Europe. Along the way we saw hundreds or more 60-storey high apartment houses for Chinese people now starting to leave the countryside. This was not the kind of farming countryside I had expected. China had exploded and buildings had grown like mushrooms out of the ground.

Although Hong Kong was now a part of China, we had to show our passports to enter. The same rule applied to people of Chinese origin. Custom controls were strict, and it appeared that it was even more difficult to enter if you were an inborn than if you were a foreigner.

The symposium at Hong Kong University was more traditional than the one in Guangzhou and no interpretation was necessary. All the Swedes and Chinese delegates spoke English. In addition to my presentation about gene therapy, I also gave one about the Nobel Prize in Physiology or Medicine. I had tried to make it exciting, without revealing any secrets from the Nobel Committee or the Assembly, keeping to the 50-year secrecy rule of everything dealt with in these bodies (Chapter 35). The final question from the auditorium was as I expected. What would China have to do to receive the Nobel Prize?

Representing someone that knew about the Nobel Prize in Physiology or Medicine, I explained that the will of Alfred Nobel stated that it needed to be awarded for a paradigm shifting discovery.

I was pressed hard on the word discovery and I told them that a long and important career with many publications would not merit a Nobel Prize. I wished them all good luck. I am sure that there will be a Nobel Prize in Physiology or Medicine for someone in China in the future, maybe even in the close future. China has rapidly developed scientific activity, not least concerning treating cancer with the new cell therapy, CAR-T cells.

It was to be another 10 years before I visited China again. This time I was invited to *BIT's first International Symposium of Hematology — challenges in the 21st century*. The conference took place in the Beijing International Convention Centre in June 2012. I gave a lecture on *Stem Cell Transplantation and Cell Therapy in Multiple Myeloma*. China now appeared more capitalist than Sweden. The conference was a failure from a scientific

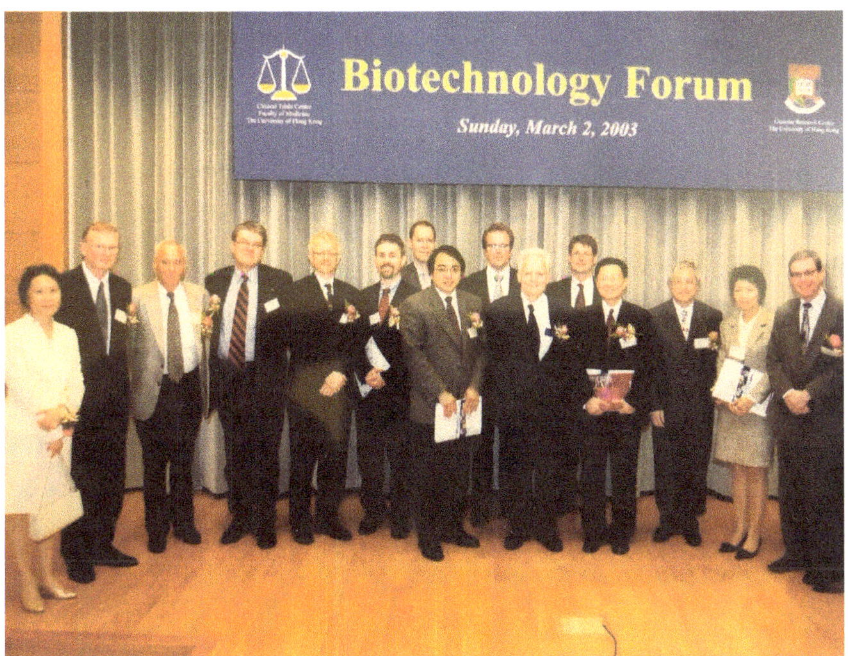

The Karolinska Institutet delegation and the hosts in Hong Kong, after my presentation about the Nobel Prize in Physiology or Medicine on 2 March 2003. The author and the two Hong Kong chairmen are seen in the middle.

point of view. Although some of the presentations were of some scientific importance, the interest from the Chinese hematologists was zero. The conference was highly commercial, and I suspect that the young Chinese hematologists could not afford the registration fee. This meant that mainly Europeans and Americans were listening to each other, and they had not needed to go to China for that purpose.

Instead, I spent much of my time admiring the economic explosion since my first visit. Crowds of modern cars were rolling along in five lanes in each direction outside our hotel. The Great Wall was absolutely crowded with Chinese tourists, in contrast to the few Chinese mixed with some foreigners during my visit

20 years ago. The Bird's Nest Olympic Stadium was one attraction our Chinese guide showed us with pride.

We queued for hundreds of meters to see the late Chairman Mao, who was displayed in the Mausoleum on Tiananmen Square. The entrance was like going through airport security, with no metal and no water allowed. Then people had to move fast, although people were allowed a short stop to buy white lilies, which had to be delivered to a designated place. The line then split, so that people passed each side of Mao, who was about 20 meters from the line. We were told that at night he was lowered into a freezer. It was a macabre way to view a mass murderer.

Although communism still prevailed, it was packaged differently. Our Chinese guide was very outspoken and told us that the law that only allowed one child per family could easily be circumvented in a number of ways. It could involve some costs, like lack of family support, but otherwise there was generally no punishment.

There were few foreigners on the streets, and they mainly disappeared in the crowds of Chinese people. Taxi drivers were reluctant to pick us up and it was hopeless trying to stop them, even if the cab was empty. They probably thought they would have trouble understanding where to go. I had a piece of paper, with the name and address of the hotel written in Chinese, that I could present to the taxi driver. When we travelled back from the Mao Mausoleum, we passed a taxi rank with a taxi that was seemingly free. We just opened the back door and jumped into it and showed the driver the paper with the name of the hotel. It worked and he drove us to the hotel.

Beijing had an excellent Metro, but unfortunately, we did not get the chance to use it. I only saw occasional cyclists, as the bicycle era seemed to have been mainly abandoned. In fact, more cyclists are seen on the streets of Scandinavian countries today. China superficially exposed itself as a capitalist country, like any western one. However, behind the scenes, it was 100% communist. We returned home after we had visited the Forbidden City and the Imperial Palace.

52 Media

When I worked as a resident in the hospital in Lund, I was sometimes called by journalists who wanted to know what had happened to patients who had been brought to the emergency room. The answer was always that we could not comment, due to medical confidentiality. Most of the time they respected this answer, but sometimes they tried to get more information, by insinuating that they already knew most of the details and just wanted a short follow-up. Sometimes I lost my patience and told them to go to hell.

However, my relationships with the press became more positive as I moved up the hierarchy and had research results that could be of interest to the broader public. The selfish side of me wanted to ensure that our scientific results were publicized, and I tended to agree when a patient wanted to speak to the press about what a magical treatment bone marrow transplantation was. After we carried out the first successful transplant on Kurt Svensson, who had aplastic anemia, his donor brother Ragnar and his other brother Pelle, who also underwent human leukocyte antigen testing, wanted to take part in press interviews. Both were celebrity wrestlers and Pelle had been a world champion (Chapter 28). We were all interviewed, and pictures were taken on the ward with Kurt in his bed, his donor brother greeting him and me and the attending doctors and nurses. The article about Kurt's successful bone marrow transplant was in Sweden's most read newspaper the next day.

We received further publicity after the first successful transplant of a patient with acute leukemia. *Svenska Dagbladet*, one of the most important newspapers in Sweden, wrote on 31 January 1981 that one out of four leukemia patients could be cured with new, fresh bone marrow. This was at a time when only sibling donors were used.

I used the press for positive publicity about our work, but there was another reason why it was so important. We wanted to get the message across to politicians that this was an important treatment that needed financial support.

However, I was still suspicious of the press and in particular of the Public Service. The latter comprised the most important television and radio channels, which were financed by taxes and dependent on the Government.

The annual meeting of the EBMT was held in Stockholm in 1992 and I was Congress President. The interest from the media was modest, both from the Public Service and the newspapers, and I wondered if perhaps I had not been active enough to engage them. However, the medical journalist from *Dagens Nyheter*, our largest newspaper, had seen something interesting in the abstract book. My friend Eliane Gluckman, the well-known transplanter and one of the founders of EBMT, had performed the first transplant with cells sampled from an umbilical cord after delivery. Gluckman was not due to arrive until the next day, and so I told the journalist about what she had done and said that she could get more information from her when she arrived.

The next morning, I read in the newspaper that the journalist had interviewed Gluckman, and she reported everything that

I had told her about the first cord stem cell transplant. She never talked with Gluckman.

Although the content of the article was true, she quoted my words and not Gluckman's, so presenting it as an interview with her was just not true. It turned out that she wanted to be first with the news and could not wait until the next day. Also, the article would not be interesting unless the famous doctor who had carried out the transplant had provided the answers. Second-hand information is not as credible as first-hand quotes.

It made me ask myself how often journalists used second-hand information as if it was first-hand? Perhaps more often than people think. Maybe this is not the most important failure of journalism, but it is still not right. My distrust of some journalists did not improve after that incident.

During my time as head of the clinical department at the Huddinge Hospital I sometimes dealt with journalists on controversial issues. Overcrowded wards were common and a great problem. Patients who had completed their specialist treatment could not be discharged from the hospital because there was no place available for them in the nursing homes in the region. Newly diagnosed patients with leukemia, heart infarctions and other severe diseases needed the beds they were occupying. Something had to be done to improve the situation. No help was available from the politicians or the administration at Stockholm County and we decided at the Department of Medicine to take action ourselves. Olle Edhag, my innovative associate head (Chapter 32), took the initiative and negotiated directly with nursing homes in northern Sweden that had empty beds and managed to reach an agreement with an excellent one about 500 kilometers north of Stockholm. Patients that only needed care, without specialists, could be accepted for some weeks. We decided to offer patients that did not need specialist treatment and care the chance to be transported to this nursing home by ambulance if they could not be cared for by relatives in their own homes. If they did not accept, they had to be sent home and cared for by social services, but often with relatives involved if possible.

A relative of one of our older patients contacted SVT, the Public Service television channel, and claimed that my department had forced severely sick patients to leave the hospital. They maintained that dangerous transport was provided to distant nursing homes. It did not take long before an SVT team with huge cameras arrived at the entrance to the Huddinge Hospital and wanted to interview the Head of the Department of Medicine, and then the patient.

I had previously participated in a course about how to handle journalists in such circumstances. The well-known previous employee at SVT who delivered the course said that it was always better to admit the media and grasp the bull by the horns rather than hide. I let them all into my office and the questions came thick and fast. How could severely sick patients be forced to leave for a distant region in the north in dangerous transports? I tried to explain that nobody was forced to go north, it was an alternative if the patient preferred it to being cared for at home by social services or relatives. Furthermore, we needed these patients to leave the hospital, as they did not need to be there, and we needed to admit seriously sick patients. It was the patient's choice what they did next, and this was just one option.

The television team then wanted to visit the ward and interview the patient and the relatives. I explained that this was not allowed due to confidentiality and for the safety of all the other patients on the ward. We said goodbye to each other, and the team left my office. But they did not, as I thought, leave the hospital. Instead, they entered the ward and the patient's room. They claimed, to the astonished ward staff, that they had the permission of the head of the department to interview the patient for an SVT news program. So, they did and the next evening there was a news report about the coercive measures being used against old patients at the Huddinge Hospital, with interviews on the ward with the patient and the relatives. I was not given the opportunity to tell the truth by SVT, even though it was part of the so-called Public Service. However, the important *Svenska Dagbladet* newspaper accepted my article criticizing SVT and explaining the facts. I was also interviewed by a second important newspaper, *Aftonbladet*, which printed an excellent and accurate version of what was actually happening and the problem of overcrowded specialist hospitals.

Eventually the Swedish Prime Minister, Ingvar Carlsson, got involved and he told SVT that the beds at university hospitals could not be used by patients that did not need their specialist care and treatment. If the patients did not agree to be cared at home, then extraordinary measures sometimes had to be taken to cope with these difficult situations, like transporting them to more distant nursing homes. Then the debate faded away.

Does the Public Service and other media have an impact on who will receive the Nobel Prize? I can only speak for the Nobel Prize in Physiology or Medicine and my answer is definitely no. Although the media often have a view on Nobel Prizes in Literature, and on the Peace Prize, they rarely discuss the scientific prizes. There may be some guesswork before the decision in October, but most of the time the media are wrong. I have tried to help them, without revealing any secrets, by telling them to look at the names and specialties of the adjunct members of the Committee. This will tell them what kind of specialists are needed for the year's nominee selections. So far, they don't seem to have adopted that approach.

53 Help to Die

You will not be awarded the Nobel Prize for ending patients' lives, even if they express that wish because of their medical condition. When the famous Swedish children's author Astrid Lindgren, who created the character Pippi Longstocking, had passed 90, she said that perhaps it was time for her to leave this life. But not tomorrow. When she died at the age of 94, she was totally deaf and almost blind. Most of us want to continue living, even in old age, frequently with quite some suffering from disease and physical problems.

However, others want to leave this life, even without any physical illness. Too many teenagers are depressed and tragically end their lives. A lot of research is very rightly being carried out to try and save young people from suicide. Many of those saved go on to lead rich and wonderful lives until they, like all of us, eventually die.

However, there are also those that suffer from incurable cancer, neurological diseases and other incurable disorders that only cause suffering despite palliative care. Some of these patients want help to die, but this is legally prohibited in many countries, like in Sweden.

Many relatives have seen their terminally sick loved ones suffer and asking for help to die. Euthanasia is permitted in an increasing number of countries, but there are strict regulations to safeguard this procedure. However, the regulations are not uniform and vary from country to country and from state to state. My view is that patients have the right to receive help, even if that help is to die under certain circumstances.

Euthanasia is not allowed in Sweden, but patients who have a terminal diagnosis do have the right to ask for specific treatment to be withdrawn. As physicians we are not allowed to treat a patient against their will, unless the patient is a child or not capable of understanding what withdrawing treatment would mean. In those cases that decision is up to their parents or the person who is responsible for them.

I will not discuss all the different regulations for active euthanasia or passive help to die in other countries. However, I will say that the Swedish Government is backwards and does not listen to the 70% of the population that support some form of help to die if people have decided for themselves due to severe suffering from an incurable disease.

I must admit that I did not get involved in this issue when I was a practicing doctor, as I was totally engaged in attempts to save patients from diseases that had previously been uncurable and deadly, like leukemia, myelomas and other hematological malignancies. But I have had second thoughts as I have got older, having seen meaningless suffering and ineffective palliative care when my parents were dying.

My mother got breast cancer when she was 40 years of age. Her breast was removed, and the operation appeared successful for many years. At 48 years of age, she was diagnosed with metastases to the lung. During about a year, she was suffering from extreme weight loss, pain, vomiting and eventually did not recognize her relatives. She had always said that she was not afraid of death, but she was afraid of dying. However, as the wife of a doctor she would never consider asking for help to die. She would know what that would have meant for my father.

My father's life followed another course. When he was 83, he was in a car accident. He lost consciousness and stopped breathing and was attached to a ventilator in the emergency room. He was still receiving artificial support when I managed to reach him a couple of days after the accident. I was able to tell the doctor, who was a colleague that I knew, to disconnect him from the ventilator. The best approach would have been to sedate him so that he died and then remove the artificial support, but that would have been defined as murder. Instead, his doctors had to remove the support and let him die more slowly, not knowing if his unconscious attempts to breathe caused him suffering.

For some time, I engaged in writing articles debating the case of a much-appreciated 50-year-old doctor who was accused of killing a baby in the intensive care unit where she worked. She had helped a brain-dead baby who was receiving palliative care to die by withdrawing ineffective treatment. A high concentration of the palliative drug had been found in the child after her death. The doctor was arrested and charged with murder. She lost her job, and the accusation destroyed her life. After five years she was cleared of all charges.

I also spent a short time in the Association for the Right to a Dignified Death. It was moving in the right direction, but after some time I decided it was too militant and left. I can only wish the Association success, but so far, they have failed to make any progress. They haven't even been able to persuade the Swedish Government to appoint a commission to analyze the pros and cons of euthanasia, which I regard as a democratic right.

Democracy is difficult to define. This is obvious when a country like Sweden, which claims to be the most democratic country in the world, has obvious deficiencies. These can be seen in these two last chapters in my book.

Maybe there should have been a Nobel Prize for promoting democracy? The right to help any person to die peacefully, without suffering, when they no longer have a dignified life, should be a reality in any democratic society.

Epilogue

There is a story that my former colleague Jan Waldenström (Chapter 18) was asked why he did not get a Nobel Prize. He answered: *"It is better to be asked why you didn't get the Nobel Prize, than why did you get the Nobel Prize?"*.

Many of the teachers, scientists and clinicians that I have met, and that are discussed in this book, have made world-class scientific contributions. Some of the discoveries have been theoretical ones, but have later been adapted by others so that they can be used in clinical practice and benefit patients. Some of the discoveries made by these frontline scientists have resulted in cures for diseases affecting millions of people. These include the new cancer drugs developed by the Nobel Prize winners George Hitchings and Trudy Elion, or the transplantation procedure to cure patients by Joseph Murray and Donnall Thomas. Some have made discoveries or developed Nobel class methods, but have never been awarded the Prize, like Torbjörn Caspersson and Jan Waldenström. Others have been luckier, like Bengt Samuelsson and Stanley Prusiner. Most of them have one thing in common and that is they have received modest or lack of interest from the media or the public, except for a few days around the Nobel Prize announcements and festivities. The lucky ones have received radio, TV and newspaper coverage, but most of them are soon forgotten, even by the medical profession.

It is clear to me that this is both expected and natural. Even famous footballers, like Pelé and Ibrahimović, will slowly fade away into the archives over time. However, I think that the media should pay more attention to those who have made the most important contributions to the benefit of mankind. Athletes, artists and politicians will not have to suffer. There is plenty of room for everyone in today's media.

Some people I have known have received attention when they have been awarded important prizes, especially the Nobel Prize, but what about those who never received a prize, despite discoveries that were close to Nobel Prize class? How many people have thought of Stig Radner when they have undergone balloon bursting and had a stent fitted to keep their coronary arteries clear and increase their expected survival by another 20 years? I obviously did, when the procedure was performed on me in 2003, but that was because I knew Radner. He was my former teacher and the first one to visualize the coronary arteries in the 1950s, which was a prerequisite for the operation.

My primary goal with this autobiography has not been to show how clever I have been during my career. It has been to show that I have met many extremely successful scientists who are worthy of more attention and publicity than they have received. Perhaps this book can contribute to making the media more aware of the fact that it isn't just athletes, politicians and artists who are worthy of their place in the spotlight.

Why not make a movie or TV show about the forgotten ones, like Torbjörn Caspersson, Sidney Farber or Inge Edler? Perhaps more should write autobiographies themselves, like me and my friend and teacher Sven Moeschlin. I found his book on Google and see it is available on Amazon. However, writing his book did not turn him into a star, either in his lifetime or in his home country of Switzerland.

Of course, it is easier to understand who the winner in the 100 meters is, as it is always one person, rather than who discovered how to cure leukemia. There are often many players in every discovery. Take curing leukemia as an example. The important figures I knew include Trudy Elion[149,150] and George Hitchings,[151] who synthesized the first useful cytotoxic drugs, and Sidney Farber,[44] who managed to treat patients in remission. Then there was Tom Frei, who discovered that combining many drugs at the same time was more effective,[52] and Donnall Thomas, who showed that bone marrow transplants could cure some patients.[152] But of course, there were many others, some that I knew and some that I did not know, who also made important discoveries that led to curing leukemia.

My hope is that my book will increase people's understanding of some of the most important medical discoveries and give credit to those that have made them. At the same time, I have talked about some of my own experiences while I have had the privilege of working with many of them. I also hope that by highlighting the important discoveries that have contributed directly, or indirectly, to curing patients with severe diseases, this will put the spotlight on those important figures in the history of medicine.

Thank You

This book has two purposes, as it is an autobiography and it highlights Nobel Prize worthy scientists. That creates some problems. An autobiography will only interest a minority, but the Nobel Prize story should be of interest to a larger group of people. I am grateful to many people if this book is a success, but I am fully responsible for any errors or inaccuracies.

I would like to thank all those important people that are mentioned in the book. Without them I would not have had anything to write about. I cannot mention all of them here, but they all deserve their place in this book.

Having said that, there are some that deserve a special mention. The first one is my former boss, Torbjörn Caspersson, who died many years ago. He probably made my professional life more exciting than anybody else. He was the reason that I moved to USA for two periods, which each lasted about a year, and that I found myself in a privileged position, where I could develop my own ideas at a world-famous institution. This, in turn, led to my thesis and my subsequent research and positions as a professor at the Karolinska Institutet and the Huddinge Hospital. All these events led to my positions in the Nobel Assembly and Committee, and meetings with the numerous Nobel Prize worthy scientists mentioned in this book.

Åsa Johansson also deserves a special mention as she had a more direct role in this book. She was my secretary from the time

I moved to the Huddinge Hospital in 1974 until my formal retirement in 1997. Åsa saved everything that was sent to me and copies of letters that I wrote during this time. She typed all my letters and the scientific manuscripts that I had dictated into my Dictaphone, most of it in English. All my correspondence and manuscripts were well organized, chronologically. She also saved dissertations from my institutions and all the abstract books from congresses, again nicely organized in chronologic order. This provided a gold mine of information and there would have been no book without it. Thank you Åsa.

I also want to mention a few particularly important people who played a role in my early research. Nils Ringertz helped me to join Caspersson's Institution. During that time, from 1961–1966, Britta Wahren, Dick Killander, Lore Zech, Anders Zetterberg, Rudolf Rigler and Lars Sörén were important friends and collaborators. Caspersson's engineers Leon Carlsson, Jan Kudynowski and Gösta Lomakka were indispensable in introducing me to the world of microspectrophotometers and microinterferometers.

Clinical translational research means direct work with patients, but it also involves intensive laboratory work with the material that has been sampled from patients. A great deal of this work is carried out manually with machines and other laboratory materials. However, the clinical scientist will, in the long run, leave a great deal of this work to technicians who may develop even more expertise than them in the laboratory.

During my first years in Caspersson's institution I did all the laboratory work myself, but I eventually received grants that meant that I could employ excellent technicians. I owe these important and clever collaborators great thanks. They include Kristina Friberg, Ann Wallblom, Birgitta Stellan, Ann-Marie Forsblom, Britt Sundman-Engberg, Monika Jansson, Eva Östling and many others. Without them I would not have had many scientific results to publish.

Numerous people participated in the clinical and administrative work during my time as head of both clinical and academic activity. The most important was Per Ljungman, Associate Head of the Clinical Department of Hematology and later my successor. The way he helped me to survive an enormous workload cannot be overestimated. During my earlier time as Head of the entire Department of Medicine, Olof Edhag and Hans Wallin played a crucial role in running the department and my numerous research collaborators were also important. These included a number of people in my department at Huddinge Hospital: Pelle Hörnsten, Karl-Henrik Robert, Gunnar Juliusson, Christer Paul, Bo Björkstrand, Jan Liliemark, Ragnhild Lindqvist, Mats Merup, Berit Lönnqvist, Eva Kimby and Eva Hellström-Lindberg. They were some of the many people who were important for my research.

There were many people in the Leukemia Group. The Professor in Pharmacology Curt Peterson was of great importance, as well as more junior colleagues like Sigurd Vitols.

Our collaboration with other departments were essential for our progress in stem cell transplants, especially the transplant surgery department headed by Professor Carl-Gustaf Groth and his collaborators Göran Lundgren and Olle Ringdén.

As well as at my own departments at the Huddinge Hospital, I enjoyed many important international collaborations that were crucially important for my research and for this book. The EBMT was my base and I made numerous friends and had many collaborators throughout the years. I will just mention a few. Professor Wolfgang Hinterberger, later Head of the Department of Medicine at Donauspital in Vienna was Secretary of EBMT when I was President. We had a fabulous collaboration at that time and became friends for life. Later Presidents also became great friends: Alois Gratwohl, Andrea Bacigalupo, Dietger Niederwieser, John Goldman, Jane Apperley, Nicolaus Kröger and Ibrahim Yakoub-Agha. In the Myeloma Subcommittee (Plasma Cell Disorders Subcommittee) I enjoyed excellent collaboration with my successors, Curly Morris, Laurent Garderet and Stefan Schönland, not to mention the indispensable statistician Simona Iacobelli, as well as Anja van Biezen, Linda Koster and the others at the statistical center in Leiden.

I have not described much of my present activity at the academic Department of Medicine at the Huddinge Hospital and Karolinska Institutet. Since my formal retirement I have been able to continue my research and have had access to the archive saved from my time as head of the department. This material has been indispensable for writing the book. My thanks go to my successors as head of the institution, Jan Palmblad and Jan Bolinder and to Klas Karlsson, who I employed many years ago and who was an excellent head of administration when I was still in office.

I also want to thank all the young researchers and clinicians who have continued to collaborate with me for quite some time after my retirement, making sure that my brain cells have kept working. They include Evren Alici, Hareth Nahi, Johan Lund, Katarina Uttervall, Michael Chrobok, Alexandra Treschow, Charlotte Gran, Göran Wålinder and somewhat earlier Sıraç Dilber, Tolga Sutlu and others. Some call me their mentor. The way they have stimulated my memory has been of great importance.

Thanks also to the Secretary of the Nobel Committee, Professor Thomas Perlmann and the administrator of its office Ann-Mari Dumanski, for helping me and giving me access to the archive of the Nobel Assembly at the Karolinska Institutet.

A great thank you to Annette Whibley for the excellent editing and correction of my English text.

I also want to thank all the patients who have given my life real value. They are the reason why everything that I have written about in this book had to be done.

Finally, I would like to thank my wonderful and supporting family, my wife Astrid, my four children and my 14 grandchildren.

References

1. Robinson D. (1952) The 100 Most Important People in the World Today. Boston, USA: Little, Brown, and Co.
2. Nobel A. (1895) Alfred Nobel's will. Stockholm: www.nobelprize.org.
3. Harnesk P, Davisdsson Å, Glimstedt G. (1966) In: Davidsson A, ed. Vem är Vem: Bokförlaget Vem är Vem, Stockholm.
4. Hillarp NA, Fuxe K, Dahlstrom A. (1966) Demonstration and mapping of central neurons containing dopamine, noradrenaline, and 5-hydroxytryptamine and their reactions to psychopharmaca. *Pharmacol Rev*; **18**(1): 727–41.
5. Bergstrom S, Eliasson R, von Euler U, Sjovall J. (1959) Some biological effects of two crystalline prostaglandin factors. *Acta Physiol Scand*; **45**: 133–44.
6. Bergstrom S, Samuelsson B. (1962) Isolation of prostaglandin E1 from human seminal plasma. Prostaglandins and related factors. *The Journal of biological chemistry*; **237**: 3005–6.
7. Carlsson A. (1959) Detection and assay of dopamine. *Pharmacol Rev*; **11**(2, Part 2): 300–4.
8. Samuelsson B, Borgeat P, Hammarstrom S, Murphy RC. (1979) Introduction of a nomenclature: leukotrienes. *Prostaglandins*; **17**(6): 785–7.
9. Paabo S, Higuchi RG, Wilson AC. (1989) Ancient DNA and the polymerase chain reaction. The emerging field of molecular archaeology. *The Journal of biological chemistry*; **264**(17): 9709–12.

10. Westling H. (2010) Erik Essen-Möller och lundapsykiatrin: Bild & Media.

11. Ehinger B, Torsten Krakau CE. (2008) In: Ehinger B, ed. Ögonkliniken i Lund under 140 år Lund: Sydsvenska Medicinhistoriska Sällskapets årsskrift: 185.

12. Svensk Biografisk (1977). Koch, Hjalmar: Vem är det. Stockholm: P A Norstedt & Söner: 545–6.

13. Fanconi A. (2015) Guido Fanconi, MD, 1892–1979 Swiss Pediatrician Life and Performance. *Pediatr Endocrinol Rev*; **12**(4): 343–6.

14. Bogliolo M, Surralles J. (2015) Fanconi anemia: a model disease for studies on human genetics and advanced therapeutics. *Curr Opin Genet Dev*; **33**: 32-40.

15. Zetterström R. (1996) The man behind Fanconi's anemia. World citizen in pediatrics (in Swedish) *Läkartidningen*; **93**(19): 1857–64.

16. Bleuler E. (1911) Dementia Praecox or the Group of Schizophrenias Leipzig,Germany: Deuticke.

17. Peralta V, Cuesta MJ. (2011) Eugen Bleuler and the schizophrenias: 100 years after. *Schizophr Bull*; **37**(6): 1118–20.

18. Moeschlin S. (1992) Rezept eines Arzt-Lebens. Autobiographie eines Weltburgers. Stäfa: Rothenhausler Verlag, CH-8712 Stäfa.

19. Moeschlin S, Wagner K. (1952) Agranulocytosis due to the occurrence of leukocyte-agglutinins; pyramidon and cold agglutinins. *Acta haematologica*; **8**(1–2): 29–41.

20. Gahrton G. (1961) ECG changes in pectus excavatum (funnel chest). A pre- and postoperative study. *Acta Med Scand*; **170**: 431–8.

21. Edler I. (1991) Early echocardiography. *Ultrasound in medicine & biology*; **17**(5): 425–31.

22. Edler I. (1961) Atrioventricular valve motility in the living human heart recorded by ultrasound. *Acta Med Scand Suppl*; **370**: 83–124.

23. Radner S. (1945) An attempt at the roentgenologic visualization of coronary blood vessels in man. *Acta radiol*; **26**(6): 497–502.

24. Radner S. (1947) Intracranial angiography via the vertebral artery; preliminary report of a new technique. *Acta radiol*; **28**(5–6): 838–42.

25. Radner S. (1955) Extended suprasternal puncture technique. *Acta Med Scand*; **151**(3): 223–7.

26. Waldenström J. (1958) Macroglobulinaemia. *Acta haematologica*; **20**(1–4): 33–9.

27. Waldenström J. (1944) Incipient myelomatosis or essential hyperglobulinemia with fibrinogenopenia-a new syndrome? *Acta Med Scand*; **117**(3–4): 216–47.

28. Gahrton G. (1970) A common therapy program of leukemia for several hospitals. *Nordisk medicin* 1970; **84**(49): 1574.

29. Gahrton G, Engstedt L, Franzen S, *et al.* (1974) Induction of remission with l-Asparaginase, cyclophosphamide, cytosine arabinoside, and prednisolone in adult patients with acute leukemia. *Cancer*; **34**(2): 472–9.

30. Turesson I. (2012) Jan Waldenström – en föregångare inom svensk hematologi (a forerunner in Swedish Hematology). In: Westin J, ed. Femtio År med Svensk Hematologi (Fifty years with Swedish Hematology). Gothenburg: Swedish Society of Hematology: 27–30.

31. Gartner I, Norden A. (1961) Studies on periodic acid-Schiff reactive material in white blood cells from the peripheral blood of patients with diabetes, polycythaemia and chronic lymphocytic leukaemia. *Acta Med Scand*; **169**: 289–302.

32. Caspersson T. (1936) Uber den chemischen Aufbau der Strukturen des Cellkernes. *Skand Archiv f Physiol*; **70**(Suppl.8): 1–151.

33. Caspersson TO. (1950) Cell Growth and Cell Function. A cytochemical study. New York: W.W. Norton and Company.

34. Watson JD, Crick FH. (1953) Molecular structure of nucleic acids; a structure for deoxyribose nucleic acid. *Nature*; **171**(4356): 737–8.

35. Caspersson T, Zech L, Modest EJ, *et al.* (1969) Chemical differentiation with fluorescent alkylating agents in Vicia faba metaphase chromosomes. *Experimental cell research*; **58**(1): 128–40.

36. Caspersson T, Lomakka G, Zech L. (1972) The 24 fluorescence patterns of the human metaphase chromosomes — distinguishing characters and variability. *Hereditas*; **67**(1): 89–102.

37. Caspersson T, Gahrton G, Lindsten J, Zech L. (1970) Identification of the Philadelphia chromosome as a number 22 by quinacrine mustard fluorescence analysis. *Experimental cell research*; **63**(1): 238–40.

38. Gahrton G, Lindsten J, Zech L. (1973) Origin of the Philadelphia chromosome. Tracing of chromosome 22 to parents of patients with chronic myelocytic leukemia. *Experimental cell research*; **79**(1): 246–7.

39. Gahrton G, Lindsten J, Zech L. (1974) Clonal origin of the Philadelphia chromosome from either the paternal or the maternal chromosome number 22. *Blood*; **43**(6): 837–40.

40. Gahrton G, Zech L, Robert KH, Bird AG. (1979) Mitogenic stimulation of leukemia cells by Epstein-Barr virus. *N Engl J Med*; **301**(8): 438–9.

41. Gahrton G, Robert KH, Friberg K, *et al.* (1980) Extra chromosome 12 in chronic lymphocytic leukaemia. *Lancet*; **1**(8160): 146–7.

42. Gahrton G. (2012) Historical note on the discovery of the Philadelphia chromosome. *Cancer genetics*; **205**(6): 338–9.

43. Foley GE. (1974) Obituary. Sidney Farber, M.D. *Cancer research*; **34**(3): 659–61.

44. Farber S, Diamond LK. (1948) Temporary remissions in acute leukemia in children produced by folic acid antagonist, 4-aminopteroyl-glutamic acid. *N Engl J Med*; **238**(23): 787–93.

45. Mukherjee S. (2010) The Emperor of All Maladies: A Biography of Cancer Scribner.

46. Schwartz R, Eisner A, Dameshek W. (1959) The effect of 6-mercaptopurine on primary and secondary immune responses. *The Journal of clinical investigation*; **38**(8): 1394-403.

47. Gahrton G. (1966) Quantitative Cytochemical studies on normal and leukemic leukocytes, with special reference to the periodic acid-Schiff reaction. Stockholm: Karolinska Institutet.

48. Gahrton G, Zetterberg A. (1966) Glycogen synthesis in normal, leukemic and polycythemic leukocytes. Preliminary report of a quantitative cytochemical study. *Acta Med Scand*; **180**(4): 497–9.

49. Gahrton G. (1966) The periodic acid-Schiff reaction in neutrophil leukocytes in untreated and myleran-treated chronic myelocytic leukemia. A quantitative microspectrophotometric study. *Blood*; **28**(4): 544–52.

50. Handin R, Braunwald E, Bunn H, *et al.* (1999) William Curry Moloney, Memorial Minutes.

51. Nathan D. (2005) George Widmer Thorne, MD, 1906–2004. *Trans Am Clin Climatol Assoc*; **116**: lxiv–lxvi.

52. Frei E 3rd, Holland JF, Schneiderman MA, *et al.* (1958) A comparative study of two regimens of combination chemotherapy in acute leukemia. *Blood*; **13**(12): 1126–48.

53. Frei E 3rd, DeVita VT, Moxley JH 3rd, Carbone PP. (1966) Approaches to improving the chemotherapy of Hodgkin's disease. *Cancer research*; **26**(6): 1284–9.

54. DeVita VT Jr., Simon RM, Hubbard SM, *et al.* (1980) Curability of advanced Hodgkin's disease with chemotherapy. Long-term follow-up of MOPP-treated patients at the National Cancer Institute. *Annals of internal medicine*; **92**(5): 587–95.

55. Hart JS, George SL, Frei E 3rd, *et al.* (1977) Prognotic significance of pretreatment proliferative activity in adult acute leukemia. *Cancer*; **39**(4): 1603–17.

56. Castle WB. (1953) Development of knowledge concerning the gastric intrinsic factor and its relation to pernicious anemia. *N Engl J Med*; **249**(15): 603–14.

57. Sullivan LW, Herbert V. (1964) Suppression Hematopoiesis by Ethanol. *The Journal of clinical investigation*; **43**: 2048–62.

58. McFadden R. (Aug 8, 2011) Bernadine P. Healy, a Pioneer at National Institutes of Health, Dies at 67. *The New York Times*.

59. Mathe G, Amiel JL, Schwarzenberg L, *et al*. (1969) Active immunotherapy for acute lymphoblastic leukaemia. *Lancet*; **1**(7597): 697–9.

60. Mathe G, Jammet H, Pendic B, *et al*. (1959) Transfusions and grafts of homologous bone marrow in humans after accidental high dosage irradiation. *Rev Fr Etud Clin Biol*; **4**(3): 226–38.

61. Jammet H, Mathe G, Pendic B, *et al*. (1959) Study of six cases of accidental acute total irradiation. *Rev Fr Etud Clin Biol*; **4**(3): 210–25.

62. Schwarzenberg L, Mathe G. (1978) Twenty years of bone marrow grafting in the treatment of bone marrow leukemias and aplasias. *Surg Clin North Am*; **58**(3): 637–54.

63. Mathe G, Amiel JL, Schwarzenberg L, *et al*. (1963) Haematopoietic Chimera in Man after Allogenic (Homologous) Bone-Marrow Transplantation. (Control of the Secondary Syndrome. Specific Tolerance Due to the Chimerism). *British medical journal*; **2**(5373): 1633–5.

64. Starzl T. (1992) The Puzzle People. Memoirs of a Transplant Surgeon. Pittsburgh, Pa, USA: University of Pittsburgh Press.

65. Thomas ED. (1991) In: Frängsmyr T, ed. Les Prix Nobel, the Nobel Prizes 1990. Stockholm: Nordstedts Tryckeri AB: 219–21.

66. Thomas ED. (1991) Bone Marrow Transplantation — past, present and future. In: Frängsmyr T, ed. Les Prix Nobel, the Nobel Prizes. Stockholm: Nordstedts Tryckeri AB: 222–30.

67. Jacobson L, Marks E, Robson M, *et al*. (1949) Effect of spleen protection on mortality following X irradiation. *The Journal of laboratory and clinical medicine*; **34**: 1538.

68. Lorenz E, Uphoff D, Reid TR, Shelton E. (1951) Modification of irradiation injury in mice and guinea pigs by bone marrow injections. *J Natl Cancer Inst*; **12**(1): 197–201.

69. Thomas ED, Lochte HL Jr., Lu WC, Ferrebee JW. (1957) Intravenous infusion of bone marrow in patients receiving radiation and chemotherapy. *N Engl J Med*; **257**(11): 491–6.

70. Thomas ED, Lochte HL Jr., Cannon JH, *et al.* (1959) Supralethal whole body irradiation and isologous marrow transplantation in man. *The Journal of clinical investigation*; **38**: 1709–16.

71. Thomas ED, Buckner CD, Banaji M, *et al.* (1977) One hundred patients with acute leukemia treated by chemotherapy, total body irradiation, and allogeneic marrow transplantation. *Blood*; **49**(4): 511–33.

72. Niederwieser D, Baldomero H, Bazuaye N, *et al.* (2022) One and a half million hematopoietic stem cell transplants: continuous and differential improvement in worldwide access with the use of non-identical family donors. *Haematologica*; **107**(5): 1045–53.

73. Hornsten P, Granstrom M, Wahren B, Gahrton G. (1977) Prognostic value of colony-stimulating and colony-forming cells in peripheral blood in acute non-lymphoblastic leukemia. *Acta Med Scand*; **201**(5): 405–10.

74. Ljungman P. (1985) Herpes virus infections in bone marrow transplant recipients. A study of transfer and persistence of herpes virus reactive lymphocytes. Stockholm Sweden: Karolinska Institutet.

75. Juliusson G. (1985) Leukemic B-Lymphocytic Malignancy. A clinical, immunological and cytogenetic study, utilizing mitogens to activate and differentiale malignant B-lymphocytes in vitro. Stockholm Sweden.

76. Juliusson G, Oscier DG, Fitchett M, *et al.* (1990) Prognostic subgroups in B-cell chronic lymphocytic leukemia defined by specific chromosomal abnormalities. *N Engl J Med*; **323**(11): 720–4.

77. Paul C. (1981) Anthracycline cytostatics in acute leukemia. Stockholm: Karolinska Institutet.

78. de Duve C. (1963) The lysosome. *SciAm*; **208**: 64–72.

79. Paul C, Tidefelt U, Gahrton G, *et al.* (1991) A Randomized Comparison of Doxorubicin and Doxorubicin-DNA in the Treatment of Acute NonLymphoblastic Leukemia. *Leuk Lymphoma*; **3**(5–6): 355–64.

80. Liliemark J. (1986) Pharmacokinetic studies on ARA-C in acute leukemia. Stockholm: Karolinska Institutet, Stockholm Sweden.

81. Kimby E. (1989) Chronic Lymphocytic Leukemia of B cell type and Monoclonal B Cell Lymphocytosis of undetermined significance. A study of the B cell clone and regulatory lymphocyte subpopulation: Karolinska Institutet.

82. Björkstrand B. (1996) Stem cell transplantation in multiple myeloma. Clinical aspects and experimental gene transfer studies. Stockholm, Sweden: Karolinska Institutet.

83. Bjorkstrand B, Dilber MS, Smith CI, *et al.* (1994) Retroviral-mediated gene transfer into human myeloma cells. *Br J Haematol*; **88**(2): 325–31.

84. Bjorkstrand B, Iacobelli S, Hegenbart U, *et al.* (2011) Tandem autologous/reduced-intensity conditioning allogeneic stem-cell transplantation versus autologous transplantation in myeloma: long-term follow-up. *J Clin Oncol*; **29**(22): 3016–22.

85. Dilber MS. (1996) Experimental Gene Therapy, with special reference to plasma cell tumors. Stockholm: Karolinska Institutet, Stockholm Sweden.

86. Rosengren-Lindquist R. (2009) Chromosome aberrations and environmental exposures in Acute Leukemia. (Doctoral thesis) Stockholm: Karolinska Institutet.

87. Merup M. (1997) Molecular Genetics of Lymphoid malignancies. (Doctoral thesis) Stockholm: Karolinska Institutet.

88. Sundman-Engberg B. (1996) In vitro studies of cytotoxic drugs and growth factors on leukemic and normal hematopoietic cells, based on in vivo intracellular pharmacokinetics. (Doctoral thesis) Stockholm: Karolinska Institutet.

89. Scherstén T, Sundkvist-Runesson I. (1992) Om användning av löntagarfondsmedel: Sammanfattning av Rådets förslag. *MFR informerar*; October 1992:3.

90. Frängsmyr T. (2001) Les Prix Nobel. The Nobel Prizes 2000. Stockholm: Nobel Foundation.

91. Wenneras C, Wold A. (1997) Nepotism and sexism in peer-review. *Nature*; **387**(6631): 341–3.

92. Gahrton G, Alvestrand A, Aperia A, *et al.* (2000) DN Debatt: Professorer protesterar mot statlig diskriminering: "Ledande forskare ratas på grund av ålder" *Dagens Nyheter*; 30 December, 2000.

93. Prusiner SB. (1982) Novel proteinaceous infectious particles cause scrapie. *Science*; **216**(4542): 136–44.

94. Prusiner SB, Barry RA, McKinley MP, *et al.* (1985) Scrapie and Creutzfeldt-Jakob disease prions. *Microbiol Sci*; **2**(2): 33–9.

95. Barnaba V, Franco A, Alberti A, *et al.* (1990) Selective killing of hepatitis B envelope antigen-specific B cells by class I-restricted, exogenous antigen-specific T lymphocytes. *Nature*; **345**(6272): 258–60.

96. Bradley TR, Metcalf D, Robinson W. (1967) Stimulation by leukaemic sera of colony formation in solid agar cultures by proliferation of mouse bone marrow cells. *Nature*; **213**(5079): 926–7.

97. Gallo RC, Blattner WA, Reitz MS Jr., Ito Y. (1982) HTLV: the virus of adult T-cell leukaemia in Japan and elsewhere. *Lancet*; **1**(8273): 683.

98. Barre-Sinoussi F, Chermann JC, Rey F, *et al.* (1983) Isolation of a T-lymphotropic retrovirus from a patient at risk for acquired immune deficiency syndrome (AIDS). *Science*; **220**(4599): 868–71.

99. Klatzmann D, Barre-Sinoussi F, Nugeyre MT, *et al.* (1984) Selective tropism of lymphadenopathy associated virus (LAV) for helper-inducer T lymphocytes. *Science*; **225**(4657): 59–63.

100. Phillips H. (1997) Ishan Dogramaci: A remarkable Turk: Bishop Wilton, York, England.

101. Tokarev YN, Spivak VA. (1982) Heterogeneity and distribution of hemoglobinopathies in some parts of the USSR. *Hemoglobin*; **6**(6): 653–60.

102. Ritter B, Safwenberg J, Olsson KS. (1984) HLA as a marker of the hemochromatosis gene in Sweden. *Hum Genet*; **68**(1): 62–6.

103. Gale RP, Canaani E. (1984) An 8-kilobase abl RNA transcript in chronic myelogenous leukemia. *Proc Natl Acad Sci U S A*; **81**(18): 5648–52.

104. Canaani E, Gale RP, Steiner-Saltz D, *et al.* (1984) Altered transcription of an oncogene in chronic myeloid leukaemia. *Lancet*; **1**(8377): 593–5.

105. Shtivelman E, Lifshitz B, Gale RP, Canaani E. (1985) Fused transcript of abl and bcr genes in chronic myelogenous leukaemia. *Nature*; **315**(6020): 550–4.

106. Hammer A, Lyndon N. (1987) Hammer — witness to history. London: Simon and Schuster Limited.

107. Gale RP, Lax E. (2013) Radiation, What it is, What you need to know. New York: Alfred A. Knopp, Random House.

108. Gahrton G, Zech L, Friberg K, *et al.* (1976) Chromosomal satellites as markers in human bone-marrow transplantation. *Hereditas*; **84**(1): 15–8.

109. Gahrton G, Iacobelli S, Bandini G, *et al.* (2007) Peripheral blood or bone marrow cells in reduced-intensity or myeloablative conditioning allogeneic HLA identical sibling donor transplantation for multiple myeloma. *Haematologica*; **92**(11): 1513–8.

110. Gratwohl A, Tichelli A, Nissen C, *et al.* (1993) Treatment of GVHD with cyclosporin A. *Bone Marrow Transplant*; **12** Suppl **3**: S32–5.

111. Gratwohl A, Hermans J, Niederwieser D, *et al.* (1993) Bone marrow transplantation for chronic myeloid leukemia: long-term results. Chronic Leukemia Working Party of the European Group for Bone Marrow Transplantation. *Bone Marrow Transplant*; **12**(5): 509–16.

112. van Rood JJ, Oudshoorn M. (2008) Eleven million donors in Bone Marrow Donors Worldwide! Time for reassessment? *Bone Marrow Transplant*; **41**(1): 1–9.

113. Gahrton G, van Rood JJ, Oudshoorn M. (2003) The World Marrow Donor Association (WMDA): its goals and activities. *Bone Marrow Transplant*; **32**(2): 121–4.

114. Van Rood JJ, Eernisse JG, Van Leeuwen A. (1958) Leucocyte antibodies in sera from pregnant women. *Nature*; **181**(4625): 1735–6.

115. Dausset J. (1959) Isoantibodies and antigens of leukocytes and platelets independent of those of erythrocytes. *Sangre (Barc)*; **30**: 634–42.

116. Kyle R. (2004) History of Multiple Myeloma. In: Gahrton G, Durie BGM, Samson DM, eds. Multiple Myeloma and related disorders. London: Arnold, Hodder Headline Group.

117. Alwall N. (1947) Urethane and stilbamidine in multiple myeloma: report on two cases. *Lancet*; **2**: 388–9.

118. Bergsagel D, Sprague CC, Austin C, Griffith KM. (1962) Evaluation of new chemotherapeutic agents in the treatment of multiple myeloma IV. L-phenylalanine mustard (NSC-8806). *Cancer Chemotherapy reports*; **21**: 87–99.

119. Gahrton G, Ringden O, Lonnqvist B, *et al.* (1986) Bone marrow transplantation in three patients with multiple myeloma. *Acta Med Scand*; **219**(5): 523–7.

120. Tura S, Cavo M, Baccarani M, *et al.*(1986) Bone marrow transplantation in multiple myeloma. *Scandinavian journal of haematology*; **36**(2): 176–9.

121. Gahrton G, Tura S, Ljungman P, *et al.* (1991) Allogeneic bone marrow transplantation in multiple myeloma. European Group for Bone Marrow Transplantation. *N Engl J Med*; **325**(18): 1267–73.

122. McElwain TJ, Powles RL. (1983) High-dose intravenous melphalan for plasma-cell leukaemia and myeloma. *Lancet*; **2**(8354): 822–4.

123. Selby P, Zulian G, Forgeson G, *et al.* (1988) The development of high dose melphalan and of autologous bone marrow transplantation in the treatment of multiple myeloma: Royal Marsden and St Bartholomew's Hospital studies. *Hematol Oncol*; **6**(2): 173–9.

124. Barlogie B, Hall R, Zander A, *et al.* (1986) High-dose melphalan with autologous bone marrow transplantation for multiple myeloma. *Blood*; **67**(5): 1298–301.

125. Kyle RA, Durie BG, Rajkumar SV, *et al.* (2010) Monoclonal gammopathy of undetermined significance (MGUS) and smoldering (asymptomatic) multiple myeloma: IMWG consensus perspectives risk factors for progression and guidelines for monitoring and management. *Leukemia*; **24**(6): 1121–7.

126. Singhal S, Mehta J, Desikan R, *et al.* (1999) Antitumor activity of thalidomide in refractory multiple myeloma. *N Engl J Med*; **341**(21): 1565–71.

127. Durie BG, Salmon SE. (1975) A clinical staging system for multiple myeloma. Correlation of measured myeloma cell mass with presenting clinical features, response to treatment, and survival. *Cancer*; **36**(3): 842–54.

128. Gahrton G, Durie BGM. (1996) Multiple Myeloma: Arnold, Hodder Headline Group.

129. Gahrton G, Durie BGM, Samson DM. (2004) Multiple Myeloma and Related Disorders. London: Arnold, Hodder Headline Group.

130. Nahi H, Chrobok M, Meinke S, *et al.* (2022) Autologous NK cells as consolidation therapy following stem cell transplantation in multiple myeloma. *Cell Rep Med*; **3**(2): 100508.

131. Sahin U, Muik A, Derhovanessian E, *et al.* (2020) COVID-19 vaccine BNT162b1 elicits human antibody and TH1 T cell responses. *Nature*; **586**(7830): 594–9.

132. Kariko K, Weissman D. (2007) Naturally occurring nucleoside modifications suppress the immunostimulatory activity of RNA: implication for therapeutic RNA development. *Curr Opin Drug Discov Devel*; **10**(5): 523–32.

133. Gahrton G, Bjorkstrand B, Dilber MS, *et al.* (1998) Gene marking and gene therapy in multiple myeloma. *Adv Exp Med Biol*; **451**: 493–7.

134. Alici E, Bjorkstrand B, Treschow A, *et al.* (2007) Long-term follow-up of gene-marked CD34+ cells after autologous stem cell transplantation for multiple myeloma. *Cancer Gene Ther*; **14**(3): 227–32.

135. Cohen-Haguenauer O, Roman N. (1999) Euregenethy/Regulation of Gene Therapy in Europe — a scientific network of users. In: Commission E, ed. BMH-4 CT 98-3894. Brussels.

136. Cohen-Haguenauer O. (2001) European Cooperation Network to collect and disperse ethical, safety and regulatory data in order to facilitate clinical implementation of gene transfer technology (gene therapy). In: Commission E, ed. Brussels.

137. Eriksdotter-Jonhagen M, Linderoth B, Lind G, *et al.* (2012) Encapsulated cell biodelivery of nerve growth factor to the Basal forebrain in patients with Alzheimer's disease. *Dementia and geriatric cognitive disorders*; **33**(1): 18–28.

138. Dilber M. (1996) Experimental gene therapy, with special reference to plasma cell tumors. (Doctoral thesis) Stockholm: Karolinska Institutet.

139. Alici E, Sutlu T, Bjorkstrand B, *et al.* (2008) Autologous antitumor activity by NK cells expanded from myeloma patients using GMP-compliant components. *Blood*; **111**(6): 3155–62.

140. Cohen-Haguenauer O, ed. (2012) The CliniBook. Clinical Gene Transfer: State of the Art. Paris: EDK/Groupe EDP Sciences.

141. Gross G, Waks T, Eshhar Z. (1989) Expression of immunoglob-ulin-T-cell receptor chimeric molecules as functional receptors with antibody-type specificity. *Proc Natl Acad Sci U S A*; **86**(24): 10024–8.

142. Gross G, Gorochov G, Waks T, Eshhar Z. (1989) Generation of effector T cells expressing chimeric T cell receptor with antibody type-specificity. *Transplantation proceedings*; **21**(1 Pt 1): 127–30.

143. Eshhar Z, Gross G. (1990) Chimeric T cell receptor which incor-porates the anti-tumour specificity of a monoclonal antibody with the cytolytic activity of T cells: a model system for immunothera-peutical approach. *Br J Cancer Suppl*; **10**: 27–9.

144. Alwall N. (1947) On the artificial kidney; apparatus for dialysis of the blood in vivo. *Acta Med Scand*; **128**(4): 317–25.

145. Kolff WJ. (1947) The artificial kidney. *J Mt Sinai Hosp N Y*; **14**(2): 71–9.

146. Palmstierna J. (2008) Jacobs stege: triumfer och nederlag i en bankmans liv: Ekerlids förlag, Stockholm.

147. Gahrton G, Habicht W, Wahren B. (1966) DNA, RNA and pro-teins in lymphoid cells from normal preleukemic and leukemic mice. Ninth International Cancer Congress. Tokyo: International Union Against Cancer and Science Council of Japan: 186.

148. Kawano M, Kuramoto A, Hirano T, Kishimoto T. (1989) Cytokines as autocrine growth factors in malignancies. *Cancer Surv*; **8**(4): 905–19.

149. Elion G. (1989) The Purine Path to Chemotherapy. In: Frängsmyr TTRSAoS, ed. Les Prix Nobel 1988. Stockholm, Sweden: Nobel Foundation: 267–88.

150. Elion GB, Hitchings GH, Vanderwerff H. (1951) Antagonists of nucleic acid derivatives. VI. Purines. *The Journal of biological chemistry*; **192**(2): 505–18.

151. Hitchings GH. (1989) Selective inhibitors of dehydrofolate reductase. In: Frängsmyr T, ed. Les Prix Nobel. Stockholm, Sweden: Nobel Foundation: 296–313.

152. Thomas ED, Buckner CD, Rudolph RH, *et al.* (1971) Allogeneic marrow grafting for hematologic malignancy using HL-A matched donor-recipient sibling pairs. *Blood*; **38**(3): 267–87.

Name Index